JAN   7 2009

A QUESTION OF MURDER

"Authoritative and thoughtful commentary on criminal cases of notoriety requires the wisdom and insightfulness of Dr. Cyril Wecht. A Question of Murder, written in collaboration with true-crime journalist Dawna Kaufmann, is another feather in the cap of this famed forensic pathologist."

–RICHARD SAFERSTEIN, PhD, chief forensic scientist
(retired) for the New Jersey State Police and author of
Criminalistics: An Introduction to Forensic Science

"A fascinating peek into the morgue and the lab. A Question of Murder *shows forensic medicine in vivid detail."*

–KATHY REICHS, PhD, forensic anthropologist and author of
the *Temperance Brennan* novels.

"Wecht, the most fearless forensic pathologist of his generation, offers a chilling study of four high-profile cases, plus a view of Hurricane Katrina and the deaths at Memorial Medical Center that many might have otherwise ignored. A Question of Murder *illustrates the power of forensic medicine and investigative reporting in such a way as to respect the science, justice, and above all, the departed."*

–MICHAEL WELNER, MD, forensic psychiatrist, chairman of
the Forensic Panel, and associate professor of psychiatry at
New York University School of Medicine

A QUESTION OF MURDER

CYRIL H. WECHT, MD, JD
AND DAWNA KAUFMANN

Compelling cases from a famed forensic pathologist,
including **Anna Nicole Smith**,
Daniel Smith—*Anna Nicole's son*—and many more!

FOREWORD BY BEST-SELLING AUTHOR
ANN RULE

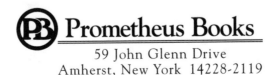
Prometheus Books
59 John Glenn Drive
Amherst, New York 14228-2119

Published 2008 by Prometheus Books

Inquiries should be addressed to
Prometheus Books
59 John Glenn Drive
Amherst, New York 14228–2119
VOICE: 716–691–0133, ext. 210
FAX: 716–691–0137
WWW.PROMETHEUSBOOKS.COM

12 11 10 09 08   5 4 3 2 1

Library of Congress Cataloging-in-Publication Data

Wecht, Cyril H., 1931–.
    A question of murder / by Cyril H. Wecht, and Dawna Kaufmann.
        p. cm.
    Includes bibliographical references and index.
    ISBN 978–1–59102–661–7
    1. Homicide investigation—Case studies. 2. Forensic sciences—Case studies. 3. Forensic pathology—Case studies. I. Kaufmann, Dawna, 1971. II. Title.

HV8079.H6W43 2008
363.25'9523092—dc22

                                                                    2008035338

Printed in the United States on acid-free paper

CONTENTS

FOREWORD

by Ann Rule

When I began writing for fact-detective magazines like *True Detective*, *Master Detective*, *Official Detective*, and their sister magazines back in the 1970s, I knew virtually nothing about forensic pathologists. I thought that coroners, medical examiners, and forensic pathologists all meant the same thing, but I soon learned there were vast differences. Coroners don't have to be medical doctors; they rule on causes of death in innumerable small towns and counties across America, and, not surprisingly, many homicides are written off as heart attacks, strokes, natural causes of old age, and accidents.

Many cases of murder thus go unsolved and justice does not always prevail.

Medical examiners are physicians. Forensic pathologists stand at the top of the ladder—medical doctors who have experience and training, and, most of all, not only a certain kind of brilliance in detecting the physical signs and clues a dead body offers up silently but also the soul and savvy of an investigator. Almost uncannily, they understand what the departed is trying to tell them, even though they never knew them in life.

I used to think that forensic pathologists must be coldhearted and unemotional in order to pursue a career that revolves around death—and, often, violent death. But I was wrong. Over three decades, I have met and come to know a few dozen forensic pathologists. Many of them—like Dr. Cyril Wecht—have become household names because the top physicians in the field are consulted to evaluate the cause of death in infamous homicide cases or in the sudden demise of celebrities. Far from being unsympathetic, these men and women are searching for justice. Usually, it's justice for the deceased, but sometimes their findings will free innocent suspects.

The word *autopsy* means "to see for one's self." And that is what a forensic pathologist achieves as he looks for both obvious and occult clues in the corpse before him. An autopsy is vital to finding the truth, and my heart often sinks when I receive mail from strangers who are the grieving friends and families of someone who has died mysteriously. They want desperately to know why and how the person perished, but it's too late. "They cremated her body the day after she died," someone wrote in an e-mail I got only yesterday. "How can we find out what happened, now?"

I have to tell them that, except for some poisons that may linger in the cremains, the cause of death may never be known. That is very hard for them to accept. And, of course, it's almost always the most likely suspect who has hastened the disposal of the body.

Although the morgue and the autopsy room are not places I prefer to be, sometimes I find myself there, observing. Almost every medical examiner's facility I've visited has a small, framed placard on the office or lab wall with remarkably similar philosophies. Below is one I copied in Washington State:

> All Who Lie Here Before You Were Once Loved;
> Respect for the Dignity of the Dead
> Will Be Maintained at All Times
> As You Are, He Was—As He Is, You Will Be.

Forensic pathologists do care about their subjects, but they learn to maintain a certain emotional distance. They have to, or they couldn't give their full attention to the mysteries that lie before them. Some cases stay with them forever, and they ponder them long after the post-mortem exams are finished, and the deceased have returned to earth.

Even after thirty-five years of researching and writing about more than a thousand true crime cases, I was fascinated by the manuscript of Dr. Wecht and Dawna Kaufmann's new book, which I read far into the wee hours. Wecht's memory and files are filled with scientific facts behind the headline cases, and Kaufmann co-authors with a fluidity that makes the pages fly by. I have long admired Kaufmann's reporting, which, like this book, is well resourced and responsible.

No other author has truly peeled away the layers of the shocking deaths of Anna Nicole Smith and her son, Daniel, the way Wecht and Kaufmann have in this book, and in such a spellbinding fashion.

Less well known, but just as gripping, is the strange murder of Stephanie Crowe, a young California girl who was found stabbed to death in her own home. Was her real killer ever found? And the kidnapping and murder case of seven-year-old Danielle van Dam by a sadistic pedophile named David Westerfield is finally illuminated by the authors. Hundreds of my own correspondents have written to ask why they haven't found a book about the van Dam case, and they will be gratified to know that the whole story is in *A Question of Murder*.

Hurricane Katrina brought New Orleans to its knees. No one was prepared for such a disaster, hordes of residents died, and it became a tragic political fiasco. Even today, I think that we have turned away from that proud Louisiana city built on water, often assailed by the weather and the sea that snakes continually from the Gulf of Mexico, the Bayous, and Lake Pontchartrain.

Cyril Wecht was one of the nationally known forensic pathologists called in to investigate deaths in New Orleans and, particularly, the deaths of ill patients left behind in Memorial Medical Center there. This book's chilling overview of those deaths will be the subject of debates for many years to come. Were patients euthanized without their permission—or were the medical professionals who treated them acting in a humanitarian way?

The one thing that is desperately important is that we need to know what happened, and the veils shrouding deaths in New Orleans from all causes must be lifted.

The world of forensic scientists—pathologists, anthropologists, and odontologists—detectives, prosecutors, defense attorneys, documentary producers, and crime writers is a small one, and we often get together at one conference or another, learning from one another. When I began writing for *True Detective*, among others, there was no DNA, no AFIS (Automated Fingerprint Identification System), no VICAP (the FBI's Violent Criminal Apprehension Program), no nationwide registry for sex offenders, and no recognition of, or definition for, serial murder. Every year, those who seek justice for those who can no longer speak for themselves—the dead—have more precise and sophisticated tools to work with.

I take pride in keeping up with all the new discoveries that help to solve crimes, but I have to admit I learned several things I didn't know as I read *A Question of Murder*. And I am sure you will, too.

I'm pleased to write the foreword to this important book in the continuing evolution of forensic investigation.

Ann Rule is the author of twenty-nine true crime books, including *Too Late to Say Goodbye*, *The Stranger Beside Me*, and *Green River Running Red*.

PREFACE

Whoever coined the phrase "dead men tell no tales" was not a forensic pathologist. As someone who has been a proud, board-certified member of that profession for forty-five years, I assure you that the dead do speak. As a forensic pathologist, or medical examiner, I serve as their voice—in the morgue, in the courtroom, or wherever I am asked to represent the interests of the departed. When there is a sudden, unexpected, or mysterious death, I go to work—scalpel in hand and with a microcassette recorder capturing my every observation.

As I perform an autopsy, the body reveals its secrets. I determine a "cause of death" by assessing injuries or maladies. After I inspect every square inch of the external body, I then surgically open it to examine the interior portions. I look for trauma or disease, and sometimes I find both. Once I measure and track the wounds, I view the organs and tissues under a microscope. Clues about the time of death come from the color and condition of the individual's flesh and, often, from stomach contents.

I send the bodily fluids out for toxicological testing to divulge whether any alcohol or drugs—licit or illicit—were ingested in the deceased's last hours. I can also have his or her scalp hairs analyzed to see how many weeks or months a particular drug was in that person's system. Since hair grows about a half an inch per month, each strand is a natural timetable for drug intake, if that is something I need to ascertain.

I get assistance from a dedicated crew of experts and the most modern scientific equipment available in my quest to find out what happened to the person on my morgue table. I do it for the deceased, for the record, and to satisfy my own abiding curiosity.

When all the laboratory results and expert analyses come in, I write an official report that can either close out a case or open it to the justice system. In that regard, the autopsy can be the end for the dead person, or the beginning of a new process.

On the way to citing a cause of death, there are many variables. For example, petechial hemorrhages, or pinpoint red spots on the eyes or skin, might suggest a death by strangulation or smothering—but that's not always the case. Strangulations also can fracture the hyoid bone, the U-shaped cartilage at the back of the throat, but some strangulations leave that bone intact. Calling the proper cause of death requires experience in assessing and giving values to everything the body shows.

Sometimes there can be many things wrong with the deceased, and more than one potentially fatal element. If someone has cancer and also gets stabbed, which was the mechanism of death? What if he was in remission and healthy but was knifed through the heart? Or what if he was in a terminal cancer ward and received a minor nick to a limb? Or what if he had cancer, and was also gravely stabbed, but actually died from a drug overdose? It's my duty to chronicle all of the possibilities and put them in a sensible order of how each contributed to the death. That's a chief reason why, after personally performing more than sixteen thousand autopsies and consulting on some thirty-six thousand others worldwide, I'm never bored in my chosen field.

Once the cause of death is established—gunshot, stabbing, drowning, asphyxiation, drug toxicity, and so forth—a forensic pathologist must classify the "manner of death." Here, I have five choices: homicide, suicide, accident, natural, or undetermined. When I declare a death to be a homicide, there usually follows a police or governmental investigation with the goal of arresting the individual deemed responsible and seeing that the perpetrator is brought to trial. But while I can state that a death is a homicide, it's up to law enforcement to decide who committed the act and to make that arrest. Sometimes I'll be brought in early and invited to the crime scene or the site where a body has been dumped. A recently deceased corpse will provide a wealth of information for my autopsy findings. But in other circumstances, I'll be presented with a body that has been mummified, skeletonized, or that is missing key parts, which usually means too few pieces of the puzzle are available.

If detectives feel there's sufficient evidence, they'll arrest their suspect and turn the case over to prosecutors. Because it may take time before I'm asked to provide deposition or courtroom testimony about my autopsy findings, the richness of detail in the original post-mortem report serves me well. Eventually a citizen jury will hear the witnesses, and the prosecution and defense theories of the case. Then the jurors will decide the defendant's fate and, if there's a conviction, the appropriate punishment.

Throughout the process, it's imperative that everyone involved be at the top of his or her game, especially when the stakes are so high. My testimony has been used to send countless defendants to jail and some to death row. But even more important to me are the times my findings have helped to free a wrongly convicted inmate. The only thing worse than seeing a guilty person go free is learning about a scientifically-proven individual victimized by the all-powerful legal system that should protect each one of us.

At any point, a closed case can heat up if something fresh materializes. There's no statute of limitations on murder in this country. So as long as somebody hasn't been tried and found not guilty, the long arm of the law can reach out and pull that alleged perpetrator into the courtroom. How many times have we heard about a just-discovered hit on the national DNA database, turning a case on its ear? Or a credible, new witness who comes forward, or a weapon that is found, or that a confession emerges? As a scientist it's my obligation to follow the evidence, as it applies to my discipline, wherever it leads. Sometimes I'll be asked to exhume a body from its burial site and conduct a secondary autopsy. Maybe I'll end up confirming what the original medical examiner found, or maybe I'll spot something that was missed before. Just because the dead are laid to rest doesn't mean they won't have to make a brief return appearance to the morgue. Cremation is the only absolute obstacle to such an event.

These days, the public has an insatiable thirst for autopsy-based media—from the nightly true crime programs on cable TV where I make frequent appearances to discuss breaking crimes and current trials, to the fictionalized depictions. There have been the weekly episodes of CBS's Crime Scene Investigation series, beginning in the year 2000 with *CSI: Las Vegas*. Two years later it spawned *CSI: Miami*, and two years after that, *CSI: New York*, all still going strong. Also on that network, *NCIS: Naval Crime Investigative Service* has been on weekly since 2003, and there are novels and movies galore in which a forensic pathologist is instrumental in solving somebody's baffling demise. But even if it seems that there's a universe of infinite scenarios from the best screenwriters in the business, nothing (in my humble opinion) is as interesting as what happens in real life. And real-life cases are what this book is about.

You may already have some awareness of the five cases you'll read about here. You may even think you know a great deal about these deaths because my work, and that of others, on each of them got a fair amount of publicity at the time. But the twists and turns of these cases are as bizarre and dramatic as that of any TV episode—yet it's all completely authentic. There's no manipulation of storytelling to accommodate a commercial break, no instant serving up of scientific results, or no predictable treatment of heroes and villains. In each case you'll walk the steps I took to decide whether a murder was committed, and you'll see forensic science at its most exhilarating as the cases unfold.

The drug overdose of twenty-year-old Daniel Wayne Smith, followed closely by the death of his mother, former *Playboy* playmate Anna Nicole Smith, got an unbelievable amount of media coverage. My vantage point from within those cases, however, is something you'll experience here for the first time. The next two cases are about the uncannily similar deaths of two young girls in a San Diego suburb, the ensuing investigations, and their wildly divergent outcomes. Twelve-year-old Stephanie Crowe and seven-year-old Danielle van Dam never knew of each other in life, but their deaths put a spotlight on the broad spectrum of forensic studies, as well as proper police procedure and suitable courtroom behavior. The final case will chill anyone who has ever gone into a hospital for treatment or left a loved one in the care of trusted medical personnel during a terrible disaster. What occurred at New Orleans' Memorial Medical Center in the aftermath of Hurricane Katrina is as vivid as any horror film, yet all the players here are not actors but real people.

As a freelance investigative journalist, my co-author, Dawna Kaufmann, gained widespread acclaim in 2002 by encouraging ex-FBI agent W. Mark Felt Sr., also known as Watergate's "Deep Throat," to come forward and tell his story, thus solving one of history's greatest enigmas. But before that, and since, Dawna's beat has been covering homicides and high-profile trials. I didn't need to bring her up to speed on the first four cases in this book, as she had written about them extensively—and, as you'll see, contributed to cracking one of them. She's as hard-boiled as any detective, with a memory for detail that always astounds me. The New Orleans case was new to Dawna, but she embraced it so thoroughly that her research eclipsed that of any news agency, according to what one of the lead investigators told me. I've consulted with Dawna on many of her published articles over the years and am delighted that we were able to work together on this book. We hope the reader will enjoy learning about these most fascinating true crimes.

Cyril H. Wecht, MD, JD

My business card reads: "Dawna Kaufmann: Crime Fighting / Joke Writing." For the first half of my career I was a successful TV producer and comedy writer, working on late-night series staffs and crafting topical gags. But in 1994, I was transfixed by O. J. Simpson's slow-speed police chase and the subsequent murder investigation and trials. I decided to reinvent myself as a true crime journalist and began covering the Simpson case as a freelancer for the tabloids, the *National Enquirer*, *Star*, and *Globe*. I soon realized that the tabloids are to the mainstream press what Delta Force is to the army—it's the elite corps for breaking the news first and best. I began specializing in stories about high-profile crimes and celebrity autopsies, and now, about a thousand articles later, I have unique insight into some of the most provocative mysteries of our times.

As my articles needed more in-depth scrutiny about crime scenes and death, I contacted Dr. Cyril Wecht, who was such a stellar expert on television. A lawyer, as well as a forensic pathologist, his comments were always mindful of the intersection of medicine and law, which I found electrifying. He graciously answered my questions, explaining complex medicolegal issues with the kind of plain-speak my readers and I could appreciate. Thanks to him, my inquisitiveness and sophistication grew, and soon I was attending the annual meetings of the American Academy of Forensic Sciences—for which Cyril was a past president—and becoming familiar with the cutting-edge facets of crime solving.

With Dr. Wecht's help, I turned out countless articles on the homicide trials of O. J. Simpson, Scott Peterson, and Phil Spector; missing person cases, including Natalee Holloway, Madeleine McCann, and Stacy Peterson; and criminal investigations of drug-addled celebrities, arrogant politicians, and abusive cops. As Cyril has noted above, four of the cases in this book we worked on respectively.

There are three cases that Dr. Wecht has involvement with that earn him, in my mind, the Most Valuable Player in the forensic science world for his tireless work to educate the public: the 1996 murder of six-year-old Boulder, Colorado, beauty queen JonBenét Ramsey; the 1963 assassination of President John F. Kennedy; and the 1968 assassination of his brother, Senator Robert F. Kennedy. Dr. Wecht has consulted on and/or written at length on all three of these brutal crimes. In each of the cases, Dr. Wecht has said that the dead body is the Rosetta Stone for comprehending how, and possibly why, the victim died. I've seen Cyril at lectures decimate people who try to debate him, but his grasp of the relevant facts, his solid logic, and the power of his presentation leave his competitors waving a white flag. Whether in a hall of academia, a courtroom, or on TV, Wecht's fearlessness and honesty shine through and make him one of the greatest living legends in forensic science.

I'm privileged to write this book with Dr. Wecht and pledge to the reader that the journey inside these cases will be well worth taking and memorable.

Please note that in most cases I have cited a mainstream news source, rather than my own tabloid articles, which, in some instances, predated the stories cited. The tabloids don't archive their articles online, so instead, I have listed URLs or information you can put into an Internet search engine to find further research.

Dawna Kaufmann

ACKNOWLEDGMENTS

We wish to thank many individuals who have helped make this book a reality, from its conception through the final edit. Your encouragement and kind words have meant a great deal.

First, we thank our families and friends for their unwavering support.

In Dr. Wecht's office, we salute Florence Johnson and Darlene Brewer, who were always helpful and full of cheer—and Sigrid Wecht's legal and administrative abilities, which provided invaluable assistance. Dawna gives a shout-out to her associates at American Media, Inc., and to Marc Wax of Wax Entertainment.

We'd also like to thank Alex Goen and Robin Bonnema of Goen Technologies; David Giancola and Mary Beth French of Edgewood Studios; Milton L. Silverman, Esq.; Dr. Frank Minyard and Rachael Gagliano of the Orleans Parish Medical Examiner's office; Arthur "Butch" Schafer and his staff at the Louisiana State Attorney's office; Craig R. Nelson, Esq., and his sister Kathryn Nelson; Dr. Bryant King; Dr. Michael M. Baden; Yvette Reyes and Carolyn McGoldrick of AP Images; and Olan Mills Photography Studios.

We also express gratitude to our executive editor, Linda Greenspan Regan, for her eagle eye and good calls, and the entire team at Prometheus Books who assisted us in making this book coalesce and those who will help promote it.

Finally, we offer much appreciation and sympathy to the loved ones of the deceased and to crime victims everywhere. You were thrust into something you never would have chosen and yet many of you have opened your lives publicly to advance the cause of justice, or turned your tragedy into activism for the good of society. Your sacrifice and grace inspires us all.

DANIEL WAYNE SMITH

s I got ready for work on Monday, September 11, 2006, I turned on
my television and saw breathless reports about the sudden and
untimely death the day before of a twenty-year-old man in the
Bahamas. I had never heard of Daniel Wayne Smith, but soon—and
for many months to come—I would find myself closely involved with
the investigation into his demise.

My understanding of what happened to Daniel combines my own
firsthand recollections, what I was told by his friends and associates,
and what I've learned from news media accounts.

Daniel was the son of actress/model Anna Nicole Smith, who was
best known to me as the twenty-six-year-old exotic dancer from Texas
who married the eighty-nine-year-old oil tycoon, J. Howard Marshall
II. When he died fourteen months later, Anna Nicole inherited Marshall's millions of dollars. Her windfall, however, was disputed by
Marshall's offspring in various legal venues, with the US Supreme
Court finally backing her right to be heard on the matter. News coverage of the zaftig blonde, dressed uncharacteristically in modest garb,
climbing up the stairs of our nation's highest court, accompanied by
her lawyer, was a memorable sight. Many of us recall that wonderful
actor Jimmy Stewart starring in the 1939 movie *Mr. Smith Goes to
Washington*, but I don't think its director, the late Frank Capra, could
have conjured such an image for a sequel titled *Ms. Smith Goes to
Washington*, starring Anna Nicole Smith!

Anna acted in several movies and, from 2002 to 2004, starred in
her self-titled reality series, *The Anna Nicole Show*, on the E! Entertainment Channel. The series also featured Daniel and Anna's
attorney, Howard K. Stern (not to be confused with the radio shock

jock Howard Stern). I had never caught any of those films or programs but can remember seeing appearances with her on talk shows and red carpet events, as she posed like a modern-day, overgrown Marilyn Monroe and made giggly and flirtatious remarks in a southern twang. I've since learned that she also had a rather remarkable career as *Playboy*'s 1993 Playmate of the Year and as a highly paid model, beginning with her print ad work for the Guess clothing company. Later Anna gained a lot of weight, and then lost a reported sixty-nine pounds after becoming the spokesmodel for the TrimSpa diet system.

Born Vickie Lynn Hogan, Anna met Daniel's father, Billy Wayne Smith, when they both worked at Jim's Krispy Fried Chicken shack in Mexia, Texas.[1] When they wed in 1985, she was seventeen, while he was a year younger. By 1987 the marriage was over and she received full custody of their son. As the small-town beauty Vickie first tried to spread her wings into local modeling gigs and later exotic dancing, her mother, Virgie, a Houston sheriff's deputy, raised Daniel until he was six. When Ms. Arthur, Virgie's now-married surname, gave the boy an unauthorized haircut, an irate Vickie took him back. Before long, Vickie would meet Marshall, who ensconced her, her son, and a nanny in a lavish home.[2]

These details were the common talking points that various TV news show hosts mulled over following Daniel's death. From the file footage of him and his mother, it certainly seemed there was a strong mutual devotion. Interviews with people who knew the duo emphasized that while Anna often seemed impaired by substances, Daniel was considered a straight arrow.

As media reports trickled in that day of Daniel's death, more intriguing tidbits emerged. Daniel, it was said, had died in his mother's private room at Doctors Hospital, where she had undergone a cesarean delivery three days earlier. The night before his death, Daniel had arrived in Nassau to meet his newborn half sister, his only sibling. Anna Nicole, then thirty-eight years old, who checked in under the pseudonym "Jean Smith," had reportedly planned to name the six-pound, nine-ounce girl Hannah. Some newscasters seemed frustrated that no one seemed to know who the baby's father was.

Anna had been living in the Bahamas for the past several months, along with attorney Stern. Apparently the pair chose the Bahamas because it offered more privacy for the birth of her child than she was likely to get in any of the typical Tinseltown hospitals with paparazzi gathered outside. Now that very privacy was slowing the news corps from getting the scoops they so desperately wanted.

None of the reports about Daniel confirmed a cause of death. They only offered that he was found deceased in the morning in his mother's maternity ward room. That would likely eliminate death by trauma, which usually results from a gunshot, stabbing, bludgeoning, or hanging.

We've all heard about seemingly hale high school or college athletes who shockingly die on the track or playing field—and I've autopsied many—only to later discover the fatal etiology or cause was a previously undiagnosed congenital cardiac defect, cerebral aneurysm, pulmonary embolism, or anaphylactic reaction from a food allergy. So I was curious about what caused this young man to expire, yet cautious not to jump to conclusions.

Statistically though, there was a good probability drugs, legal or illicit, were involved. This, despite a public statement released by Mr. Stern that family members did "not believe that drugs or alcohol were a factor" in Daniel's death.[3] Daniel's autopsy was performed on September 11, at the morgue in Princess Margaret Hospital, with the country's chief forensic pathologist, Dr. H. C. Govinda Raju, conducting the procedure. Although I was soon to meet Dr. Raju for the first time, I was no stranger to that department of pathology.

Having consulted for both the prosecution and the defense on a number of cases in the Bahamas—and being on the winning side for each trial, I might add—I was familiar with many of the key personnel in the coroner's office and government. I was especially delighted to renew my acquaintance with Mr. Quinn W. McCartney, the chief superintendent and director of the forensic center of the Royal Bahamas Police Force, with whom I had worked on two homicide cases in the past.

In the late 1990s an eighteen-year-old Bahamian named Tenel McIntosh was arrested for the vicious rape-murder of a British teacher's assistant named Joanne Clarke, twenty-four, who was visiting Paradise Island. Police went to a spot where they believed he had buried her in a shallow grave and dug up the body—only to discover that the corpse was someone else. The second victim, also murdered, was an American second-grade teacher named Lori Fogelman, thirty-two, from Richmond, Virginia. Clarke's body was about eighty feet from Fogelman's. The cases were extremely complicated, with McIntosh tried for each murder, the juries deadlocking, and both cases being retried, eventually winning convictions. I testified for the prosecution during all four trials and apparently made a big impression on the defendant. "Hey, Dr. Wecht," he spoke to me in open court as I took the stand in the final trial, "Good to see you! How have you been?"

Now a sovereign nation, the Commonwealth of the Bahamas was originally a British colony and is still governed by laws similar to those in the United Kingdom. Nassau, the capital city, is on the island of New Providence. The subtropical climate is gorgeous in the winters, but in late summers and autumns, it often gets slammed by hurricanes and flooding.

I appreciate the Bahamian court system, with its magistrates wearing powdered wigs, which are so incongruously formal for a country whose citizens generally wear beachwear all year round, even as courtroom spectators. It was a nice change of pace to be able to do business at a morgue without having to wear a tie and starched shirt under my scrubs.

That evening I watched CNN's *Larry King Live*, which featured a panel about Daniel's mysterious death. Dr. Hubert Minnis, Anna's obstetrician, described the cesarean birth of Anna's daughter as "uncomplicated," helped by an epidural anesthesia that enabled the new mother to be in an upbeat mood during and after the surgery. Dr. Minnis had no inside information about Daniel's passing, but local reporter Inderia Saunders of the *Nassau Guardian* did. She had gotten an anonymous tip Sunday morning that Anna Nicole Smith's son had died at Doctors Hospital hours before, presumably from an overdose of antidepressants. When she arrived to investigate, a security lockdown was in force. That afternoon a press conference was held, declaring that a twenty-year-old male had died at the hospital. However, the victim wasn't named, and no cause of death was given. But by the time of the CNN broadcast, everyone knew the victim's identity.

Assistant commissioner of the Royal Bahamas Police Force Reginald Ferguson was another guest. He confirmed an investigation was in process and that no cause of death had yet been determined, adding, "No foul play is suspected in this matter." *People* magazine staff editor Larry Sutton countered that his reporter had heard Daniel died of "unnatural causes." But the editor also warned that any twenty-year-old's death might be considered "unnatural," and only the full autopsy would reveal the facts. He floated the notion that Daniel might have had a "heart problem" a couple of years back, though it was "nothing major," and downplayed Saunders's tip about the antidepressants, saying he thought "it would take an awful lot of them to cause a death" and "that would be obvious to his doctors earlier."[4]

As a frequent panelist on many news-breaking programs myself, I understand the tap dance of trying to contribute to a vigorous discussion before substantive details are known about a matter. I'm generally comfortable saying that I don't yet have all the facts if I'm asked about something I don't know. Some other individuals, perhaps afraid they won't be invited back on the programs, toss out tidbits just to hear themselves talk. The hosts should know what a panelist's area of expertise is so that nonmedical guests don't have to comment on matters beyond their abilities. But a guest can also dig his or her own hole. Sutton was more in his element when he spoke of the terrible irony of Daniel's death coming so shortly after the joyous birth of Anna's daughter. It was, he explained, a "classic *People* story."

Over the next couple of days the hunger for news was so intense that a series of shocking items were leaked: that Daniel died of a "massive heart attack" in front of his mother's eyes, that he vomited uncontrollably and left bloody sputum all over the hospital room, that the medical team that tried to revive him was unable to find a supply of oxygen, that Anna wouldn't allow doctors to touch her son's lifeless body, and that her voice was overhead screaming at another person in the room, "You caused this!" All very dramatic developments, if true. But as we came to learn, there was little truth to these so-called facts.

Banks of TV, radio, and print reporters from around the globe were camped out in front of the medical examiner's office, and Her Majesty's Coroner Linda P. Virgill endeavored to feed the beast. She knew what caused Daniel's death, she said, but was holding back the information until toxicology results and a full autopsy report were released by the end of the week. "The cause of death is not natural," she told the crowd, and to an Associated Press reporter she used the term "suspicious."[5] She added that a coronial inquest was set for October 23, where her staffers would interview Anna Nicole Smith, hospital workers, customs officers, and anyone else relative to developing an accurate time line of events. The inquest could lead to the filing of criminal charges, she explained.

A third person was in the room when Daniel died, Virgill said, but she wasn't going to reveal the individual's identity now.[6] One needn't be Agatha Christie to connect those dots and assume that she might be hinting at foul play, even as other officials patently denied it.

Of course, panelists on the American nightly crime-news programs repeated this information with great abandon, speculating about who might be arrested, what could be the charge, and what kind of prison sentence might be warranted. I could only shudder at the disaster I was watching unfold.

I imagine part of the reason for Virgill's tough stance was so that the Bahamas could stand apart from its Caribbean cousin, Aruba. The May 2005 disappearance of Alabama teenager Natalee Holloway—still unsolved, despite help from investigators from the acclaimed

Netherlands Forensic Institute and our world-class experts from the Federal Bureau of Investigation—ripped a hole in that country's tourism business when the investigation appeared botched from the get-go. Aruba consequently got the undesired reputation as "*the* spring break location for American blonde girls who never want to be seen again."

Virgill was the coroner—a political position—and not a doctor, much less the doctor who performed Daniel's autopsy. But as the designated spokesperson for the office, some felt she was going beyond disseminating solid information and inviting wild conjecture. And why was the thrust of her message open to the interpretation that a crime may have been committed? If a physical ailment was responsible for this young man's death, why would an inquest even be necessary?

Anna Nicole's Nassau attorney, Michael R. Scott, of the prestigious law firm Callenders & Co., appeared on news clips, denouncing reports that Daniel had antidepressants in his system. "It's sheer speculation" and "it's irresponsible speculation," he blasted.[7]

Scott also endeavored to protect his client by saying that Anna was in seclusion at her home and might not want Daniel's lab results made public. "Would you want your son's toxicology report released to the media? Of course not," he asked and answered.[8]

Scott named Anna's personal attorney and companion, Howard K. Stern, as the other person in the room when Daniel was found dead, but maintained there was nothing untoward about him being there and that he was now with Smith at her house, sharing her grief.[9]

Assistant Police Commissioner Ferguson also went on record to affirm that no drug paraphernalia or traces of illegal drugs were found on Daniel Smith, in the hospital room, or near the room. He also gave a thumbs up to the staff at Doctors Hospital and police personnel, saying that everybody had performed professionally on the morning of Daniel's death[10]

Later, Magistrate Virgill took to the airwaves again, stating that

Daniel's body would be released for burial as soon as the toxicology report was in. Then, apparently feeling some pressure from within the coroner's office, she clarified her previous remarks about the death being "not natural" and the need for an inquest. Sudden deaths are usually classified as "suspicious," she said, and an inquest is not an unusual occurrence. Then she added: "[First there is an] initial autopsy and then you must have a second, just to confirm the findings."[11]

In fact, most coroner cases get closed out with just one autopsy performed; it's only when a dispute is in progress or expected that a second opinion becomes necessary. Linda Virgill's comment signaled where the Daniel Smith case was going. Shortly thereafter, it was announced that I would be flying to Nassau to perform that second autopsy.[12] When my secretary told me there was a call from the Bahamas, I picked up the phone to find Howard K. Stern on the line. I expressed my condolences and asked that he pass them along as well to Anna, which he said he would do. He said Anna's Nassau attorney, Michael Scott, would like to be part of the phone conversation, which I of course welcomed.

To be honest, I never asked what caused Stern to call me, although perhaps he had seen me giving TV interviews about some of the high-profile cases I had worked on. Just months before, I had been a frequent commentator about the second autopsies I performed on missing California mother-to-be Laci Peterson and her unborn son, Conner— a case that ended with her husband, Scott, being convicted of murder and sentenced to death row.

I had also performed a second autopsy on Chandra Levy, the twenty-four-year-old Washington, DC, intern who went missing in 2001, and whose partial, skeletonized remains were found a year later. Despite an intense investigation that proved her death was a homicide—which I concurred with—and the media's fascination over her romance with the married and much older US congressman Gary Condit (now retired), there were never any arrests for the crime and the case remains unsolved.

Stern and Scott were pleased to know that I was up to speed on the reports of Daniel's death. When asked if I would conduct a second autopsy on Daniel, I said I could, provided they understood that I'd call the facts as I saw them, no matter where that might lead. Due to the insatiable media curiosity, whatever I found would have to be shared with the public. They agreed, so I quickly packed a bag as my assistant made my travel arrangements.

Before I would be allowed to perform any procedure in Nassau, I had to get a "Short-Term Work Permit" from the Department of Immigration and approval from the Bahamas Medical Council. Attorneys at Callenders & Co. handled the paperwork, which was requested on an urgent basis, and they paid the $144.23 fee. I only had to supply two passport-sized photos of myself and bring my valid passport. The permit was granted for a three-day period, allowing me to "perform the necessary forensic procedures relating to the deceased, Daniel Smith." Signed by Dr. Baldwin Carey, the chairman of the Bahamas Medical Council, with a copy to the chief of staff at the hospital morgue, I was promised "renewed assurances of the highest consideration of this office."

Soon word got out that I was headed to Nassau, and the news machine kicked into overdrive. I wasn't interested in putting out some kind of "spin." My job was simply to gather the facts and present them to the interested parties and the media. If my findings echoed those of Dr. Raju's first autopsy, fine. If they were wildly disparate, that would also be revealed, along with my reasoning.

Anna and Howard were both convinced that Daniel was an upstanding kid who didn't do drugs, so they probably hoped I'd defend his honor and find some other reason—*any other reason*—for his death.

I was concerned that the coroner seemed to be focusing on Howard K. Stern as a suspect in some nefarious dealings and was offended that this seemed to be done without suitable cause or a proper investigation. Nevertheless, if my work somehow shored up Virgill's notion and a real link could be drawn between Daniel's death and Howard, I'd tell Stern and Scott to hire a criminal defense attorney at once. But that determination was a long way off, and so was any decision as to whether I would participate in the inquest the coroner seemed intent on pursuing.

On Sunday morning, September 17, I flew into Lynden Pindling International Airport, the Bahamas' leading gateway, named for the commonwealth's first prime minister. I was mindful that just a week before, Daniel Smith had walked through the same short terminal, on what turned out to be a one-way trip for him. Though he arrived late at night and my arrival was early in the day when the sun was bright, he would have found the same clean air and helpful airport employees similar to the ones I met.

Michael Scott picked me up and checked me into the Atlantis Hotel and Casino on Nassau's Paradise Island. The resort is one of the most luxurious in the Caribbean, but I'll have to go back to bask in the amenities some other time—on this trip I barely saw my room, let alone anything else there. Next we drove to a private beach club where we joined Stern; his attorney, Anthony McKinney; Scott's colleague at Callenders & Co., Ms. Tracy Ferguson; and an attorney named Wayne Munroe, who I learned was the president of the Bahamian Bar Association. We spent a couple of hours having brunch while they oriented me about the events of the past few days. I would also learn background information about Howard, Daniel, and Anna. It would be a continuing education.

Stern, then thirty-seven years old, earned his juris doctorate at the University of California at Los Angeles and became a member of the California state bar in 1994. By the time the E! series began airing in 2002, Anna had become Stern's sole client. He negotiated all of her business and merchandising contracts and accompanied her to court when she faced off against the family of her billionaire late husband.

Daniel's death was a total shock to Howard, who admitted being the lad's father figure for the last several years. Daniel barely knew his real father and hadn't spoken to him since 1996, so Stern was more than willing to step in as Daniel's father figure.

During the years the trio starred in the E! Channel series, they lived in a home Anna had purchased in Studio City, California—an upscale suburb of Los Angeles, in the San Fernando Valley. Daniel was a straight-A student who attended private institutions when he wasn't home-schooled. After high school graduation he contemplated what to do with his life, deciding he'd take some film and philosophy courses at a local junior college. But when he seemed to fall under the sway of some kids Anna suspected were into drugs, and after Daniel once stayed out all night, his furious mother kicked him out of the house, I was told. He moved into the spare room of a family friend named Raymond Martino, an actor who also wrote and directed a few feature-length videos with and about Anna. I eventually found out that, as aggressively overblown as Anna Nicole was, Daniel was her polar opposite, so shy he barely looked people in the eye. Intelligent and well spoken, he was a gentle kid who always said "please" and "thank you," but wasn't much of a gabber.

A casual dresser, Daniel usually wore clothes from the Gap and an ever-present baseball cap. He liked surfing, snowboarding, playing with his Xbox video console, and the game *Mortal Combat*. He collected Japanese animé cartoons and kept abreast of the latest movies, particularly comedies. *Zoolander*, starring Ben Stiller as a male model, could make Daniel double over with laughter. Howard told me that weekends were usually spent on Anna's bed, with Daniel, Anna, Howard, and their four yappy little dogs munching popcorn and watching the latest DVDs.

Daniel never flaunted his mother's celebrity, nor recoiled in embarrassment at her crazy lifestyle and bosom-busting clothing, though there were plenty of opportunities. Together they were the Dynamic Duo—the wacky mom and the boy she called "Pumpkin" or "Pumpkinhead." When she'd go on TV shows or make personal appearances, he was in the wings, cheering her on. He even appeared in one of her films, 1997's cheesy action flick *Skyscraper*. Even after Howard started handling Anna's business, Daniel was still her touchstone.

The threesome had had a pleasant bonding experience in the late summer of 2005 when Anna starred in a movie titled *Illegal Aliens*, with Daniel and Howard present for the filming. An outer space spoof, which also starred the ex–World Wrestling Federation star Joanie "Chyna" Laurer, Anna invested money in the project with the provision that Daniel be brought on board and made an associate producer, a title she shared. The film shoot in Vermont was delayed when Anna said that Daniel was going to do an uncredited rewrite on the script. Director/co-producer David Giancola, already working on a shoestring budget and schedule, was panicky until he got the script back and saw that Daniel had actually improved it. He had an absolute knack, Giancola later said, of knowing just how to make his mother better in the project, and he represented a Generation-Y sensibility that the filmmakers found priceless. Throughout the shoot, Daniel kept his mother focused and productive and got the chance to experience hands-on moviemaking that suddenly made going to college a less important goal.[13]

While the film was being edited and readied for a 2006 release, Howard told me he, Anna, and Daniel returned to California. But shortly into the New Year, Anna learned she was pregnant, which excited them all. In July, Stern explained, he and Anna had moved to the Nassau home—a gated property called Horizons—so she could get ready to have a calm and private birth in a few weeks. Daniel chose to stay behind in Los Angeles because he didn't like the sweltering climate. It was rough on everyone, Stern said, as they'd never been apart for such a long spell. Daniel—or "Danny" as he called him—had been having regular stomachaches and back pain and had even been briefly hospitalized on two occasions. Once, he had checked into an intensive care unit when his heart started racing. A male cousin in the family had suffered a fatal heart attack at age fourteen, and Daniel was aware of his family's genetic history, so going to the hospital was his way of being proactive.

The second time Daniel sought help was for mental health reasons, following the breakup with a girl he had been dating. Anna knew he was battling depression, but he assured her that he was okay and the two phoned each other often, Howard said. In December 2007, while the inquest was under way, Stern told *Entertainment Tonight* that he only learned of Daniel's full medical history through testimony that came out during the proceedings. He hadn't known before, he claimed, that Daniel's July 2006 hospitalization was to help him beat a Valium addiction.[14] I surmise that had Stern known of that detail when he and I were discussing Daniel's background, he would have told me. Following the birth of her daughter, Anna called Daniel, broke the cheery news, and asked him to come meet his baby half sister. According to Stern, Daniel was thrilled at the prospect and knew he could help his mom in the hospital too, where she would be recovering from her major surgery for the next couple of days.

Because there hadn't been enough time to plan the trip, Daniel couldn't find a direct Los Angeles–Nassau flight. He ended up booking Burbank–Fort Worth, Texas; Fort Worth–Miami; Miami–Nassau, a long journey for someone who never much liked flying under the best of conditions. His friend Ray Martino drove him to Burbank's Bob Hope Airport and made sure he had a healthy breakfast for what would be an exhausting travel day. Daniel's stomach was acting up, but it wasn't going to stop him from traveling.

American Eagle flight 5005 arrived in Nassau at 10:25 p.m. that Saturday night. Daniel was cleared through Immigration by Officer Marva Gibson, who said later that the youth appeared normal and was "very quiet and conservative at the time." He asked for and was granted a ninety-day stay, telling Gibson he would be staying with his mother at the Horizons home on Eastern Road, although he could not recall the street address. She let him through even though his form wasn't completed.[15]

Howard told me that once Danny had arrived, he was taken aback at how thin Danny looked; he must have dropped twenty-five pounds since the summer. But he was in good spirits and so eager to see his mother and the infant, they didn't even stop at Horizons to drop off Daniel's luggage. At Doctors Hospital, Daniel practically ran into room 201 and gave his mom a big hug. She was still in much discomfort from the C-section of two days earlier, but shed happy tears at the sight of the people she loved most in the world all in one place. Howard brought over the baby, who had been asleep in her bassinet, and Anna held up the tiny pink-wrapped bundle. "Here's your brother, Daniel," she cooed to the little girl. She let Daniel hold the child—he had never before seen a baby that young—and he softly stroked her head and let her tiny hand encircle his finger. Any jealousy he may have felt went out the window, Stern said. Daniel's heart was won over and he couldn't stop grinning about it.

Howard snapped a few photos of the blissful occasion, not realizing the importance of what he was chronicling, he told me. These photos were later brokered by the Getty Images photo agency, which sold them to *In Touch Weekly* magazine and the TV show *Entertainment Tonight*, for a combined $650,000, reportedly. A spokeswoman for *In Touch* said at the time: "There is an incredible amount of emotion attached to this story and the photos, and our story will be a tribute to Daniel's life as a well as a celebration of it." *People* magazine supposedly got beat with its bid of $350,000.[16]

First photos of a celebrity baby always command top dollar. It's a common business practice and a nice way to start a newborn's trust account. Howard was only doing what many a savvy lawyer or manager would do under the same circumstance. Also, it was reported that Anna had plans to use a portion of the money for a Daniel Smith memorial.[17]

Anna's friend G. "Ben" Thompson, a former beau and the millionaire owner of the Horizons home, had also been visiting that night. He watched the poignant family get-together, then excused himself to go home; he'd see them all tomorrow, he said.

After he left, Anna felt hungry and asked Howard to go get some food. Not much was open in town after midnight, so he and Daniel drove to a nearby twenty-four-hour mini-mart and bought chicken strips, chips, and soda. They returned to the hospital and shared the food. The fellows drank the soda, while Anna stuck to water and juice;

she had never developed a taste for carbonated drinks. Everything seemed great, Stern said, even though Daniel once wondered aloud why he was so tired. Howard told me the comment later haunted him, that perhaps he should have seen it as a sign that something was wrong.

The room had two beds—a now-drowsy Anna was in the one by the window, and Howard was sitting on the other one. He offered Daniel the bed, but Daniel said he was fine in the armchair he was camped out on and that he wanted to watch some TV. Howard lowered the lights and dozed off. Over the next several hours, he was vaguely aware of Daniel occasionally walking his mother to the bathroom. Nurses who made hourly rounds noted the trio was asleep for most of the night. A notation at 6:20 a.m. showed Daniel helping his mom resettle in her bed; subsequent checks stated that all three adults were asleep.

Just after 9:30 a.m., Anna woke to find Daniel snuggled up in her bed. He appeared to be sleeping, but was cold to the touch. She shook him but got no response. "Howard, wake up!" she yelled. "Daniel's not breathing!"

"I put my fingers on Daniel's neck, but there was no pulse," Stern told me. "I tried shaking him, as we screamed for help. Anna was hysterical, not understanding how this could be."

At 9:38 a.m., the nurse's station heard a buzzer go off in room 201. The responding nurse saw the patient crying and shouting that her son was not breathing. Daniel's lips and skin were pale and there was no respiration noted, according to hospital notes. His pupils were fixed and dilated, and his fingers had turned blue, indicating that his blood had become deoxygenated.[18]

A "Code Blue" emergency was called, and the crash cart was brought in. Medical personnel flooded the room. The response team—led by Dr. James Iferenta, head of the hospital's emergency room—consisted of at least two nurses, an anesthesiologist, a pharmacist, a radiologist, and two security guards. Doctors began CPR on the prone lad, while Stern told them that Daniel had no known serious medical conditions.

Anesthesiologist Dr. Reginald Neymour would later testify at the inquest that the boy's body was "cool to the touch" as he embarked on his resuscitation mission. "I placed a face mask on him. He had no pulse and no heart beat," he said. Daniel was intubated with an endotracheal tube into his windpipe, and an IV was inserted into the backside of his left hand. Dr. Neymour administered medicine—epinephrine, sodium bicarbonate, Atropine, vasopressin, and Narcan—through both devices in an attempt to start the heartbeat and increase blood pressure. Chest compressions continued, and the pressure bag was commenced on fast flow. A second dose of epinephrine was given, then a third, fourth, fifth, and sixth. But it was all to no avail. At 10:05 a.m., Daniel Wayne Smith's death was called.

Anna grabbed Daniel's leg and wouldn't let go, Howard told me. "She was screaming, 'No, No! Please Jesus, take me instead! Don't take Daniel, don't take my Pumpkin!'" She kept trying to revive her son, pumping on his chest and telling Howard to blow into the tube that went into Daniel's mouth and down his airway.[19]

Dr. Iferenta would testify that Anna was highly emotional and was fighting off several males who were trying to get her to let go of the decedent. "There were difficulties in getting her out of the room and she clung on to him [Daniel] during my time in the room," he said.[20]

Nurses collected 50 cc of urine via a Foley catheter and drew blood from Daniel's groin; these items were given to lab workers. A priest was requested and police arrived in the room, then Anna's obstetrician, Dr. Minnis, joined them.[21]

Howard phoned Ray Martino with the awful news, he told me, and then he called Ben Thompson, saying only there was an emergency and telling him to come back to the hospital. When Ben arrived, a nurse told him Daniel had passed away. He saw the boy on the bed, with Anna holding him, practically falling off the mattress. Ben was afraid that the new mother might fall off the bed and open up her surgical wound. She was sobbing so loudly she had to be sedated; it was the only way the doctors could separate her from Daniel.

A local funeral home was contacted to transfer the body to the morgue at Nassau's Princess Margaret Hospital. Once there, Dr. Caroline Burnett tagged the body and officially pronounced Daniel deceased.[22]

Right before Daniel's body was removed, Howard snapped a final photo of Anna cradling her son's head. Her tear-stained, puffy face showed absolute pain while Daniel's skin was deathly pale, his eyes were at half-mast, and the airway tube was still sticking out of his mouth. The photo later proved to be roundly criticized by the media, but Howard told me that Anna had wanted him to take the picture so that she would really accept that he was dead. A photo was also shot and sold of Daniel in his coffin, although I don't know who took it or profited from it.

It was a lot of information to take in, but I couldn't process it all then because it was time to go to the morgue. Michael Scott once again did the driving, and while he and Tracy Ferguson waited in an outside room, I went into the examination area. Dr. Raju introduced himself and Magistrate Virgill. Both were very gracious, as were the members of their staff. I was never given a copy of the original written autopsy report, so I made my own rough notes and did not prepare a formal autopsy report at that time.

Daniel's body was brought in from the cold storage. He was slight and slender—probably about five feet nine and one hundred fifty pounds, an estimated antemortem, pre-autopsy weight. His organs and fluids had already been removed in the previous procedure, so my body weight measurement was an approximation. I was presented with the organs, so I could take samples.

He had uncombed sandy brown hair, about four inches in length, and around two days' worth of facial stubble, with a scruffy Vandyke beard. His irises were light brown, but because vitreous humor—eyeball fluid—had been removed for toxicological testing, the eyes appeared shrunken. There were no petechial, or pinpoint, hemorrhages on the conjunctivae, or the mucous membranes that line the inner surface of the eyelids and the forepart of the eyeball.

Daniel's teeth were natural and intact, and he had no tattoos or piercings. Seven loops of a black soft leather or plastic were on his right wrist, and one loop of dark orange, hard plastic was on his left wrist. No clothing was present. Fingernails and toenails were short but intact, with cyanotic nailbeds, a post-mortem condition signaling no blood circulation.

Four intravascular puncture sites were present, all having been done at the hospital, according to Dr. Raju. There was some post-mortem greenish discoloration, plus a couple of small bruises, and four superficial scratches spread around his body. There was no evidence of injury or needle puncture marks from self-inflicted injection sites.

To remove the organs, the Y-shaped thoraco-abdominal and bitemporal incisions had been made appropriately and were closed with a thick white string.

For about three hours I reviewed Dr. Raju's findings. He had ruled out foul play, cancer, infection, blood clots to the heart or lungs, or any other natural disease process, and I concurred. Though we both knew about Daniel's stomachaches and back pains, there was nothing at autopsy that suggested a reason for them. We also looked at the boy's stomach contents, but there was nothing noteworthy there, such as undigested pills or capsules.

Raju attributed cause of death to "accidental multiple drug toxicity," and I agreed that's what it looked like. Initial screening—sent by Raju's team to LabCorp, an excellent basic toxicology lab in Tampa, Florida—showed that Daniel's system had no traces of alcohol, opiates, amphetamines, cocaine, marijuana, or any other illegal drugs. What he did have, however, was methadone—a painkiller that's been around since the 1940s—and two antidepressants, Zoloft and Lexapro. Daniel had no known addiction to morphine or heroin, so the presence of methadone was a puzzler. While it is a powerful analgesic, methadone's first-line usage is for weaning heroin, oxycodone, or opiate addicts from their substance abuse. It's not a standard drug of choice, but we medical examiners are seeing more methadone than ever in drug death cases. I wanted to learn the reason Daniel had it in his system.

Zoloft and Lexapro are both SSRI medications—selective serotonin reuptake inhibitors. They are highly effective psychotropic pharmaceuticals that provide depression relief by affecting the neurotransmitters in a person's central nervous system. No sensible doctor should prescribe both medications at once for a patient, in any dosage. If one doesn't work well, a doctor should switch the patient to the other drug, but only after cautioning him or her to stop taking that first drug. Also these SSRI drugs take some time to begin working—usually days, but sometimes weeks. Someone feeling especially depressed one day would not take an extra dosage and expect to feel an immediate mood leveling. It also made no sense to me why someone would take two drugs intended to elevate his mood and top it off with a "downer" like methadone.

Still we all know of patients who hoard drugs, self-medicate, and even "doctor shop" to get different prescriptions from different doctors, without revealing their full pharmacological histories.

All three of these medications in Daniel's system were of high therapeutic levels, but the combination of the two antidepressants was akin to taking a double dose—and the methadone, on top of that, guaranteed to send him into a fatal downward spiral.

First, we eliminated the idea that Daniel might have committed suicide for various reasons. One was the documented glee he displayed when he was with his mother and half sister. There were many witnesses and photos that showed him beaming as he held the newborn. He'd have to be an award-winning actor to fake that kind of enjoyment. This is a family that should have been looking forward to the approaching holidays together, instead of having one of them dead and the others left to defend themselves against baseless charges.

Second, no note was found, not that that is always a bellwether of suicide.

Third, few people commit suicide by taking small doses of a variety of drugs; generally, a person determined to purposely overdose tries to empty a bottle of whatever is the chosen pharmaceutical. Sometimes, a plastic bag is slipped over one's head to halt the breathing process faster and accomplish the goal, making it less likely that the individual will vomit up the pills and revive. Often the manual on the subject, the book or DVD of Derek Humphry's *Final Exit: The Practicalities of Self-Deliverance and Assisted Suicide for the Dying*, is present.

Daniel's death had none of the markers of suicide and had all the features of an accidental drug fatality. But could he have been killed? That is a more complex question, and it would take a while before we would have that answer. While Dr. Raju found no attributable physical ailment, he understood that I would want to perform my own studies. Myocarditis, or inflammation of the heart, may be caused by an infectious agent, usually a clinically silent virus that is asymptomatic.

I took blood samples and representative sections of various body organs and tissues, each measuring approximately a quarter inch to a half-inch. I put each into a screw-topped plastic container, filled with formalin, the universal chemical preservative, and brought them back to Pittsburgh. The blood was sent to the National Medical Services lab in Willow Grove, Pennsylvania—founded by my late friend Dr. Fredric Rieders and now run by his sons Michael and Eric, and other family members—the premier forensic toxicology experts in the country, if not the world. Its equipment and personnel can probe deeper than the basic toxicology screening labs.

The tissues were sent to my local histology lab. There, the samples were sliced paper-thin, treated with the dyes H&E (hemotoxylin and eosin), put onto glass slides, and returned to me. Then I studied each slide under my high-powered microscope to rule out myocarditis and other subtle evidence of an infectious disease process.

There are special cells along the right side of the heart that transmit the nerve impulses that control the heart's normal rhythm. A small nidus, or nest, of inflammatory cells, so few in number as to be invisible to the naked eye, can seed out and interrupt the conducting mechanism, producing a fatal dysrhythmia.

Leaving the quiet sanctum of the morgue that Sunday evening, I stepped outside the building to a hive of buzzing reporters, at least fifty strong. With attorneys Scott and Ferguson behind me, and the permission of them and Howard K. Stern, I became the focus of an impromptu press conference that was beamed around the world. Questions were shouted at me, and cameras and microphones were aimed at my head, almost knocking me over. In more than four decades of doing this work, I had never seen such a constant and intense barrage of news media inquiries, all of which I endeavored to respond to with patience, information, and discretion. Little did I realize that just five months later, when Anna Nicole died, there would be all this kind of chaos and much more.

After the press conference, we drove over to the Horizons home, where Anna, Stern, and some staffers were staying. Later I would learn that the ownership of the waterfront property was in question and there were problems with Anna's and Howard's residency, but those issues were not germane to my visit.

The gated, million-dollar estate was lovely, with a yacht slip in the back, a tennis court, a swimming pool, and a multistoried neo-Mediterranean house. It wasn't the most sumptuous residence in the area, and fell short, in my mind at least, of earning the title of "mansion," the term bandied about in the media. What mattered more was that I might hopefully obtain some answers to what I could see was a household in crisis.

If the many photos on the walls of Anna and Daniel in happier times weren't reminder enough of why I was there, the red-rimmed eyes of the home's inhabitants were. Anna was sleeping, I was told. She was understandably destroyed by her son's death and still recovering from the cesarean section birth of a week ago. She came into the room once, wearing a pink chenille bathrobe over pajamas, her face stripped of makeup—hardly the glamorous image I had seen in photographs.

Walking over to me, she said in a trembling voice: "Hi, Dr. Wecht, I'm Anna." I offered my hand to shake, but she grabbed it and squeezed it for dear life. "Thank you for coming here," she said, misting up. "I don't know how this happened. Daniel was a good boy—he wasn't into drugs."

"I'm sorry that you lost your son," I told her. Then vowed to do whatever I could to find answers. She nodded and let go of my hand; then she went upstairs and presumably back to bed.

An older nanny was in charge of the baby, whose name I now learned was Dannielynn Hope Marshall; the first name in tribute to the half brother she would never know and the surname because it was Anna's legal, married name. Stern said Anna called herself "Mamalynn" and liked to add "lynn" as a term of affection to those in her inner circle. The newborn was already a little beauty and seemed well cared for and healthy. Stern spoke of the child as his daughter, and I was told his name would be on the birth certificate. Months later that would change as the child's biological father was revealed to be someone other than Howard.

Stern confessed that he and Anna had been a romantic couple for some time, but kept it hush-hush as he feared it might be perceived as inappropriate, given that he was still her attorney and primary adviser. He told me that he and Anna had plans to marry legally down the line, but in the near future, they were going to hold a commitment ceremony in the Bahamas to go public with their love affair.

I pressed Stern for answers about where Daniel might have gotten the drugs that were in his system—in particular, the methadone—but he assured me he didn't know. Anna had a prescription for that drug, Howard said, but Daniel didn't, as far as he knew.

While we sat around the dining room table, attorney Scott made a conference call to a Los Angeles-based internal medicine physician, Dr. Sandeep Kapoor, who had treated both mother and son. Kapoor told me he had written a methadone prescription for Anna when she was eight months pregnant—methadone being an effective painkiller for someone used to strong medication, yet relatively safe for a developing fetus. No one saw Daniel take his mother's methadone, however; nor can anyone really say if that prescription was the source of what he ingested.

Dr. Kapoor told me he had treated Daniel for stomach cramps and depression after the romantic breakup that landed him in the hospital. The doctor prescribed a low dosage of Lexapro, with only a limited quantity of tablets, a staggered regimen, and the intention of weaning him from the drug. He couldn't account for the Zoloft. He never would have prescribed two competing antidepressants to someone at the same time, he said.

Much later I learned that Daniel's landlord and friend, Ray Martino, might have insight on that matter. Two weeks after the death, Martino is said to have told Bahamian authorities, as he went through Daniel's belongings, he supposedly found a half bottle of Zoloft. As far as I'm concerned, this is still uncorroborated information, and there was no report of which doctor wrote such a prescription, for whom it was written, or why.

I knew there was a good likelihood that Daniel's death was entirely prescription drug–related, but it would take a couple more weeks for all the lab results to come in, even with the fast-tracking I had requested. Unfortunately, no one was paying me to spend those weeks sunning myself around the pools at the Atlantis Hotel or playing high-stakes baccarat in the casino, so our meeting ended with pledges to keep each other informed of new developments.

Michael Scott dropped me off at my hotel. A producer for *Larry King Live* spotted me going into the restaurant, and we had dinner together. Then I went upstairs, got a few hours' rest, and headed to the airport the next morning, having spent just one night at that marvelous resort.

Back in Pittsburgh, the news coverage was still 24/7, and my phone was still ringing off the hook. One item piqued my curiosity: On September 20, Bahamas chief justice, Sir Burton Hall, stripped Magistrate Linda Virgill of her designation of "coroner" and abolished the "coroner's court." No reason was given.[23]

The next day, Daniel's preliminary death certificate was issued, "pending chemical analysis." Signed by Dr. Raju and myself, before I left Nassau, it cleared the way for Daniel to be lawfully buried. But it would take Anna and Howard nearly a month to hold the funeral—first came their "commitment ceremony," a non-legally-binding wedding that took place on a friend's boat on September 28, for which *People* magazine paid more than a million dollars for exclusive coverage.[24] There was a separate major sale of a reported million dollars for Dannielynn's birth photos and footage from her birth[25] and I was told plans were being made for Anna's first taped interview after Daniel's death—for what I deduced would be a large fee—to *Entertainment Tonight*. Again, as a responsible lawyer and manager to a celebrity whose important events are chronicled in the media for a price, Howard doesn't deserve condemnation for making these sorts of deals. Public curiosity drives the market.

The question of murder was still on everyone's lips when an episode of FOX News Channel's *On the Record with Greta Van Susteren* tackled the subject. One of the show's guests was Tampa-area assistant state attorney Pam Bondi, who said, "Whenever you have a twenty-year-old who's relatively healthy and he dies in his sleep, of course, that's going to be suspicious. I think Bahamian authorities think there is some kind of crime involved."[26]

That might well be her opinion, but it's not one I agree with as it pertained to this case.

In many jurisdictions, someone who gives a drug to an individual who ends up dying of an overdose can be charged with negligent homicide or manslaughter, even if the deceased person had voluntarily requested the drug.

Also on that Greta Van Susteren program was former Los Angeles police detective Mark Fuhrman, most famous for working the homicide case against O. J. Simpson—and getting caught on tape using the "n" word. He added that the drug doesn't need to be illegal. Any person who has prescription drugs and passes them to someone else is "equal to being a drug dealer and is contributing to whatever happens to the person the drug was given to," he said

Bondi explained: "In Florida, it's first-degree murder—we've used this statute very successfully."

But she also admitted that most of those prosecutions were to build cases against drug traffickers, where throwing the book at a defendant might be more understandable.[27]

That didn't seem to be in play here. Stern strongly insisted that neither Anna nor he had furnished Daniel with the drugs. Could the youth have found the drugs himself and taken them? That seems a valid option to me. Proving there was malicious intent on Howard's or Anna's part that caused them to give Daniel drugs with the intention of ending his life—and that goal being met—just seems outlandish. And how could that possibly be proven to a reasonable degree of medicolegal certainty, let alone reasonable doubt, the higher level of evidentiary proof required in a criminal case?

I knew that Bahamian detectives had interviewed the immigration officer and people on the flights with Daniel, presumably to see if anyone saw him being given drugs or if he might have been drinking alcohol, which had metabolized by the time of his death but could have enhanced the effect of the drugs. If Daniel was imbibing on a flight that originated from California, there might be an issue of his being a year too young to legally drink alcohol, so could someone have bought a drink for him, or might he have used a false ID?

As far as I could determine, nothing of any value came from these interviews, except to show that the Bahamian police were diligent in trying to find answers. But alas, good intentions don't always provide answers.

The startling reality is that two out of every five coroner cases that I encounter these days are what I would call "acute combined drug toxicity" deaths, or accidental overdoses. But in order to put that on an autopsy report or a death certificate, all other possibilities need to be considered and negated. I continued to be booked on TV to discuss the case, always with Stern's blessing, but by no means did he have input on what I would say. Whenever asked, I would explain that there was nothing to suggest foul play or suspicion, nor was there anything of a furtive or clandestine nature involving some third party, directly or indirectly, in the death of Daniel Smith.

But other people close to the case had their own viewpoints. A well-discussed one was told by Anna's friends, Ben Thompson and his son-in-law Ford Shelley, about the night Daniel died. While Howard stayed at the hospital and spoke to police, a wheelchaired Anna, the baby, Ben, and a friend named Theresa Laramore left for Horizons. Ben's son Gaither and son-in-law Ford Shelley were at the home already and witnessed what they said was an odd event. When Howard later returned to the house, carrying Daniel's clothing, Ford and Gaither watched him go through the jeans' pockets. Both men have said that two odd-shaped white pills fell out of the front pocket and that Howard picked them up, went to the bathroom, and closed the door. Concerned, Ford walked to the bathroom door and heard a flush. Howard, he claimed, exited the bathroom, saying, "I took care of a problem."[28]

Howard has flatly denied to me that this alleged incident occurred.

There were two other sets of mysterious pills. Nadine Carey, a nurse present during the lifesaving attempts on Daniel, apparently discovered two white tablets, one smaller than the other, resting on the bedcovering where Stern had been sleeping. Following protocol, she gave them to the doctor, who handed them to a supervisor, who forwarded them to Bahamian detectives.[29] The tablets were then put into plastic bags and sent for lab testing. They were later determined to be the muscle relaxant carisoprodol and methadone.[30] Anna had prescriptions for both medications. While three nurses gave statements that only Howard was seen in that bed, on a *Larry King Live* show two weeks after that frantic morning, Stern said that Daniel had spent time in the bed, as well.[31] But there is no proven link between those pills and Daniel.

Another report of pills came from Ray Martino, Daniel's friend who took him to the airport. Martino reportedly told Los Angeles private eye Jack E. Harding that he had given the youth two Valiums for antianxiety and another pill—which Harding says might have been the over-the-counter motion sickness medication Dramamine—to help him handle the long flight. But neither medicine was in Daniel's bloodstream when his toxicology results came back.

Harding, whose company is titled Nemesis, Ltd., and who also works with US military intelligence with an Above Top Secret clearance, had a direct encounter with this case when a few weeks after Daniel's death he received an at-home visit from four Bahamian plainclothes detectives and two local policemen. The detectives wanted to know why Harding's business card was found among Daniel's belongings, which had been confiscated before the items were given to Stern. Harding told them that shortly before Daniel made the trip to Nassau, he had met with him twice—once with Martino when he was introduced to the young man and gave him the business card, and a second time when Daniel called and asked for a private meeting, making it known that he didn't want word getting back to Martino. Over coffee Daniel told Harding that he was worried about his mother. Harding alleges the youth told him that Anna was being kept on "mind-bending drugs" by Stern. Howard, Jack was purportedly told, would hang up the phone when he caught Anna speaking to Daniel. "Howard hates me and keeps me away from her," Daniel supposedly said, adding, "He's made her a prisoner. I want to get her out of there."

Harding told the detectives that Daniel also allegedly said that Stern dispensed drugs to him, too, although the private investigator found Smith to be "clear-eyed and absolutely coherent" during their two get-togethers. According to Harding, Daniel asked him to go to the Bahamas and save his mother, but lacked the funds to hire Harding or anyone to travel to a foreign land, investigate, and stage a rescue operation. When Harding learned of the boy's death, he felt terrible that he hadn't been able to help him, he told the detectives—but he was prepared to repeat his anecdote to the coroner's inquest jury.

Some months later, my co-author, investigative journalist Dawna Kaufmann, played a video clip for Harding of an interview Anna Nicole and Howard gave to *Entertainment Tonight* a few weeks after

Daniel's death. Anna tearfully explained a phone call she had made, telling Daniel she had just given birth.[32]

"I have a baby sister? I have a baby sister?" Daniel asked. "Oh, Mama, can I come down? Can I come down? Can I come down right now?"

Anna said she told Daniel, "Yes, Pumpkin, you can come down," and he replied, "Really, Mama? Really, Mama?"[33]

The clip mystified Harding. Here was Anna herself talking, not some third-party account of what went down. "It sounds like someone, perhaps Stern, was blocking Daniel's access to his own mother," Harding told Kaufmann. "It's hard to imagine that someone in the loop wouldn't know his own mother was pregnant with a daughter, and his gushing about being allowed to visit makes it seem as if he had been deprived of the company of his mother for some time.

"Daniel's isolation from his mother was very real and heart-breaking," Harding said.[34]

Were Daniel and Anna out of touch during her pregnancy? Not according to Stern, who said they spoke on the phone frequently. But Harding's allegation about Daniel asking him for help was certainly compelling. I would have to file this under "imponderable"—impossible to calculate.

These are examples of how cases often have strings that never get properly tied into a pretty package. Why did the Bahamian police going through Daniel's pockets find Harding's card but miss the two white pills? Who knows? And why did assistant police commissioner Reginald Ferguson state that no drug paraphernalia or traces of illegal drugs were found on Daniel Smith, either in the hospital room or near the room?

Stern, at least to me, always professed a deep attachment to Daniel and never intimated that there was any chasm between Anna and her son. But there is another source for Stern allegedly shutting people out of Anna's life. Her mother, Virgie Arthur, bitterly complained that Stern isolated Anna in the Bahamas from Virgie's family members in Texas. Arthur heard about Daniel's death from TV news accounts, and days after received a phone call from Anna. "She was mumbling like a drunk," Virgie said of her daughter's slurred speech, which she attributed to drugs. "All I got out of it was, 'Mama, he's gone, he's gone—but he's coming back!'" Virgie told a reporter. Then there was a click and the line went dead. She never heard from her daughter again.[35]

Former pals and employees have described Stern as the keeper of Anna's floating pharmacy, allegedly filling a Coach bag with all the medications she'd take in a day and doling them out in little paper cups, every four hours: painkillers, muscle relaxants, diet drugs, sleep aids, antidepressants, antihistamines, antibiotics, antivirals, anti-inflammatories, antiseizure meds, and more.[36]

Everybody seemed to have an opinion on whether Anna was a puppet of Stern, or if she was pulling his strings—and how they each fit into Daniel's death. Many sought me out to express themselves. One e-mail I received appeared to be from someone purporting to be "Coldwater," the moderator of a Court TV (now called TruTV) Internet discussion forum. The message—which was also copied to thesmokinggun.com, a Web site owned by that cable network and dedicated to posting legal documents—stated (in caps): *"WE WILL PAY YOU THE SUM OF TEN THOUSAND ($10,000) DOLLARS FOR PICTURES OF THE POST MORTEM OF DANIEL WAYNE SMITH."*

When I complained about this to Court TV, I received another e-mail—this time from the actual Coldwater, stating that the first message was a hoax. I suppose this crude ploy was someone's idea of a joke, but the humor escaped me.

Throughout this time I received at least twenty phone calls from Stern, making specific requests, seeking information, and urging me to communicate with the toxicology labs, hospital pathologist, and others. He called at all hours of the day and evening, at my office and home, weekdays and weekends—and I responded promptly to every one of his calls, always following through with his requests to the fullest extent possible. I had no problem receiving these calls and appreciated being kept up to date on the latest events.

Howard seemed to be aware of every comment about the case on every cable TV news program and in every magazine and newspaper, and expressed gratitude when I was interviewed and able to disseminate accurate information in those fast-talking, sound-bite environments.

On September 25, I sent a letter to Dr. Raju thanking him and his administrative staff for their warm hospitality and professional collegiality. We had handled a complex and highly sensitive matter in a mature and responsible fashion, I felt, and the Nassau crew deserved a pat on the back. I also made the point that we would shortly know the cause and mechanism of Daniel's death, pending microscopic examination of tissues, toxicological analyses, and a review of pertinent medical and hospital records. When those reports came in, we discussed them on the phone. Some months later, when Dr. Raju came to Pittsburgh for a family function, we were able to have an enjoyable luncheon, still marveling a bit at what a whirlwind we had shared.

In the vacuum created by having to wait for information, rumors and ideas flew at warp speed. One PhD who works in the realm of sexual abuse even wrote me to suggest that Dannielynn's DNA be compared to that of Anna's and Daniel's in case there was something "about the nature of their relationship and the bearing that might have on the son's untimely death."

A woman from Germany also e-mailed my son, Ben: *"Hello, my English is not so got, but maybe I can something help. Please give to Cyril Wecht the information, importend is what Daniel exactly 24 hrs bevor exitent has drink and the person wth him. Maybe test her hair for this time."*

Another person wrote me a scathing letter about how Anna's "toxic parenting" was the sole reason for Daniel's death.

And yet another person wrote me an e-mail and enclosed a photo of Daniel, smiling. She suggested that since the young man's gums appeared to be "red and swollen," he might have had periodontal disease. She also included recent literature that linked an increase risk of heart attacks with bacterial infection spread by vigorous teeth cleaning. Teeth are rooted in bone, and it is possible for bacteria to enter the blood circulatory system, leading to arterial damage.

Most of the people were trying to be of assistance, as were others of a more scientific nature who submitted abstracts, Internet URLs, and studies of similar cases or aspects of the medical issues. I wrote them all back, saying I would carefully consider their information in my review and analysis of this matter, and thanked them for their communications.

Over the next several weeks, Anna was still heavily medicated and inconsolable, Howard told me. She would wake from a nap and ask for Daniel, then crumble all over again when Howard explained that the boy was gone. So severe was Anna's anguish, friends feared she might take her life, and there were two reports of her trying to do so. But baby Dannielynn seemed to soothe her pain.

Even in Anna's sober moments, she could never quite remember what happened the morning when she lost her Pumpkin. Howard told me she felt as if someone had "*Punk'd*" her—referring to the Ashton Kutcher–produced TV show that is based on pranks. (On that series after a celebrity is the victim of a practical joke, Kutcher or one of his cohorts jump out and yell: "You've been 'Punk'd!'")

Later Anna posed for photos wearing colorful tattoos she had emblazoned on her back—one showed her with Dannielynn, and the other showed her and Daniel, with his birth and death dates, and the caption: "My Pumpkinhead." Both turned out to be temporary tattoos.[37]

Interest in whether Daniel's death was murder was ratcheted up on October 12, when Cable Headline News host Nancy Grace convened a panel that included the boy's grandmother, Virgie Arthur. Virgie called Daniel "a blessing" and consistently referred to her daughter's given name of "Vickie Lynn." She said there was no sign of Daniel taking "any kind of drug, other than a sleeping pill and an anxiety pill." And she insisted her grandson didn't use methadone: "Somebody had to give it to him. He had to get it somewhere," she stated, adding ominously, "There were only three people in that room. Danny was one of them."[38]

Grace, a former Atlanta prosecutor whose "hang 'em high" style makes defense attorneys cringe and crime victims cheer, was repeating the rumor that the levels of Lexapro and Zoloft were "seven times" the expected dosage. This unsubstantiated rumor was later proven false when the National Medical Services toxicology lab results were revealed.

Arthur went on to say she was happy to be a grandmother again, but when she tried to inquire about Dannielynn by phoning her daughter and Stern, she discovered their unlisted number had changed. And she complained, "I'm very upset that my grandson is still laying in a cold room and hasn't been buried yet. The last bit of respect you get in this world is at a funeral, and my baby's not had one."[39] She had a point there—it had been more than a month since Daniel's death. I'm sure the morgue personnel were also wondering when he was going to be moved.

Anna Nicole's wealthy late husband had set up a trust fund for Daniel, Virgie told Nancy Grace, but she didn't know what happened to that money. But it was the money Anna hoped to inherit—more than a half billion dollars—that Virgie suggested might be a motive for getting Daniel out of the way: "If Howard marries Vickie and Daniel's gone, that leaves Howard and the baby, to inherit whatever money she has.

"If Howard Stern marries her and she ends up dead, then who does the money go to?" she asked. "Danny's not here."

Throughout the show Virgie wiped away tears and seemed in authentic distress about her helplessness to connect with her wayward daughter, so when Grace gave her a chance to speak out to Anna, the no-nonsense Texas mother took it with a chilling shot that made headlines from coast to coast:

"Vickie Lynn, you know I love you, always have," Virgie said, looking straight into the camera. "Be very careful about who you hang around with, because you may be next."[40]

Grandma Arthur had no way of knowing how prophetic her words would be as she gave public notice that she'd be paying close attention from now on. I couldn't help but feel sympathy for a woman who lost her beloved grandchild and feared for her daughter's well-being. But I also felt sympathy for Howard Stern, whose sincerity seemed genuine. After all my years in the business, I think I've become a fairly accurate judge of character, and I'd like to think both persons here had the best of intentions. But I also wasn't forgetting the enormous pot of gold these people might be chasing. Greed has a way of ruining relationships, sometimes with even deadly consequences.

After much debate as to whether Daniel should be buried in the United States or the Bahamas, Anna and Howard decided to pursue permanent residency in the islands and agreed that Daniel would stay close to their new home. On October 19, thirty-nine days after his death, Daniel was finally laid to rest in a brass-trimmed mahogany casket at the Lake View Memorial Gardens and Mausoleum in Nassau. Concerned that the funeral might be disrupted, and to avert prying eyes, planners arranged for the casket to be taken from the funeral home in a van. The driver then rode to a meeting point, switched the casket to a gold-colored hearse, and motored on to the burial site. Anna, Howard, and a select few followed in three white limousines. The gravesite, which overlooked the picture-perfect blue waters of Lake Cunningham, was near a grove of palm trees and by a pavilion called The Citadel. The mourners gathered underneath a large green tent, where Baptist bishop Neil Ellis conducted the service.

The open casket showed Daniel in his favorite outfit of blue jeans, green T-shirt, and trucker cap, with a spare white Nike "Swoosh" cap set on the pillow under his head. Anna was dressed in a demure black dress and black hat and veil; she wore dark sunglasses throughout the ceremony.

No one from Anna's family was invited to attend the services, including her mother, Virgie Arthur, and Daniel's biological father, Billy Wayne Smith.[41]

A reporter in attendance allegedly heard a woman's voice, ostensibly Anna Nicole's, wailing: "I don't want my husband, I want my son back. Leave me alone, leave me alone. Don't touch me!"[42] And a former nanny, Quethlie Alexie, who attended the funeral, told a TV host that she saw Anna yell at Howard, "I trusted you, I trusted you! Stay out of my life. Go, go!"[43] When I asked Stern about these remarks, he said that Anna was justifiably hysterical, but that she directed no ill comments toward him.

Mourners received a program with photos of Anna and Daniel in happier times—and there was also a message Anna wrote to her son:

> My dearest son Daniel, you were my rock. You were the only one that could keep me solid. Why God took you away from me I do not understand. Perhaps someday I will. It is so hard to think of you, but I do every second.

Just before the coffin was lowered into the ground, Anna demanded it be reopened. Crying loudly, "I'm sorry, I'm sorry!" she grabbed her son and hugged him. "If Daniel is gonna be buried, I wanna be buried with him!" she shouted, as she tried to climb down into the grave. Howard and another man caught her before she fell in, and Howard embraced her.[44] She wanted nothing more than to be with her son forever. Just three and a half months later, that wish would come true.

By September 27, the toxicological and histological results came back, allowing me to advise Dr. Raju to term Daniel's official manner of death an "accident." National Medical Services lab, which has more sophisticated testing than was available to the Bahamian coroner, found a total of seven prescription drugs in Daniel's body. My esteemed colleague Dr. Robert Middleberg, the NMS chief of forensic toxicology, personally supervised the testing and apprised me of the results.

The methadone was at a relatively high level for someone unaccustomed to taking the drug, although we really don't know what his experience was with that medicine. The Lexapro was at a high therapeutic level and the Zoloft somewhat higher—in the toxic, but non-lethal range. But again, it was the combination of these three drugs that caused the problem.

There was also Benadryl or diphenhydramine, an over-the-counter antihistamine, at a subtherapeutic level; pseudoephedrine, an over-the-counter decongestant mostly marketed as Sudafed, also at a subtherapeutic level; and a very tiny trace of Ambien, a prescription sleep medication. There was also a hint of Elavil, a mood elevator, at a subtherapeutic level.

When I gave my press statements about these drugs, I held back from naming the final drug, stating that its presence was very minute, and it had nothing to do with Daniel's death. I felt that revealing it might abrogate his privacy, but declared, "It was not for a venereal disease or leprosy." But now that time has passed, and especially after the February 2007 death of his mother, I will name that medication, exclusively. Daniel had a very trace amount of Topamax, an antiseizure prescription medicine, also taken for migraine headaches. Anna Nicole had a prescription for Topamax and it was present in her system when she died. Why Daniel had it in his bloodstream is unknown.

The physiological mechanism of the three main drugs led to a condition called "torsades de pointes," in which there's a prolongation of the QT interval of the heart's rhythm, producing a fatal dysrhythmia. "QT" refers to two different spikes—the Q wave and the T wave—as seen on an electrocardiogram when measuring the pace. The faster the heart rate, the shorter the QT interval. The simplest explanation for it is "Sudden Adult Death Syndrome." Methadone can cause it, and so can Lexapro and Zoloft, and when the three are taken together, a cardiac arrhythmia can easily follow.

The next few months were filled with squabbling over the paternity of Dannielynn—with Howard refusing to forfeit the child he insisted was his and ignoring requests to prove it by taking a DNA test. Larry Birkhead, a Los Angeles-based photographer who had had a turbulent dating relationship with Anna prior to her leaving the country, was certain he was the baby's father. He retained California attorney Debra Opri to argue the matter in Nassau, but this line of inquiry was slow going.

Somewhere along the way Howard Stern severed ties with the Callenders & Co. law firm and made his primary counsel Wayne Munroe, possibly the single most powerful advocate in the country. He would be behind every important move Howard and Anna made from then on.

Munroe knew the law and, as a prominent defense attorney, operated with derring-do bordering on showboating. Just months before when prime minister Perry Christie's Privy Council ruled that the country's death penalty was unconstitutional, Munroe told the *Bahama Journal* he was in favor of capital punishment—and public hangings.

Claiming there is proof that executions don't deter crime, the bar association president said they are "cheaper than keeping people in jail for an extended period of time. That's a consideration when you look at the government having limited resources. Do you spend those resources to house people who really should be put to death, who aren't fit to live in society, or do you spend [those resources] on education and health for the rest of society?"

Munroe also said the death penalty should stay lawful because it satisfies the revenge sentiment in people. Then he upped his own ante: "I personally think that the way the Taliban used to do it in Afghanistan is to be preferred—public executions by members of the aggrieved families. I don't think the Bahamian people would have the stomach for that. I think if you do that the death penalty would be off the book fairly quickly."

Referring to the then twenty-eight men on death row: "If you can't sit and watch what is being done on your behalf, it's because you fundamentally have a problem with it. I could sit and watch it because I fundamentally do not have a problem with it."[45]

On January 11, 2007, police were finished investigating Daniel's death and director of public prosecutions Bernard Turner announced that a decision would be forthcoming as to whether it remained necessary to convene a coroner's inquest. Turner denied that the probe had taken an excessively long time. "Every matter has to be investigated based on the peculiarities of that case. You have to keep in mind that although he died in the Bahamas, he had only arrived here a few hours earlier, so this ended up not being an entirely local matter."[46]

On January 16, chief magistrate Roger Gomez stated publicly that there would indeed be an inquest, and it would begin on March 28.[47]

In a series of closed-door meetings with Gomez, Munroe tried to get Daniel's inquest tossed. Anna Nicole Smith had died in early February 2007 while visiting Florida, and Howard was left in the Horizons home with the baby and a nanny, recovering from the trauma of losing his best friend and client. Making him a target of a coroner's inquest into Daniel's death was unnecessarily cruel at this point, his attorney argued.

But it didn't work. Only a miracle would stop the inquest—and the miracle came the night before the inquest was to begin.

FOX News's Greta Van Susteren had taken a camera crew to Nassau in hopes of picking up some bombshell on the spot. Although cameras were banned from the actual proceeding, and the likelihood was good that only local reporters would be permitted to sit inside the small room during the hearings, she was given a live tour with the affable Chief Magistrate Gomez. Smiling as if he were hosting a television special, he introduced Van Susteren's viewers to the "Coroner's Court in Royal Victoria Gardens, Nassau, Bahamas—the most beautiful country in the world."[48]

In reality the courtroom looked more like a bungalow that an errant high schooler might have to sit in during detention. Folding chairs were supplied for the jurors, the press, and the small number of public observers. The witnesses would stand while giving testimony.

Gomez related that he was one of fourteen permanent magistrates in the system, all of them coroners. Witnesses don't generally bring their own attorneys, he said, but if any of Daniel's witnesses wanted to, they could. The magistrates already knew when and where Daniel died—September 10, Doctors Hospital—so the question they needed answered was "how he died, the circumstances under which he died." To that end, he said "fact and expert witnesses" would take the stand, under oath.

Seven citizens, taken from the voters' registry and all with previous jury trial experience, would hear the testimony, Gomez said. They then make a recommendation to the attorney general whether criminal charges should be filed. Van Susteren, also an attorney, guided him to describe what possible options there might be for the jury.

"Quite a few. Accidental death," he replied. "You can say murder, manslaughter, suicide, death by misadventure."

And if the death were ruled accidental, "Could the attorney general veto that?" Greta asked. Gomez responded: "Yes, the attorney general still has the power to continue with the investigations and overrule the decision, but they normally accept the decision of the coroner. Only if new evidence comes up afterward would they look into it more."

VAN SUSTEREN: If it's murder, does the attorney general have the ability to reject that as well?

GOMEZ: Yes. And they can decide, for example, if—I'm not talking about this particular case now, but in general. . .

VAN SUSTEREN: Right.[49]

Too late!, I thought, as I watched with my eyes popping out of my head. What happened to the inquest secrecy I had heard so much about? I don't know what gets into people when they see a television camera and feel compelled to talk. Without that, I suppose Jerry Springer and Dr. Phil would have no careers.

This guy was yakking like there's no tomorrow—and, in fact, his yakking caused there to be no tomorrow. Apparently Wayne Munroe and Howard K. Stern were watching the program too—and they weren't at all pleased that the chief magistrate hearing their case was telling the broadcasting world how his legal realm worked.

Gomez went on to say that the attorney general could reduce a murder charge to manslaughter and that jurors are advised to only consider testimonial evidence brought before the court. They would get a "double warning," he said, "due to the great media attention that's happening."[50]

The next day Wayne Munroe appeared in Gomez's court and argued to get the inquest stalled, if not canceled.[51] It became a closed-door hearing, so it's impossible to know exactly what was said by both parties, but cameras caught Munroe grinning as he left the building.

There was a standoff for the next several months while Munroe petitioned the Bahamas Supreme Court to pull the plug on the inquest. He also challenged the constitutionality of the coroner's court and the way in which its jury was selected. It was also suggested that fast-tracking this inquest was unfair to all of the other cases waiting patiently for their chance for a hearing, setting up a two-tiered system that seemed to favor wealthy nonresidents. During this legal back-and-forth, tongues wagged about whether Daniel's body should be exhumed. Of course, there was absolutely no medical reason for an exhumation, but there's something about that word that seems to excite certain journalists beyond any rationale. Already Daniel's body had undergone two thorough post-mortems, and there were tissue and fluid samples galore, as well as photographs and written reports. If there was a legitimate medical question, the answer could be found in someone's drawer or on a shelf. Even if somebody came forward with an accusation that Daniel had been poisoned by a heavy metal, such as arsenic—a highly doubtful notion—the samples were already preserved and could be resubmitted to National Medical Services lab. The only possible reason to dig him up would be if his next of kin might want to rebury him somewhere else, like in the United States. But with his mother now deceased, who was his next of kin? Some of this was actually discussed during a strange court hearing that occurred in Florida following Anna's death (as you'll see in the next chapter).

In July, Supreme Court Justice John Lyons turned down Munroe's request to cancel the inquest and he set a new date for the end of October. Lyons also yanked Roger Gomez from the case and replaced him with magistrate William Campbell.[52]

Finally, after more than a year's delay, on October 29, 2007, the coroner's inquest into Daniel Smith's death began. A four-woman, three-man jury was sworn in and then excused until November 19, because tropical storm Noel was threatening the entire Caribbean. Flooding was widespread and the courthouse was leaking—but this time the leaks were from Mother Nature, not chatty personnel.[53]

Magistrate Campbell told the panel there was a new mission. Because police had turned up no evidence of homicide, the jurors were solely to decide what was Daniel's cause of death.[54] After a bit of a rough start, including one morning when a juror forgot to show up, a couple days of testimony occurred—only to get halted again for the Thanksgiving holiday and other scheduling.[55] While Thanksgiving isn't a legal holiday in the Bahamas, the magistrate accommodated Virgie Arthur and her lawyer, who were in attendance.

In December there were several days of testimony until the Christmas holidays hit, then a few more days in January. Witnesses from the United States could not be compelled to testify, although I understand there was an open-door policy for those who wanted to be heard. About three dozen witnesses—mostly hospital personnel and police—spoke about the hours leading up to and following Daniel's death, with questioning allowed by the coroner, as well as Stern's and Arthur's attorneys.

Dr. Raju's testimony was that Daniel died because of the lethal combination of drugs, taken between four and six hours prior to his passing. Raju based his opinion on the two US toxicology reports, he said. During his time on the stand, Daniel's grandmother, Virgie Arthur, was seen dabbing her eyes with a tissue. A woman named Carolyn Nairn, who was a patient in room 202 on the day of Smith's death, testified that she had heard a lot of commotion coming from the room next door to her—presumably Anna Nicole, crying and screaming, "My baby boy."[56]

Two other witnesses' testimony caused me some concern. Forensic chief Quinn McCartney, who is a very competent detective, was asked about the pills found in the bed after Daniel died. Then Magistrate Campbell asked him whether Daniel might have had "cumulative buildup" of methadone in his system from before he came to Nassau, and read to him from a report that stated how dangerous the drug was. McCartney admitted that a buildup was "possible." When it was Wayne Munroe's turn, he suggested that maybe the carbonation in the soda pop that Daniel drank might have sped up the reaction of the drugs, and McCartney said more study was needed. A fanciful theory, if true, but I have never heard of any study, abstract, or scientific presentation regarding carbonation's potential effect on drug absorption. McCartney stated the obvious—that the red, frothy material in Smith's lungs was proof of a drug overdose. Then he added that even if there were no other drugs present in Daniel's system, "the methadone level alone would be enough to set off alarms."[57]

I don't know why the coroner and Stern's attorney asked these medical questions of a law enforcement officer, rather than of Dr. Raju, who is a forensic pathologist—but I believe in his sincere desire to be cooperative, McCartney overstepped his area of expertise. Once that door was opened, a theme sprouted that methadone was the sole drug that caused Daniel's death. It was as if the Lexapro and Zoloft were never in the picture. Dr. Raju could have been recalled to set the court straight, and I could have backed him up: The three drugs in concert caused Daniel's demise—methadone, Lexapro, and Zoloft. Deaths from acute combined drug toxicity are at epidemic levels in morgues these days, and Daniel was another sad statistic.

To further complicate matters, one of Stern's attorneys—the news item I read didn't identify which one—said that Daniel had been taking methadone "to treat either depression or a bad back."[58] Was this just unfortunate reporting or an accurate quote? Where did this concept come from that Daniel had been taking methadone? That's in conflict with what I was personally told by Howard and Dr. Kapoor, who had been Daniel's physician. Kapoor had prescribed methadone for Anna, but not for Daniel.

Even more vexing to me was the testimony from Dr. William

"Lee" Hearn, the chief toxicologist of the medical examiner's office in Miami-Dade, Florida. He told the court, "Clearly the methadone was the key in understanding this death. But for the methadone he would not have died." While Hearn acknowledged the presence of the Zoloft and Lexapro, he zeroed in on the methadone, saying, "Based on the amount in the stomach, it was not an attempt to get high. There's a high degree of probability it was an intentional ingestion."[59] Suicide!

I immediately sent an e-mail to Stern, citing my "strong disagreement with the opinions expressed by some witnesses (including nonmedical individuals) that Daniel's death was due solely to methadone, and that his death was a suicide." I pointed out that the Zoloft and Lexapro were at high therapeutic/low toxic levels, which could not be ignored or dismissed as having contributed to the overall central nervous system depressant effect that led to Daniel's death. "Evidently, it appears to me that someone is attempting to create a suicide scenario by focusing solely on methadone and excluding the other two drugs," I wrote. "It is extremely rare for a sane, fully conscious person to commit suicide by taking three different drugs." Howard e-mailed me back, saying he was "surprised and disappointed" in the toxicologist's opinion regarding suicide. Stern didn't think that Daniel would have killed himself, much less in the hospital where his mother had just given birth. Howard also wrote that Dr. Hearn did not feel the Lexapro and Zoloft were in high amounts—so I faxed Stern the reports from the two labs, which belied that theory. Howard told me he would forward my thoughts to Wayne Munroe, who then contacted me to say they may indeed want me to testify before the inquest jury.

Testimony was heard sporadically until the end of March 2008, but I was never called to attend the hearing or offer an opinion. Jurors were presented with the case on March 31 and needed less than two hours to reach their verdict—that Daniel died of an accidental overdose.[60] No criminal charges would be filed against anyone—and the jurors wisely did not go along with the theory that Daniel committed suicide.

That night, Howard Stern phoned me to say he was pleased by the outcome and to thank me for my assistance.

As I reflect on the case, I remain in accord with Dr. Raju that this was simply a tragic accidental drug overdose. Any idea that this was suicide, murder, or manslaughter is absurd. No matter what one thinks of Anna Nicole, there can be no doubt she was a devoted mother to her son and that she was devastated over his demise. Yet there are still loose strings that may never be tied together.

Since we know the Lexapro was prescribed to Daniel, I've tried to envision how the Zoloft, the Elavil, and the methadone, and even the Topamax, got into his system. I come up totally blank on the Zoloft and the Elavil. They are not medications connected with his mother, and Howard told me neither he nor Anna had any clue where these came from. Could Daniel have brought them from Los Angeles, thinking they were sleep medications, the kind you gulp down so you can rest on an airplane? That's doubtful because he had ingested a substantial amount of the Zoloft. There's no way to know how much he took and over what period of time. So that's just a question mark.

The methadone and the Topamax were both medications his mother had in her life. Daniel was the only person still awake in the hospital room. Could he have grown bored watching TV and felt he needed to go to sleep because he had a big day of family fun ahead? Might he have spied the Coach bag that reportedly held Anna's prescription containers and decided to help himself?

According to a report released in December 2007 by the National Drug Intelligence Center, record numbers of people are dying from methadone overdoses, as doctors are dispensing more prescriptions of this powerful painkiller. The study stated that in the years between 2001 and 2006, there was a 715 percent spike in usage, with people between the ages of fifteen and twenty-four suffering the most fatalities.[61] And recent research from the National Household Survey on Drug Abuse & Health confirms that the fastest-growing group of new prescription drug abusers are people under the age of twenty-five years old.[62]

I also have to consider that the information I was given by Howard Stern was inaccurate. Perhaps he had his own prescription for these alien medicines but didn't feel the need to tell that to me or anyone else. Daniel could have found them in Stern's belongings and taken them on his own, to Stern's horror when he later found out. But Stern assured me he didn't know where those medications came from.

One disturbing trend among young people these days is a "pharm party," or a gathering when the adults in a home are away and the youngsters invite over friends, find the parents' prescription medications, dump them into a candy dish, and play games where they grab and swallow the pills, randomly. I know it's the "duty" of youth to find more ways to assert their independence and worry their parents, but of all the possible choices, from tattoos to piercings, from goth music to punk rock, and even inclusive of sexual high jinks, there is nothing more frightening to me than to imagine a kid ingesting a pharmaceutical medication because it looks alluring or matches his or her outfit.

Whatever motivated Daniel Wayne Smith to overmedicate himself will not be resolved by an autopsy report or an inquest. At twenty years old, he died just when he should have been relishing his first jolt of independence, creative satisfaction, and true love. But he left a mark on the people who cherished him. Hopefully, when they think of him, they will remember the joy of his life, rather than the mystery of his death.

ANNA NICOLE SMITH

nna Nicole Smith was only thirty-nine years old when she died on February 8, 2007. But that gave her three years more than her idol Marilyn Monroe. Marilyn died in Los Angeles on August 5, 1962. My colleague Dr. Thomas Noguchi, then the deputy medical examiner for Los Angeles County and later its chief coroner, performed the autopsy and sometime later asked for my personal opinion as an unpaid consultant. This is in contrast to the times in later years where he contacted me for official assistance in the Tate/LaBianca murders (committed by the Manson family), the Symbionese Liberation Army shootings (related to the Patty Hearst kidnapping), and the assassination of Senator Robert F. Kennedy. In the Marilyn Monroe case, he ruled, and I concurred, that the legend's death was a "probable suicide," due to "acute barbiturate poisoning."[1] I saw the autopsy photographs of Marilyn; her blue eyes were wide and vacant, her face mottled and puffy. It was quite a different view of the sex symbol who so famously sang "Happy Birthday, Mr. President" to her rumored lover, John F. Kennedy, at Madison Square Garden in May 1962, while wiggling around in a flesh-colored, sparkling designer dress that was so tight she had to be sewn into it.

As you will see, Monroe and Smith shared many similarities not only in death but in life as well. Marilyn was the iconographic inspiration for Anna's career and lifestyle to such a pervasive degree that Anna had a short-term rental of the Brentwood, California, Spanish hacienda where Marilyn died.[2] Both women came from humble beginnings and achieved superstar status due to their magnetism and ambition. Anna's birth name was Vickie Lynn Hogan, and Marilyn's was Norma Jeane Mortenson, although coincidentally her maternal grandmother's maiden name was Hogan. Both Anna and Marilyn grew up with light brown hair, went blonde at the start of their careers, and died with bleached tresses. Both women were head-turning teenagers with perfect features and smiles, whose wholesome good looks would later shine through even when Hollywood slathered them with makeup. And both had cosmetic surgery procedures—Marilyn had rhinoplasty and scars removed from her chin, and Anna had numerous breast enhancements and, reportedly, liposuction.

Both adopted a high-pitched, breathy voice to use in their professional lives, a throwback to the 1960s view of womanhood, which was even employed by former first lady Jacqueline Kennedy; only close associates would ever hear their normal speaking voices. Marilyn took an art appreciation class in her youth; Anna was a gifted painter, whose works hung on her home walls and included a portrait of Marilyn. And while women of Marilyn's era seldom got tattoos or body art, Anna's body was a virtual canvas; among her tattoos was an inked image of Marilyn's face on her lower right leg. Both were fans of animals, especially dogs; Anna even had a white silky terrier named Marilyn.[3]

Both women found early success as local print models and then realized they could make more money by exposing their shapely bodies. Marilyn posed nude for calendar photographer Tom Kelley, who sold the images to aspiring publisher Hugh M. Hefner as he was about to launch a saucy magazine called *Playboy*. Subtitled "Entertainment for Men," the black-and-white cover photo of Marilyn, waving and wearing a dress with a plunging neckline, promised and delivered nude photos inside. The scandalous issue came out in December 1953, without a date on the cover since Hefner wasn't sure there would be subsequent issues. The inside photos of Marilyn, resplendently posed on red velvet, were used for the magazine's centerfold, crowning Monroe as *Playboy*'s "Sweetheart of the Month." Instead of pretending that the photos of her had been doctored, Marilyn proudly owned up to them, delighting fans with her bold embrace of sexuality. Overnight, the tastefully elegant display jump-started her career from cameos and minor parts to starring roles in major films. The photos also created a magazine dynasty for Hugh Hefner that continues to this day.

As a teenager, Anna Nicole pinned Marilyn's *Playboy* spread to her bedroom wall in Mexia, Texas, and drifted to sleep wondering how she could follow in Monroe's footsteps to fame. Her chance came later when she moved to Houston and began exotic dancing in strip clubs. The southern lovely was considered too chubby to get on the prized nighttime schedule, so she was relegated to the afternoon shift. But it was there she met the elderly man who would change her personal life forever—and get her one step closer to living like Marilyn.

In 1991, a twenty-four-year-old Anna—then known as "Vickie Lynn Smith"—spotted an ad in the newspaper. *Playboy*, which is always on the hunt for new talent, was looking for nude models. She asked a local photographer named Eric Redding to take some naked snapshots of her, which were then mailed to the magazine. Redding, who would later become the beauty's manager for a while, was bemused by her awkwardness about taking off her clothes. It was one thing to dance naked, she told him, but she had never even had sex in a room with the lights on.[4]

Playboy editors get about one thousand amateur submissions per year but were sufficiently impressed by Vickie Lynn's pictures that they flew her to Los Angeles for a face-to-face meeting. Senior contributing photographer Arny Freytag took some Playmate test shots but rejected them. Although her face was "great," she was—at one-hundred-sixty pounds on her five-foot eleven-inch frame—overweight by the magazine's standards. Lose a few pounds and try again, he told her. But Marilyn Grabowski, the longtime West Coast photo editor, was mesmerized by the small-town girl's star quality and overruled Freytag. Grabowski was intrigued that this curvy innocent who worked as a stripper back home was so shy at the photo shoot, she'd bundle herself in a robe when the camera stopped clicking. During her session, the company's photography director, Gary Cole, found that

Anna had "camera charisma," a quality that can't be taught. She never blinked or had a bad expression, he said.

Anna debuted as a cover girl for *Playboy*'s March 1992 issue, for which she was paid the grand sum of $500. She sat demurely on a brocade chair, in a strapless blue satin ball gown, with long gold gloves, and holding opera glasses. Two months later she made her nude appearance as a *Playboy* centerfold, under the name "Vickie Smith," and for which she earned $20,000. On the data sheet, she fibbed that she weighed one-hundred-forty pounds and proclaimed her goal "to be the new Marilyn Monroe."

"She felt a great affinity for Marilyn, the first *Playboy* centerfold," Grabowski recalled. "While we were shooting she would put on Marilyn's music to get in the mood, and she'd sing along. She had a high little voice like Marilyn's but with a Texas twang." And Bill White, the manager for the magazine's studio, added: "Marilyn Monroe didn't make many records. We would rotate two CDs, playing an endless loop of 'Diamonds Are a Girl's Best Friend,' 'Some Like It Hot,' and a few others—show tunes that would drive you crazy after a few hours."

But the way Anna connected with the camera was worth all the effort. Hugh Hefner described the magic as "sexuality, plus vulnerability" and said both Anna and Marilyn had it. Anna Nicole would do four more covers for *Playboy*, starting in June 1993, when she was named "Playmate of the Year" and pocketed $100,000. The cover pose was a black-and-white over-the-shoulder shot, and inside was a color homage to Marilyn, including one photo where her white skirt billowed up as Monroe's did in the famous *The Seven Year Itch* publicity photo. In February 1994, she was wrapped in a crimson robe as the magazine's "red-hot Valentine." In February 2001, she was bathed in diamonds and wearing a fuchsia gown and gloves, the only cover where she showed her wide, unrestrained smile. And in May 2007, for the post-death "Anna Nicole: The Playboy Years" remembrance, she was shown in a white fur and diamonds.[5]

Anna's and Marilyn's personal lives were marked by countless romantic encounters. Affairs with wealthy and powerful men were a natural extension of their highly charged sexual energy. Marilyn coveted children and was known to have had miscarriages and abortions—and there was a rumor that as a teenager, while in an orphanage, she was raped and gave birth to a son whom she never saw again. I don't know how much of that is true, but her autopsy report shows a well-healed five-inch horizontal suprapubic scar along the escutcheon line—or, below the navel, at the bikini line. That could have been from a cesarean delivery but was more likely from an appendectomy since her appendix was missing at autopsy.[6]

Anna lived in a time when women finally had better family-planning choices; still, mistakes could happen. According to a handwritten diary entry from 1992, Anna had gotten pregnant by an unnamed lover and was considering an abortion. "He will only support me if I have it," she wrote. "But if I decide to go the other way he won't. I'll be on my own. I think that's tacky. I'm scared."[7] We can't know whether Anna was writing truthfully here, but her only son was born in 1986 and no other pregnancy is known to have gone to term until she gave birth to her daughter in 2006. In other passages she conveys that while she enjoyed being a sex symbol, at times she detested guys: "I hate men! They suck, there [*sic*] scum. There [*sic*] not worthy."[8]

Marilyn had had a long history of depression, as well as alcohol and prescription sedative abuse. On the night she died, she added the sleep medication chloral hydrate to the Nembutal she was taking and she expired. According to her autopsy report, she had been under a psychiatrist's care for a while with the goal of lessening the amount of drugs she had become dependent upon and she had been making some progress in that regard. There were, however, pill bottles found in her home for medicines that were not in her bloodstream at autopsy. Coroner investigators brought in a team of outside psychiatric experts to review her medical files and speak with her doctors; they learned she had felt disappointed and "wanted to withdraw, give up and even to die." On more than one occasion in the past she had attempted an overdose with sedative drugs, including one recent try, only to call for help and be rescued. Three factors made the psychiatric consultants agree with the medical experts, including myself, in determining that Marilyn Monroe's death was a suicide: first, the high level of barbiturates and chloral hydrate ingested over a short period of time; second, the completely empty bottle of Nembutal, which had just been filled the day before; and third, that she had locked her bedroom door, delaying help from her live-in housekeeper or any doctor who might have been phoned.[9]

The similarities between Marilyn's and Anna Nicole's deaths are significant. Could this have been on purpose, based on what Anna Nicole knew about her idol's final days? I will leave that to you to decide. One big difference though is that Anna Nicole lived her life of excess in the public eye—on her reality series, as an awards show presenter, as a talk show guest, or just in her daily life as she would go into stores and restaurants. She would leave tongues wagging at her bizarre antics or slurred speech. The extent of Marilyn's decadence, at the time, was mostly known only to people on the movie sets, when she would show up late or not at all. It wasn't until years after her death that the public learned of her rampant unprofessionalism.

To this day, Marilyn is considered Anna Nicole's superior, mostly due to her stellar film career and widespread popularity as an actress. Her marriages to baseball great Joe DiMaggio and playwright Arthur Miller also put her in a more prestigious category. Marilyn was the subject of much discussion over her friendship with prominent politicians and the show business elite, such as the "Rat Pack" of Frank Sinatra, Dean Martin, Sammy Davis Jr., and Peter Lawford. Stories abound of her intellectual cravings and crushes on Albert Einstein and other scholars. How much of that was press agent talk, we'll never know. But had Marilyn lived in today's era of round-the-clock celebrity news, paparazzi stalkers, gossip blogs, and cell phone cameras, perhaps we'd have a more realistic view of what this troubled and needy woman was like as she drowned in substance abuse and melancholy.

While Marilyn was largely kept away from her fans, Anna Nicole was unpretentious, down-home, and approachable. Rock concerts, casinos, and boxing events were her forms of entertainment, along with the strip clubs she would visit as a customer instead of as a worker. She had a purple-haired assistant, hung out with flamboyantly gay designers, and washed down her fried chicken dinners with champagne.

Vickie Lynn Hogan was born on November 28, 1967, in Mexia, Texas. The dusty town, in Limestone County, is about forty miles east of Waco and ninety minutes south of Dallas–Fort Worth. Locals call it "Me-hay'-a," for the Hispanic general it was named for, and they tout the good-natured city slogan: "A great place no matter how you pronounce it!"[10]

Virgie Mae Tabers was the single mom of a year-old son named David when she married Donald Eugene Hogan and gave birth to their daughter, Vickie Lynn; Virgie was sixteen years old, with Donald not being much older.[11] A *London Observer* article from 2007 stated that they were poor and miserable, and, according to Virgie, he was an alcoholic thug who beat her black-and-blue while she was pregnant. In that same article, she also claimed he raped Virgie's ten-year-old sister and another girl, and served a ridiculously slight sixty-day jail sentence.[12] By Vickie's second birthday, the two were divorced, and he had nothing to do with his daughter for the next twenty-four years, until 1993, when she flew him to Los Angeles for her Playmate of the Year celebration at the Playboy Mansion. An uncomfortable reunion was aired on *Extra*, the syndicated newsmagazine.[13] Virgie and Donald went on to various marriages, and Vickie ended up with scads of half siblings. Virgie's current husband, James Arthur, is her fifth; they've been married since 2000.[14]

Virgie went to work for the sheriff's department and tried to raise her daughter with Christian values, even if that meant the occasional belt whipping on her rear end. According to a *Dallas Observer* piece from 1999, the family lived in a house that seldom had heat, survived on food stamps, and encouraged its kids to swipe toilet paper rolls from restaurants and bring them home.[15] Aunt Elaine and Uncle Mel Tabers helped with the young ones when Virgie was at work. Vickie Lynn was a handful, with her head in the clouds and always scheming about how she could blow town and make a name for herself. She balked at Virgie's strict rules, and the two tussled a lot until Vickie ran away from home. After flunking out of her freshman year of high school, she worked at a series of low-paying jobs, including waiting tables at Red Lobster and cashiering at Wal-Mart. While employed at Jim's Krispy Fried Chicken, she fell for the cook, Billy Wayne Smith. They wed in 1985, when she was seventeen and he was sixteen. Their baby, Daniel Wayne, was born that year. He was a planned birth—at least for Vickie. Unbeknownst to Billy, she had flushed her birth control pills down the toilet in hope of getting pregnant. Within two years, Vickie and Billy's marriage was kaput, although they didn't officially divorce until 1993. "My husband was really physically abusive and jealous, and would never let me go out," she told R. Daniel Foster of *Los Angeles* magazine in 1994.[16]

In 1989 Vickie Lynn Smith was arrested in Houston for driving under the influence.[17] And while Vickie might have planned her pregnancy, she wasn't a very responsible parent: For Daniel's first six years—until 1991—he lived with his Grandma Virgie, although his mother visited frequently. During that time, Vickie struggled to earn a living so she could reclaim her son. She decided that she needed a big infusion of cash—more than she could find with grunt work around Mexia. She moved south to Houston, where she spied a gentleman's club and got a job dancing. At first she feared that showing her nakedness would be sinful, but when someone explained that God created her beautiful body, Vickie found her salvation. It might even fast-track her to heaven, she later rationalized to the *Los Angeles* magazine reporter.[18]

Wearing only a G-string and a smile, she was soon pocketing up to a thousand bucks a day at clubs around town. Virgie learned of one job and used her police authority to get Vickie fired, but the young stripper moved on to other joints, like Baby O's and Leggs, fooling her mother by dancing under the names of "Miss Nikki" or "Miss Robin." At one upscale chain of clubs called Rick's, owner Robert Walters put her onstage. "She was rather plump to be working here, so we put her on the afternoon shift," he recalled to *People* magazine in 1995. Today, there's a photo of Anna Nicole Smith on the wall of the club. Her ample rear end is prominently displayed with her autograph: "Remember Sweet Cheeks."

It was at Gigi's Cabaret in 1991 that the big-boned ecdysiast met J. Howard Marshall—known to all as "J. Howard"—who would make Anna's life so much easier. Marshall was a Yale-educated, lawyer-turned-oil magnate who, in the 1930s, helped write laws that would shape the petroleum industry. Now wheelchair-bound, he had been down in the dumps over the Alzheimer's-related death earlier that year of his second wife, Bettye Bohannan, with whom he had had a thirty-year marriage. He also hadn't recovered from the death of his mistress two years prior. She was a Houston topless dancer-turned-socialite, Jewell Diane Walker—or, as she was nicknamed, "Lady"—who passed away while getting a face lift. During their ten-year relationship, he lavished her with millions to paint her fingernails with real gold and tool around in Rolls-Royces color-coordinated to match her outfits. When he found out that her will named a young male lover as her heir, *People* reported, he sued her estate for the gifts he had bestowed upon her, eventually settling out of court.[19]

His driver, Dan Manning, figured the best way to cheer up the old codger was to get him back in the game, so when Miss Nikki bent over and said hello, shaking her best features, he found an eye-popping reason to go on living. He invited the twenty-three-year-old to lunch the next day and handed her an envelope filled with cash, persuading her to quit her cabaret gig and become his private dancer.[20]

Within days, Marshall began asking Vickie Lynn Smith to be his wife, but she turned him down—for more than two years. As she later told Larry King: "I wanted to try to make something of my life," which Marshall reluctantly accepted. Luncheons would be spent at the

River Oaks Country Club or at Red Lobster, where she used to work; whenever they'd see her old friends there, she'd introduce the mogul as her grandfather. After one Red Lobster lunch, with her half brother Donnie watching, Marshall presented her with a gift-wrapped box. She opened it to find $50,000 in crisp one-hundred-dollar bills. He also paid to get Vickie's teeth fixed and for a series of breast enhancements—her going from 36A to 38DD just gave him more to love. Much later, after gaining a lot of weight, she expanded to a size 42, but Marshall was gone by that time.

In the evenings she would keep the octogenarian very satisfied, even though she has said there was no "physical attraction" on her part and the pair never lived together. When her friends told her to date someone her own age, she'd joke: "It just happens I get turned on by liver spots." She made him feel young again, and he gave her security. "I loved him so much for what he did for me and my son," she said. "No one has ever loved me and done things for me and respected me and didn't care about what people said about me. I mean, he truly loved me, and I loved him for it."[21]

Marshall's son, Everett Pierce—known as E. Pierce, or Pierce—was none too pleased about his father's affair with "Miss Cleavage," as he called her, but there wasn't much he could do as long as his dad remained healthy and sane.[22] The family fortune would remain relatively safe as long as they didn't marry, so Pierce was forced to ignore the presents his father gave the bombastic blonde, which included a new Toyota Celica (soon to be upgraded to a Mercedes) a fifteen-acre ranch in Tomball, Texas; a brick mansion in Houston; designer clothing; endless piles of cash and jewelry, including one Harry Winston shopping spree that left Marshall two million bucks lighter; and later, the Marilyn Monroe rental in Brentwood, California. He paid for a nanny for young Daniel and even won over Virgie, who felt her daughter was finally with someone who could provide for her.[23]

Vickie Lynn demanded sufficient time to devote to her career, which included taking modeling and voice lessons. Evenings were free to pursue her own fun that, it's been said, included flings with her chauffeur. But when she got the call from *Playboy* to shoot the magazine's cover, she dropped everything and flew to Hollywood. The accompanying questionnaire that she filled out stated that her life's ambitions were to be a Playmate and to have a daughter. "The people of [Texas] won't believe it when these pictures of me hit the newsstands, because I was considered a goody-two-shoes nerd in high school," she told a Lone Star State friend.[24]

Marshall was proud of his pretty baby's magazine cover and tolerant of the trips she had to take to promote it. She'd send handwritten, girlish postcards to her "Paw-Paw," as she called him, signing with her trademark flourish and happy face. As she spent more time away from him, he would fly to either of the coasts to see her.[25] According to a legal document Marshall's son filed, on one trip to Los Angeles, Vickie had told J. Howard that her leg was broken and showed him the cast. But when he took a nap, his nurse Betty Harding spied Vickie without the cast and her limbs wrapped around the housekeeper as the two giggled and rubbed noses. During that same visit, Harding accompanied Marshall to a jewelry store where he purchased gifts for his "Precious," but when he showed them to Vickie, she demanded to look at the receipt. Not feeling he had been generous enough, she sent him back to the store for more pricey baubles. On a trip to Manhattan, she made him wait in his hotel room for days before she would see him, then when she agreed to meet him at Harry Winston's, she allegedly fed him a Valium. While Marshall crumpled and drooled in his wheelchair, Vickie was said to have shopped for a sixteen-carat diamond engagement ring, Harding stated in the legal filing. On the trip back to Houston, Marshall suffered from heart palpitations, which his nurse felt might have been brought on by the Valium. She was concerned that the old man's life was in jeopardy.[26]

While Vickie's greed reportedly grew, so did her public image. Paul Marciano, the president of the trendy Guess clothing line, saw her *Playboy* cover and called Hefner, asking "Who is that girl?" Marciano then decided to replace his corporate model Claudia Schiffer with Vickie Lynn Smith and commissioned a sizzling set of black-and-white photos in a style that was reminiscent of Jayne Mansfield. "I didn't know what Guess jeans were," she laughed. "I just shopped at Wal-mart and Kmart, and stuff like that." Marciano signed Vickie to a huge contract and changed her name to "Anna Nicole." In what was perhaps an unprecedented launch, her gorgeous image soon exploded onto the best magazines and on billboards around the world. The Swedish fashion company Hennes & Mauritz, better known as H&M, shot seductive posters of her in underwear; the posters caused eighteen car accidents in major European cities and are still collector's items today. "I finally feel like I'm becoming somebody. I really think like I can do something. I just know I can be an actress. I want it so bad," she told *People* magazine in 1993, as she looked back on her Guess work and forward to her future. "I've tried so hard my whole life. I'm kindhearted, and I give, give, give. I think maybe it's my time to receive."[27]

But there was a price to pay for her rags-to-riches tale. In her barely literate, and often misspelled, handwritten diary of the time—which went on the auction block after her death—she fretted about her relationships with Marshall, Marciano, and food: "O my Gosh!! Paul Marsiano [*sic*] called today to see if I got his books also I'm gonna go to San Antonio to do photo shoot," she wrote on June 23, 1992. "I'm so excited!! I can't believe this. This could be it." The entry ends with five smiley faces. "I've been really stressed out lately and depressed and I can't quit eating. I feel like a pig," she penned in August. "Howard has been buying me som [*sic*] jewelry but he call [*sic*] me 15 or 20 times a day. . . . I don't know [*sic*] what to do about Paul. I hate for men to want sex all the time."[28]

Personal appearances and talk shows followed, and more money than she ever dreamed of making on her own. Anna and Daniel moved into an iron-gated mansion, provided by Marshall, and Anna paid back the favor by getting "Papas"—presumably for Paw-Paw's—tattooed on her groin area. According to the *Dallas Observer* article, getting tattoos was a meaningful art form to Anna. She expected her family members and friends to go to Bubba's Skin Pin Studio in Houston and get Anna's face tattooed on their bodies, and most complied. Daniel and Marshall were exempt from having to be inked. Around this time, Anna was also reportedly doing a lot of binge eating and then purging to keep her weight down; when stronger methods were required, she would have liposuction, wrote the reporter Randall Paterson.

One Christmas, Paterson wrote, a Neiman Marcus truck showed up, courtesy of Marshall, and models swanned around while Anna pointed at whichever outfits she wanted, and there was a no-expense-spared trip to Bali for the old man and his beauty. To amuse her pals, Anna would play phone messages that J. Howard would leave on her answering machine. "Precious, this is your man," was one, and another said: "If there's someone else, you need to tell me." Days would pass before Anna would call him back, then when she couldn't stall him any longer, she'd have him over, wheel him into the bedroom, ply him with baby talk and bosom thrusting, and send him on his way, the article stated. He was still pestering her to marry him, and she was still refusing.[29]

By March of 1994, Anna could add "actress" to her modeling résumé, thanks to a hilarious role in the Peter Segal-directed spoof *Naked Gun 33-1/3: The Final Insult.* Written and produced by the creative team that turned out the *Police Squad* TV series and its *Naked Gun* film spin-offs, the movie starred a brilliantly deadpan Leslie Nielsen as Lieutenant Frank Drebin, and, as his costar, O. J. Simpson as Detective Nordberg of the LAPD. In the third and final sequel—and in what became Simpson's last released movie before going on trial for the violent stabbing deaths of his wife, Nicole Brown Simpson, and her friend, Ronald Goldman—Drebin had to foil a terrorist plot at the Academy Awards. Anna Nicole portrayed Tanya Peters, a sexy nurse in a fertility clinic and the villain's moll. In a nod to her magazine work, a character in the film is seen perusing one of the *Playboy* issues with Anna Nicole on the cover.[30] Casting Anna in the role was a stroke of genius, and she nailed the humor perfectly.

In 1994 Anna had a small role in the quirky Coen brothers' comedy *The Hudsucker Proxy*, which starred Tim Robbins, Jennifer Jason Lee, and Paul Newman.[31] But the hope of her early movies gave way to the sad truth that she just wasn't very versatile as a performer. If she wanted to star in films, they would have to be low budget and forgettable. Anna made a few R-rated movies of the straight-to-video or DVD variety. Most were directed by Raymond Martino, the family friend with whom Anna's son Daniel was staying before his fateful trip to Nassau. The first Martino/Smith collaboration was 1995's *To the Limit*, a clunker where Anna played an ex-CIA agent who links up with a mobster to bring down the assassin who killed her husband. The taglines for this movie were: "Her code name was Colette. Her mission was danger" and "This agent bares all in the line of duty."[32]

Their 1997 film *Skyscraper* starred Anna as a charter helicopter pilot who lands on a building controlled by terrorists and faces rape to save hostages. Her young son, Daniel, played one of the captives. The film's tagline, "86 Floors of Action-Packed Terror!" was more ambitious than accurate. The film's minuscule budget forced the production to take place in a building only twenty-six stories tall, and when there were shots of a police helicopter flying around, the ID number painted on its side matched that of the charter helicopter, meaning both copters were one and the same. So that Anna could boast that she had made a movie with Marilyn Monroe, the film briefly showed a photo of the screen goddess right before Anna's character strips down for a shower scene.[33] In 1999, there were a few respectable TV guest stints, including the courtroom series *Ally McBeal* and the sitcom *Veronica's Closet*.

People seemed to like Anna best when she portrayed herself. She and Martino made two quasi-documentaries about Anna, both in 1998: *Portrait of a Pinup Queen* and *Anna Nicole Smith: Exposed*. The latter video, which was co-directed and co-written by Anna, included a lesbian fantasy with the star in a bathtub with soft-core star Ahmo Hight. And Anna starred in the 2003 film *Wasabi Tuna*, a silly story about

Halloween pranksters who steal her little dog Sugar Pie, and how a team of drag queens dressed as Anna rescue and return the pup. In 2005, she had a bit part, again playing herself, in *Be Cool*, which featured John Travolta, Uma Thurman, and a star-studded cast in a music industry crime caper, based on the Elmore Leonard novel. The film was a sequel to the book and movie *Get Shorty* but was not nearly as popular with the critics or audiences. Blink and you'll miss Anna as she kisses Danny DeVito on the Jumbotron screen at a Lakers game.[34]

Throughout the 1990s, Playboy Enterprises kept Anna busy by starring her in a half dozen of their video documentaries. These projects were essentially centerfold pictorials set to music and put out on videotape, which paired many of the Playmates in soft-focus romps and inch-deep interviews. And up until the time she began her own series, she was also a regular on the talk show circuit and appeared in celebrity roasts for Jeff Foxworthy and Pamela Anderson. She also starred in British crooner Bryan Ferry's music video of "Will You Still Love Me Tomorrow?" a classy piece even though all she did was walk around and look delectable.[35] There were two other notable TV and film appearances, which I'll get to later.

Nineteen ninety-four was a challenging year for Anna. The drugs she had been popping since her dancing days were starting to take their toll. She carried around bottles of prescription tranquilizers that she'd wash down with alcohol. Cocaine, ecstasy, sleeping pills, wake-up pills—she had medications for every occasion. In February, while staying with a boyfriend named Daniel Ross at the Peninsula Hotel in Beverly Hills, she overdosed on prescription drugs mixed with alcohol and spent three days at Cedars-Sinai Medical Center.[36] It wouldn't be her last brush with death. Later that year her bodyguard Pierre DeJean claimed he saved her life when she tried to slit her wrists[37]—and her autopsy report did show healed scars there.[38]

She described a later episode in a 1997 interview with the *Extra* television program: "I woke up in the hospital with a coma. That kinda got me scared, because I had to learn to do a lot of things over, like walk and talk. I mean, it was really bad. . . . I was just sitting in bed, watching TV and I woke up in a coma, from a coma. . . . It was the most painful thing because I had pneumonia also and I had these respirators. It was like a fifty-fifty chance. They didn't think I was gonna pull out, and when I woke up it was like, ugh! I had these tubes down me and I'm freaked out because I don't know what is going on."[39]

In May, Anna's twenty-three-year-old housekeeper, Maria Antonia Cerrato, sued Smith for $2 million, claiming the model had sexually assaulted her the previous year; Anna's attorneys filed a counterclaim, saying Cerrato's filing was an extortion attempt, according to *People* magazine.[40] Around that time, according to the legal document prepared on behalf of Pierce Marshall, Anna filed a police report stating that much of the jewelry Marshall had given her had been "stolen." Then she claimed she had given the items to another employee, a man whom the Marshall family learned had allegedly had a record for multiple felony convictions. She later amended her report, stating that she had left the jewelry in a taxi. The police stated her stories were "unfounded," no arrests were made, and the jewels were never recovered.[41]

J. Howard Marshall was still urging his "Precious" to marry him, and Anna finally agreed. Their ceremony, on June 27, 1994, was held at Houston's White Dove Wedding Chapel, but it wasn't an event for the *Social Register*. Only eleven guests were in attendance, including Anna's eight-year-old son, Daniel, who was the ring bearer; Marshall's assistant, Eyvonne Scurlock; and his nurse, Charlotte Fade. A new driver by the name of Arnold Wyche waited outside. No one from Marshall's family was there to toss confetti; they weren't invited. It would be more than a month before Pierce Marshall was informed that he had a new stepmother, and that she hadn't been given a prenuptial agreement to sign. Anna marched up the aisle on a carpet of white rose petals, and met Paw-Paw, who was in his wheelchair and already in place. At the reception, Marshall, wearing a white tuxedo, announced to the crowd how much he adored his brown-eyed girl. Anna, wearing what was described as a veil and a "very, very, very low-cut" white hand-beaded, heavy satin gown, bent down to kiss him. Then she whispered that she had to leave immediately so she wouldn't miss her flight to Greece. She gave him a peck on the cheek, waved to the assembly, and exited the chapel as Mrs. J. Howard Marshall II.[42]

There was no European travel though; she returned to Los Angeles and spent her honeymoon with another man. Soon after, she was spotted having sex in the pool of the Playboy Mansion where she lost her wedding ring. A security guard found it, but Anna didn't bother retrieving it until six months later. "I know people think I married Howard for his money," Anna told a reporter who wondered about their odd marriage. "But it's not true. I love him." She even said they were hoping to have a baby together. "We had sex a lot," Smith told another reporter. "He could not exactly satisfy me, which is to be expected. But he was very satisfied himself. That's really all that mattered to me. He satisfied me in other ways. He cared about me. He never looked down at me."[43]

One advantage of Anna's association with Marshall was the confidence it gave her to protect her legal interests. A case in point was the suit Anna filed against *New York* magazine when she claimed they misrepresented their intentions in a photo shoot. Her lawyer, T. Patrick Freydl, brought the action in Los Angeles Superior Court, which was now Anna's home turf, seeking a $5 million remedy in damages to her reputation, plus punitive damages: "She was told that she was being photographed to embody the 'All-American women look' and that they wanted glamour shots." But while she was goofing around on a break, he said, a photo was shot that was decidedly ungainly. It showed the voluptuous blonde squatting in a short skirt and cowboy boots, with her knees apart, scarfing down a bag of Cheez Doodles. It became the cover for the magazine's August 22, 1994, issue with the caption: "White Trash Nation." Kurt Andersen, the magazine's editor, said that the photo was one of dozens taken for the cover, adding, "I guess they just found the picture we chose unflattering." Apparently so. The magazine settled the lawsuit for an undisclosed amount.[44]

That same month, when Marshall flew to Los Angeles for a visit, she refused to let him lie next to her, purportedly telling him he'd urinate in the bed. Before he left she took all the money from his wallet and made him write her a blank check, according to Nurse Harding, who was there. On another occasion at the Tomball ranch, Anna asked Harding to leave Marshall alone with her. When the nurse returned she stated that she found the elderly man disheveled, with the buttons torn from his shirt, and in a state of anxiety. He wouldn't describe what had happened but made the nurse promise to never leave him alone with Anna again. He also said his marriage to the beauty was a mistake and that all she wanted him for was his money.

During the Christmas holiday, Marshall gave Anna a stuffed teddy bear with an emerald pendant. She cooked breakfast for him, allegedly insisting he eat raw bacon, which made him sick. That night, they went out for dinner, but Anna left Marshall in his wheelchair in the rain, while she went dancing with her bodyguard, according to an employee. Yet, as a Christmas gift, her loving hubby gave her an envelope filled with cash and several inches thick. All of these assertions were made in a later appellate court filing by Pierce Marshall, who benefited by seeing Anna in the most hideous light. Anna is not around to give her side of the story—nor is Pierce, for that matter—but if these claims are true, Marshall's last year must have been nightmarish.

In January, Marshall became seriously ill in Houston, and Anna flew in to see him. She allegedly spoon-fed him chicken soup, even though he couldn't swallow, and he choked until he lost consciousness, according to that same legal document. Luckily he was revived by his driver. In March he was hospitalized for gall bladder surgery and soon after diagnosed with inoperable, terminal stomach cancer. On May 26, 1995, according to his staffers, Anna visited Marshall at his home, climbed into his bed, exposed her breasts, and asked him, "Do you miss your rosebuds?"[45] Then she requested that he repeat on videotape what he allegedly "said last night"—that he wanted her to get half of all his assets. He refused, although he did mutter: "Vickie Nicole

Smith shall receive the house, which she calls the ranch, and the town-house, and her Mercedes automobile. . . . and everything else that I have ever given her now and forever. I love you. . . . I want my wife to be supported by me."[46]

On August 4, 1995, Marshall died of heart failure and pneumonia at the age of ninety. Anna had not seen him for more than a month, partly because she had spent a few days in the hospital in July after she had had seizures. The night before his death, he had declined to take a phone call from her, said his nurse. He told Nurse Harding his year-long marriage had been "a total long, lonely, frustrating, miserable existence."[47]

Pierce Marshall, his brother J. Howard Marshall III, and other family members set August 13 as the day they'd hold a dignified, private funeral. But the winsome widow wanted her own funeral, one that would come before Pierce's. On August 7, Anna staged a memorable ceremony at Houston's Geo. H. Lewis & Sons funeral home. She wore her low-cut wedding dress and veil, and Daniel wore a white tuxedo and carried a tiny black dog. Marshall was laid in a flower-draped expensive casket, adorned with a glittery banner that read: "From Your Lady Love." Photos of the lovebirds dotted the parlor. Harp music played, and about thirty mourners were present, all of them friends of Anna. After a eulogy from the Methodist Hospital chaplain, Anna rose to read a Bible passage but only got a few words out when she collapsed in tears. Other people rose to give comments, including one man who admitted not knowing J. Howard but said he believed that the Marshalls had an inspiring love story of a marriage. When the group began singing the Bette Midler anthem "Wind Beneath My Wings," Anna ran out of the room, sobbing. "She wanted to take the coffin out to her ranch and set him up on the patio deck," said an employee of the funeral home. "I had to talk her out of it—I could just see him sliding into the swimming pool."[48]

When it was Pierce's chance to hold the family funeral, he had his dad cremated. He sniped, "Smith spent so little time with my father that she had no idea that he was a Quaker and that he wanted his remains cremated," in accordance with traditions of that religion. A judge would later rule that the "cremains" should be split between the two warring sides, but Anna, angry about not being able to bury her husband, waited five years before she picked up his container of ashes. And when she did, it was chiefly to use as a prop for her reality TV series.[49]

Anna would be even more livid later as she learned that Pierce had been granted power of attorney for and legal guardian of his father's money and had no plans of seeing his half-his-own-age stepmother waltz off with hundreds of millions of Marshall family money. Pierce's first move was to pull the plug on the $50,000-per-month allowance his father had been sending Smith. Then he filed a series of motions that made it obvious he had had excellent sources that could swear to her adulterous affairs and mistreatment of J. Howard. Pierce tried to evict her from the ranch, citing she couldn't prove she held the title and that she had never lived with Marshall as man and wife. He also claimed she had a history of defrauding the elderly gentleman of real estate and other goods. But Smith responded with a letter from her husband that read, in part, "I don't object to [Pierce] being guardian for my affairs, matter of fact he runs a lot of businesses and does very good. But he has no business coming between my wife and myself. She is the light of my life. . . . maybe he's a bit jealous. . . . I have been a successful businessman, and I am not broke. I want my wife taken care of." In the absence of a will or trust that named her as an heir, what exactly did "taken care of" mean?[50]

Anna lost more than her Sugar Daddy when Marshall died—she also lost her drive. She had the occasional film or TV gig, but she spent most of her time in bed, watching television, and eating herself into a tizzy. Mashed potatoes and brown gravy. Pizza with everything. Pickles and salt. Fried baloney and cheese. Whole packages of biscuits. Colossus burgers, so juicy they'd stain her bedspread. And for dessert? Twinkies and Ho-Hos and creamy Dream Pies. When she couldn't fit anything else in her gut, she'd go in the bathroom and vomit.[51] I'd call this the "Modified Elvis Diet," except Elvis threw in the occasional banana, even if it was fried. Having consulted on Mr. Presley's autopsy, and seen photos of his bloated corpse, I can tell you how well his habits served him. And both Anna and Elvis had another tendency in common—popping vast quantities of prescription medicine like they were breath mints. In Elvis's case, he fooled himself into thinking his addiction didn't count because his medications were legally prescribed; he was very against illicit drugs, even famously volunteering to be a narcotics agent for President Richard Nixon.

But Anna didn't discriminate against illegal drugs. She still enjoyed a snootful of cocaine now and then, especially when it seemed to kill her appetite, and she liked taking ecstasy before sex. I understand she was not a smoker of any kind. Cigarette smokers in her company would be forced to go outside before they lit up. That November she spent another six days in the hospital, drying out after a near overdose. Shortly thereafter, she checked into the Betty Ford Center in Rancho Mirage, near Palm Springs, California, a respected alcohol and drug dependency treatment clinic and a familiar stop to many celebrities who are serious about stopping their addictive behavior.[52] Anna's mother, Virgie, was there to help her daughter through the intensive thirty-day regimen.

As Anna's size grew and her work with the Guess corporation ended, she became the spokesmodel for Lane Bryant, the fashion outlet for plus-sized women. Footage from one of the company's events shows her—and there's no other way to describe it—waddling down the catwalk, but she smiled as if she were having a blast. At home, things weren't so chipper. The sexual assault lawsuit by the former housekeeper was getting nasty. Anna's attorney T. Patrick Freydl, of Freydl & Associates, had filed a countersuit, asking for repayment of a $25,000 loan, but she lost both suits, and Maria Cerrato won an $850,000 judgment against Anna. According to an Anna Nicole fan Web site,[53] and confirmed by the California state bar,[54] Freydl suffered his own humiliations on other cases, including suspensions from the California state bar and disbarment in 2002 for misusing a client's funds. Anna was also engulfed in a long legal battle with publicist David Granoff, who had sued her in 2003 for $155,000 in unpaid fees, plus $25 million in lost revenues; she countersued for $1.5 million for using her image after she left his agency. It's unknown how those suits were settled, but after Anna's death, Granoff, in an online interview with Hollywood writer Mark Bellinghaus, allegedly stated that he had seen her demise coming, adding: "Anna Nicole had no spark anymore."[55]

Meanwhile Pierce Marshall and his ace legal team were letting Anna know they were not about to give up one extra penny of J. Howard Marshall II's purported $1.6 billion estate. Their position was she could keep the money and property her spouse gave to her when he was alive, but since he made no provisions for her in a will or trust, she was out of luck for anything else. For a brief time, she partnered up with J. Howard Marshall III, who had been disowned by his father and not named as an heir in the will, but neither of them much benefited from the other's involvement. In an interview with *Extra*, Anna described how she reacted to the pressure: "My husband got sick and I got thrown into all these legal battles, all these legal affairs. I had people suing me from here and there, and I just got so overwhelmed. I'm just this one little girl, I'm this one little person, and I've got fifty things thrown at me. And I'm like, 'What did I do? What did I ever do but take pills?' (laughs) Well, 'take pills and drink alcohol.' But I've never hurt anybody."

Continuing on, she stated: "It's hard, and for one little person to survive, if you're by yourself and you've got all this power and money around you and you've got all these legal affairs around you. . . . And I was just taking more and more pills and I just wanted to be by myself, you know? I was scared. . . . See, I was still going through mourning. 'Til this day I'm still going through mourning. I had all that, the legal, the mourning, the litigation, all this, and I had nobody. I had my son and you can't just dump all this on your child."[56]

By now, Daniel was becoming an old hand at caring for his mother. "He's kind of like my little man," she told *Extra* on another occasion.[57]

He was there to bring her pills and pillows for her ever-present back pain, a result of her center of gravity being compromised by her excessively large breast implants. At one point she had had two silicone pouches inserted into each breast. She spent a lot of time depressed and sleeping. One burden was removed when she filed for bankruptcy protection in February 1996, although it didn't absolve the lien she owed Cerrato.[58]

In 1997, she recorded a CD version of "My Heart Belongs to Daddy,"[59] partly because Marilyn Monroe had done a version in the 1960 film *Let's Make Love*, but mostly to stick it to Pierce. It didn't sell many copies but was a minor hit in the gay disco clubs, and she made a vampish video of the tune. The Web site TMZ.com would later post a video of a 1997 bar mitzvah that Anna crashed. Although not Jewish, Anna invited herself to the festivities of thirteen-year-old Evan Weiss when she saw people go into a ballroom at the Beverly Hills Hotel and followed them inside. Dressed more conservatively than usual, Anna made a beeline for young Evan and dirty-danced the hora with him and his father for fifteen minutes, as bubbies and zadehs can be heard on the video, gossiping about her. My own bar mitzvah experience was much different, but I'm sure Evan will forever tell the story of the night he became a man.[60] In 1998, Anna also appeared in music videos for Supertramp's "You Win, I Lose," and Third Eye Blind's "Jumper."

During these years she made frequent appearances on Howard Stern's syndicated radio show, which was basically a raunch fest where the overtly sexual and often comical host baited and belittled Smith. She grew to hate going on the program because he attacked her weight mercilessly, but the show was so popular she couldn't resist the chance to promote whatever she was doing and let showbiz executives know she was ready, willing, and able to work.[61]

In April 1998, she was crowned Miss Republic of Cuervo Gold, out of a field of six contestants. The beauty pageant officials chose Anna over the other, mostly unknown, women because "her party spirit won out." The tequila company that sponsored the gala owns an

eight-acre island in the West Indies that it had christened CuervoNa-
tion, and the rinky-dink pageant consisted of bikini girls strutting their
stuff while showing off "talent," such as margarita balancing. Anna
won, even though she was the only girl who wore a wrap the whole
time, ostensibly to cover up her beefy body. When her name was
announced, the emcee heralded her as the emissary who will "spread
the word of life, liberty, and the pursuit of a good Cuervo Gold margarita." There's a YouTube.com clip of the highlights, including a
straight-faced Anna speaking backstage, after the crowning: "This is
something that I've always wanted as a kid. I've had these fantasies,
dreams. I've had every dream come true so far and this tequila pageant
is the same to me as any other pageant, and I won. Even if I didn't win,
I got to be in it, so it's a dream."[62]

Anna was soon to get a another dream fulfilled, in the form of a man
who vowed to protect her for the rest of her life. And beyond.

Howard Kevin Stern, born in 1968, one year and one day after
Anna Nicole, wore several hats in their relationship. He was her
attorney, her friend, and, apparently, much more. Born and raised in
Los Angeles, and one of three children, he graduated from the University of California at Berkeley with a BA and went to law school at the
University of California at Los Angeles. He was admitted to the California state bar in 1994 and partnered with a pal, Dave Shebby, in a
law firm specializing in entertainment, corporate, and personal injury
matters. Stern met Anna in 1996 when his firm handled some of her
modeling contracts. They hit it off and soon he was her frequent escort
at parties and premieres. Anytime Anna spotted a camera and would
run after it like a heat-seeking missile, Howard would stay a few steps
off to the side, holding whatever she tossed at him, from her coat, to
her purse, to her little dog. Howard even brought her home for his
family's 1998 Thanksgiving feast, delighting his sister, Bonnie, who
took photos with the ebullient celebrity.

For a guy who was so frugal he drove a twenty-year-old car and
had a style that was exceedingly low-key, Anna brought pizzazz to

Stern's life. He learned how desperately alone and frightened she was from all of the legal maneuvers she was facing and presented her with a wise approach in dealing with one thing at a time, instead of letting all of the issues stack up into a tower she couldn't see over. She was sick of paying lawyers big fees and not seeing results, so when he offered to help her fight for the Marshall millions on a contingency basis, she hired him as her personal counsel. He severed his law practice with Shebby because Stern wouldn't be bringing in any income. He had become an attorney with just one client: Anna Nicole Smith.[63]

Howard represented Anna in court against the Marshall family, questioning her on direct examination. Her lead attorney, however, was Phillip Boesch, who was referred to "as my main nemesis," by Rusty Hardin, Pierce Marshall's first-chair counsel. In computing possible assets she might derive from a win in the Marshall case, the bankruptcy court took over jurisdiction of the case. Anna's team filed motions in California and Texas, asking for half of her late husband's estate. In November 1999, Howard walked Anna into a Los Angeles courtroom; she leaned on him for relief from a back injury, reporters were told. More slender than she had appeared in a long while, she wore a conservative blue suit, little makeup, and maintained the appropriate demeanor of a widow in mourning. She dabbed her eyes with tissues and spoke clearly when questioned by Marshall's attorneys. She had not claimed J. Howard's ashes, she testified, because cremation was "really disgusting," and she denied being unfaithful to her husband. When asked on which day she was wed, she couldn't recall, but stated it was one of the most important days in her life. "I believed when I married my husband that I was entitled to half of what he had," Anna told the court.

Boesch and Stern presented evidence that Marshall had loved his wife and resented his son Pierce's intrusion into their domestic bliss. And they argued that there was a verbal agreement that ensured her half of the fortune. While Anna might have been Marshall's trophy wife—and while he was undeniably very, very wealthy—such partnerships are not unusual in high society and it wasn't the court's job to pass judgment on a marriage it might not approve of or understand. There were also charges that Pierce Marshall had forged and altered documents, surreptitiously formed a new trust that he alone would control and that he alone would inherit, and tried to hide the true value of his father's stock holdings, so the Internal Revenue Service would charge him less. Anna strode out of the courthouse with her head high and wearing dark shades.[64]

On September 27, 2000, the California judge awarded Anna $450 million, later upping it to $474 million. It was a legal ruling that topped every news broadcast and caught my attention, big time. However, the Marshall family was not ready to write a check just yet. They appealed to a Texas court, which agreed to hear the case. But in November, a Houston court became the scene of "The Anna and Rusty Show," as local reporters called it. For five grueling months, Anna went from manic to panic as Rusty Hardin and the rest of Pierce Marshall's attorneys worked her over on their home territory. She claimed Pierce made her go bankrupt because he withheld monies due her. And on the stand in January 2001, she seemed self-assured in a pretty cerise top, and even funny, when she responded to grilling about how Marshall would give her funds. "I don't care how he sent it," she giggled. "Cash or check, it's all fine with me." And when asked to explain how she spent Paw-Paw's liberal monthly cash allowance, she testified: "I go to premieres, like every week. I've got to buy gowns, and they're like $30,000. You've got to buy shoes, and hair and makeup. It's very expensive to be me."[65]

Over the next weeks she would accuse Pierce Marshall of trying to have her electrocuted; possibly ordering an anesthesiologist to kill J. Howard's former mistress, Jewell "Lady" Walker; and killing his own father by keeping her from him. But perhaps the best-remembered moment of the trial came during a six-day cross-examination where Pierce's attorney bore down hard on Anna. When Hardin asked whether she'd been taking new acting lessons, she snarled: "Screw you, Rusty!"

None of Anna's testimony went over well with jurors. In an interview with ABC's *Primetime*, one male panelist said she was too far-fetched: "At the end of the day, some of us had headaches from trying to keep up with what she was saying." And a female juror added, "It's not possible for her to be telling the truth and twenty other witnesses are lying." Another woman said what troubled her was Smith's obvious "dumb blonde" act: "So she goes, 'Well, I'll play the part. Then I can lie and get away with it, you know, because I'm just dumb.'"[66]

On March 7, 2001, the Houston court ruled that Anna was not a legal heir and not entitled to half of Marshall's assets. The same court also walloped J. Howard Marshall III with $35.3 million in damages for bringing a baseless claim into court and willfully knowing it was false. But before Pierce could breathe easily, he had to win an appeal of Anna's bankruptcy court ruling. Two months later he did just that when a US District judge in Los Angeles overturned the $474 million award.[67]

But in the courtroom equivalent of a tennis match at Wimbledon, the following March, the US District Court held that Anna deserved half of the investment income Marshall earned during their fourteen-month marriage, as well as punitive damages due to Pierce's malicious attempts to cut her off. The Marshall family was ordered to pay Smith $88.5 million. Anna Nicole was the only person who ever testified that Marshall promised her half his estate, and her video of J. Howard wanly providing for her was never played before a jury. But federal Judge David O. Carter, in his 2002 opinion, found that the old man had made some preliminary inquiries of his lawyers to draw up a new trust that would buoy Anna's interests. And there was evidence that Pierce was so worried about it that he sent a private investigator to tail his father in California to make sure no new will would be drawn up on the visit.

In December 2004, a federal appeals court in San Francisco over-turned that order, deflating Anna's hopes once again. But there was still one place to go. On March 1, 2006, wearing a chic black outfit and sitting silently in the back of the courtroom, Anna attended a hearing in Washington, DC, before the US Supreme Court. She exited through a side door, avoiding the press, for once in her life. Nobody seriously expected that she would prevail; in fact, the late-night talk shows had a field day on the subject, including a joke about Anna being invited into the private chambers of the supposed ladies man Justice Clarence Thomas, so she could "inspect his briefs." But there were no quips inside the hallowed courtroom as the justices argued the merits of the case. Chief Justice John G. Roberts Jr. noted that the case "involved a substantial amount of assets," and Justice Stephen Breyer remarked that the battle between Anna Nicole and Pierce was "quite a story." When Marshall's counsel argued that Smith, after losing in Texas, was shopping for a new venue in the federal courts, as if she were at Neiman Marcus, Justice David Souter cut to the chase: "She's saying, 'I just want some money from this guy.' That's all she's saying. 'I'll assume the will is valid, just give me some money.'"

"No matter how you dice it or slice it," Marshall family attorney G. Eric Brunstad told the justices, "she is trying to make an end run around the probate court." But Justice Ruth Bader Ginsburg didn't seem to buy that. "You're suggesting an extraordinary setup where a state court can bar all the other courts from dealing with a similar and related issue. I've never heard of that," she said. Their decision on May 1, 2006, written by Justice Ginsburg for the unanimous panel, remanded the case back to the Ninth US Circuit Court of Appeals, which had dropped the ball before. Anna would be able to pursue the windfall from her late husband after all. She didn't win the case; she just won the right to have the federal court hear the matter again.[68]

It was great news for the five-months pregnant performer.

A disgruntled Pierce pledged to "fight to clear my name in California federal court" and "to uphold my father's estate plan." And in a written statement he declared, "The fact that my father gave Vicki [sic] more than $7 million is absolute proof that no one was interfering in his business. . . . If Vicki [sic] had just acted responsibly she would be financially set for life." But after a brief but aggressive infection, Pierce Marshall died the next month at the age of sixty-seven, before he was able to learn to spell Anna's birth name. His widow, Elaine, was left to continue the legal skirmish, and with Anna's own death in February 2007, her estate will be going into the next round, presumably with Howard K. Stern still involved.[69]

By 2002, Anna was broke, overweight, and bored. Howard had incorporated her company, Hot Smoochie Lips, of which she was president and Stern was the registered agent. Anna was paid through that entity, and it held the title to her California home. Years later, though, it was purported that Stern never filed or paid taxes on the corporation and it was $30,000 in arrears. The Franchise Tax Board put the corporation into "suspended status."[70]

Anna needed a new adventure and she got it after a meeting at the Hollywood offices of the E! Entertainment Channel, a popular and ambitious low-budget cable network that is known for producing celebrity biographies. Ozzy Osbourne and his family had just had a hit season on the channel's competitor, MTV, so the E! executives asked Anna about doing a similar program. The show would follow her around with a camera crew, videotaping her as she went about her business, doing whatever it is that she did. A reality series with no scripts, no lines to memorize, just Anna being herself, with the cast of characters in her life playing themselves on the show. And they'd pay her a lot of money. "I finally got to a point where I could work again," Smith told a reporter. "I was like, 'Hmm, I love cameras.' So why not? Let's go for it."

The Anna Nicole Show debuted in August 2002 to unprecedented ratings—7.6 million viewers, making it E!'s best numbers ever and the best debut for any reality show in cable history. With a colorful animated title sequence and a snappy theme song with lyrics: "Anna Anna Anna Anna Anna Nicole, you're so outrageous!" it seemed fresh enough to be a hit. In an interview with *Entertainment Weekly*, Mark Sonnenberg, E!'s executive vice president of programming, explained:

"Here's a single mother who's been struggling to make it while taking on the rich and powerful to make a better life for her and her son. She's also a grieving widow. When you watch and spend time with her, she's very captivating." The series tagline was: "It's not supposed to be funny. It just is."[71]

The half-hour episodes were slices of Anna's life and nothing was too trivial. Anna's ulcer acts up after she takes part in an eating contest. Her straight-A student son Daniel, sixteen, plays video games. Anna goes to the dentist. She and Howard travel to Las Vegas and cavort with strippers. Anna learns to drive. Her tres fey designer Bobby Trendy wants to change her décor. Her toy poodle, Sugar Pie, humps a stuffed animal and gets put on Prozac. Anna brings home the urn containing the ashes of her late husband. Howard briefs her on Middle East politics, urging her to support the Israelis, and Anna replies, "I'm just gonna keep my mouth shut. I know nothing about nothing."[72] And so on.

One common theme was that her twenty-three-year-old purple-haired, androgynous assistant, Kim Walther, seems to have had a crush on her. She gets a tattoo of Anna on her arm and, in one odd episode, while driving Anna around, she and Smith slug each other every time they spot a Volkswagen on the road. Another theme is that Stern is there like an obsequious valet, taking her orders and insults. Foul language is bleeped and nudity is pixilated, but otherwise, anything goes. Sex is discussed endlessly, as Anna runs off to masturbate or bounces on a friend's bed to see how sturdy its headboard is.[73]

Critics, who got an early preview of the series and a question-and-answer session with its star, were dumbfounded when Anna wouldn't answer questions about her late husband, the seven-year legal quest for his money, or even the content of the series. She talked about "breast transplants" but wouldn't admit to having implants, and she used what was described as "barely audible girly speak" to express a hope that the show would allow viewers to "see that I have a little talent and maybe they'll take me seriously." Even Tim Goodman, a reviewer for the *Chronicle* in the very tolerant city of San Francisco, titled his column "Anyone Home?" when he griped about her "hammy vacancy" and his fear that E! was exploiting her, and that she was exploiting her son. In a clip Daniel was heard saying, shyly, "I love my mom, but I hate the cameras."[74] But Anna replied that it wasn't a problem—then, emulating a dim-bulb Marilyn Monroe, she pretended not to understand subsequent questions.

The pans only got worse when the series began airing. But an argument could be made that a program like this isn't made for the critics—it's escapist entertainment for folks who just want to come home, pop open a beer, put their feet up, and have a chuckle. From what I hear though, even those people soon had their fill of Anna's inane antics. "It's like watching a train wreck," was one oft-mentioned remark. The first few times she stumbled over furniture and slurred her speech might have been acceptable, because you might think it wasn't how she really was and maybe there was an editor making her look bad. But when it sunk in that this was all too real, that she was really a mess, the talk became more about what was wrong with her and why a TV network would allow a person with an apparent substance abuse issue on the air. The show was renewed for another season, but Anna seemed to get spacier, nastier, and more obese with each episode. To date, only the first year is available on DVD. It was not an act she put on for the cameras; at a *Vanity Fair* magazine Oscar party, she was barely able to walk and had lipstick smeared all over her face.

To promote the first season, Anna made a stop at the New York City station where shock jock Howard Stern and his morning crew hosted their nationally syndicated radio program. Despite the way he often teased her, she couldn't resist his massive audience that she wanted to watch her TV series. His program was also simultaneously videotaped and edited for broadcast on E! for its overnight schedule. Corporate symmetry be damned, things went bad, fast, once she entered the studio, with her own Howard K. Stern by her side. The brutally honest radio clown began berating her about her weight, calling her a "big, fat porker," and bringing out a scale he demanded she step on. She ran out of the studio in tears, with lawyer Stern behind her.

Instead of apologizing for hurting the feelings of a loyal friend, the radio star turned up the heat, telling guests for days what a chunky diva she had become and arguably damaging her reputation. He used the clip on his TV show, further embarrassing her—then she used it herself on her own program, emphasizing his bullyboy tactics.[75] The taboo was broken; suddenly Anna Nicole's weight became fodder for late-night comics to "weigh in on." Anna was mortified. But someone at the radio station, who had recently lost one hundred pounds, called her with a suggestion to check out a diet supplement that was a sponsor on the show. The product was TrimSpa, and its connection to Anna was kismet for both her and the company.

TrimSpa X32 is an appetite suppressant whose active ingredient is *Hoodia gordonii*, a plant that grows wild in three southern African countries. For hundreds of years, San tribesmen would chew on it to stave off hunger when going on long hunting expeditions across the Kalahari Desert. Anna, who had tried countless other diet plans with no lasting success, began researching the product and liked what she read. The company, established in 1993, was the official weight loss product for the Hawaiian Tropic, Mrs. America, and Mrs. World pageants, and an associate sponsor of some NASCAR Busch series races. Anna also liked that the company worked with the Susan G. Komen Breast Cancer Foundation, the American Cancer Society, and the Make-a-Wish Foundation, which helps terminally ill children. According to Alex Goen, TrimSpa's founder and chief executive officer, the company had conducted an eight-week double-blind placebo-controlled study that demonstrated that users of X32—who also were on a diet and exercise regime—lost two and a half times more weight than those who just used diet and exercise alone.

Anna was ready for a dramatic change and began a daily campaign of exercise, better eating habits, and TrimSpa—two tablets before each meal. When her series stopped production, Anna went underground and worked hard to get back into shape, said Goen. What happened was nothing short of astounding. She signed on as TrimSpa's first celebrity spokesperson and made a series of TV commercials and print ads that showed her looking younger and more elegant than ever before. From head to toe there was a difference—in time, it was revealed that she had lost a whopping sixty-nine pounds. Tight jeans and sleeveless evening gowns could come back into her wardrobe. She purred the catchphrases "TrimSpa, baby" and "Do you like my body?" as often as possible. The company stock soared, and her old swagger came back. Goen and his wife, Monique, became close friends with Anna and Howard and would be valuable assets in the troubled times ahead.[76]

On the eve of the 2004 Kentucky Derby, Anna, Daniel, and Howard attended the Barnstable Brown Party, the chic annual bash thrown by society twins Patricia Barnstable Brown and Priscilla Barnstable. Patricia's husband had died the year before of diabetes, so the sisters were co-hosting a fund-raiser for research at the University of Louisville and the University of Kentucky. The gala drew numerous celebrities, but Anna Nicole was the talk of the party and not just because of the pink, frilly frock and hat she wore. She had brought along a camera crew, which bad boy recording artist Kid Rock didn't like. He asked if she had to have cameras follow her every move, and she snapped that, yes, she did. With escalating voices and insults, they flipped their middle fingers at each other. The singer later apologized to Daniel for having made the obscene gesture in front of him. By that time Anna was greeting fans who were breaking down barricades, trying to get her to pose for photos and sign autographs. She even upstaged then-married singers Nick Lachey and Jessica Simpson, who were the current darlings of MTV with their reality series, *Newlyweds*.

Getting into embarrassing celebrity contretemps was nothing new to Anna—over the years she had called director Oliver Stone a "fucking asshole," waved a naked breast at Bruce Willis, and vomited at Dolly Parton's feet. But this night in Louisville, her biggest win was catching the eye of a local photographer by the name of Larry Birkhead. They flirted and began an on-again, off-again romance, and he would eventually move to California to be near her.[77]

In May 2004, Anna was again booked as a guest on the Howard Stern radio show. She brought along a crew from the syndicated TV gossip-news show *Extra* to capture what should have been her triumphant return. But the radio host, well-known for not giving up control, would not give the crew access. Anna and Howard could enter the studio alone, but the TV cameras had to stay outside, explained the show's producer, Gary Dell'Abate. While Dell'Abate and Anna's attorney had a public hissy fit, which was caught by *Extra*'s cameras, Anna returned to her white Hummer limousine and called in to the Stern program, where she was put on the air, live. She demanded that the host apologize for demeaning her, both when she was heavy and now. But instead he made himself the hero: "Who helped you lose the weight?" Anna replied, "Does that get you off, to call people fat?"— and then hung up on him. She turned to an *Extra* camera and defiantly stated: "I did not lose weight because of Howard Stern. It wasn't because of him. I lost it for myself. What he said to me was very hurtful. I don't think it's right, and I wanted to go in there and tell him that." Then she signed a few autographs and gave a parting shot: "I'm not even going to give him the respect of being angry." But she was furious, and so was Howard K. Stern.[78]

Over the summer, mega-selling hip-hop artist Kanye West had hired Anna to appear in a music video for his just-recorded song, "The New Workout Plan." The playful song featured West as an exercise guru, addressing women in the gym about how to slim down and catch a rich suitor. One line where he sings about "working on the stomach," took on new relevance in November 2007 when his mother, Donda West, famously died after complications from a tummy tuck. The video's almost slapstick humor used before and after photos of Anna Nicole Smith, and graphics that identified her as "Former Trailer Trash," "From Whoa to Yo!" and "Ultimate Trophy Wife." Anna actually rapped a line about being a poor gal from Mobile, Alabama, whose life improved since using Kanye's workout plan.[79] It's a cute video and she looks terrific in it. So when the *Thirty-Second Annual American Music Awards* rolled around on November 14, 2004, it seemed like a bright idea to invite her on the program to introduce West. This would be her first live TV appearance anywhere since sporting her new shapely figure.

From her entrance, she looked beautiful, in a floor-sweeper with a low-scooped neckline. But as she approached the microphone, she was waving her arms in the air and seemed to babble. On the close-up, it was plain to see that she was in some altered state. Was she drunk? Drugged? About to pass out? The director in the booth must have wondered if he would have to ditch the shot and go to a commercial. Anna clutched the podium, tried to focus her eyes, and slurred, "Like my body?" Then she pointed to her neck where she was wearing a gold letter necklace that read "TrimSpa." For people who couldn't read the letters it looked as if she were slitting her own throat. "I was honored to be in our next performer's new video, and if I ever record an album I want this guy to produce it," she shouted, drawing out the syllables. "'Make me beautiful' duets, 'cause he's a freaking genius!" With that she clapped her hands like a seal, and then yelled, "Make some noise for my boy, Kanye West!!!"[80] A collective sense of horror rippled throughout the studio audience and across America. Backstage, Anna allegedly staggered around and had to be held up by two bodyguards. She told people there she had lost too much weight and was sick of the constant taunts about appearing stupid: "I liked me better bigger because now I'm too bony. I'm just portrayed as some bimbo and never taken seriously."

Anna's career was in a freefall for the next several months, as she concentrated on stabilizing her out-of-control habits. She appeared in an ad for the animal rights group People for the Ethical Treatment of Animals, or PETA, spoofing Marilyn Monroe's "Diamonds Are a Girl's Best Friend" number from *Gentlemen Prefer Blondes*. "To kill an animal for a coat is crazy," Anna told a magazine, emphasizing that while fur in Monroe's era was fashionable, it's now a social liability. "My late husband gave me two fur coats years ago, but I've never worn them, and I never will," she said. After Anna's death, the organization issued a press release that read, in part: "PETA and animals lost a good friend and outspoken supporter, Anna Nicole Smith. She used every opportunity to speak out against senseless cruelty to animals, and she will be greatly missed. We always thought that Anna Nicole was a perfect fit for PETA because, just like us, she not only hated cruelty to animals but also couldn't be ignored and because, no matter what people thought of her, they always had an opinion one way or another."[81] In 2005, Anna lightened things up as a presenter at *Australia's First Annual MTV Awards*. In a nod to the 2004 Super Bowl half-time show where singer Janet Jackson had the so-called wardrobe malfunction and exposed her breast, Anna pulled down her dress, revealing that both of her breasts were plastered with MTV logos.[82] The press reported this as if it were a horrendous scandal, but it seems to me that it was a written bit that Anna did for a laugh. Someone from MTV had to give her the logo stickers.

That year she also took on a job no one could see coming—as a columnist for the weekly *National Enquirer* after one of the magazine's editors called Stern, telling him they wanted a celebrity who would speak her mind about the world of showbiz. Anna's column, with her hand-drawn doodles, debuted in April and ran until October. "I know I'm not a writer. I don't even know how to spell," she cracked at the launch party. "What better way to get an education, right?" Explaining why she signed on, she said: "They did a poll on me, and I found out that there's a lot of people that don't like me. And I thought, well, maybe if I have my own column, you know, and people know me, then maybe they'll change their opinion." Her breezy style was assisted by an in-house editor who cleaned up her text. Praising the May-December relationship of actors Demi Moore and Ashton Kutcher, she wrote: "Go, Demi! Go, Ashton! Go, age difference!" When TV gossip anchor Pat O'Brien checked himself into rehab for alcohol addiction, she gave him advice from the heart: "Rehab sucks.

There's no special treatment." And when singer/actress Jessica Simpson criticized her, Anna hit back: "I heard that Jessica Simpson is running her mouth again about not wanting to be compared to me. Well I've got news for you, honey—the feeling is mutual. Let's see how you react when the media turns on you—and they will!" She also yammered on about her own weight, her dogs, her son, her search for a good man, and hinted that she would soon be starring in a new movie.[83]

Illegal Aliens began shooting in Vermont, in September 2005, by a small but active production house called Edgewood Studios. Its president, David Giancola, directed and co-executive produced the film, and Anna and Daniel were co-associate producers, after she put up some funding for the project. By Hollywood standards the $3 million budget was microscopic, but for Edgewood, it was a major investment, with expensive special effects and computer graphics. Anna, Daniel, and Howard spent a few happy weeks on the set, and with Giancola and co-executive producer John James, who once starred as Jeff Colby on TV's prime-time drama *Dynasty*. The film, which was written by Ben Coello but received an uncredited rewrite from Daniel Smith, was a campy sci-fi salute to the *Charlie's Angels* flicks, with Anna as one of three outer space hotties who save Earth from a villain played by former pro-wrestler Joanie "Chyna" Laurer. Edgewood's publicist puckishly described it as if "Mel Brooks directed a Monty Python movie, edited by George Lucas, who was forced to work with Woody Allen as the screenwriter and Marilyn Monroe as the star." It's full of broad comedy, bodily function jokes, and sexy shots of the women. In other words, it should have had no trouble finding an audience. The movie was finished and looking for distribution when Daniel died in September 2006.[84]

It should have been an ideal chance for Anna to get back in the swing of show business, with East and West Coast premieres, and promotion on the TV talk show circuit, but suddenly everything was on hold. Anna and Howard were catatonic over Daniel's tragic demise, and Giancola knew it wasn't the time to press them about the film's next step. He inserted an "In Loving Memory" dedication card to Daniel, right before the closing credits, and then slowly realized he'd have to scrap his plans to release the film in theaters and, instead, just issue it as a DVD. "Danny was a full creative partner in the making of this movie," Giancola told my co-author, Dawna Kaufmann. "He had an on-the-nose sensibility about comedy and music, and he knew how to handle his mother. He did a full rewrite on the script, to make the best of Anna's skills, and he was there on the set, watching and learning. I think in time he would have ended up a writer/director because he had innate talent, plus business acumen. On the set, and in the editing process, when we'd send them edited footage, his notes were excellent. If Danny liked something, we knew it would work." There were no signs, Giancola said, of Daniel's being ill. "He was vibrant and healthy the whole time."

But if Daniel's death wasn't enough of a blow for Giancola and his team, Anna's death totally crushed them. Edgewood got offers to rush the film into theaters while Anna was big news, but Giancola demurred: "I want people to have some time pass so they can laugh freely, which is what Anna would have wanted them to do." John James added: "At first look, *Illegal Aliens* appears to be just another low budget sci-fi comedy poking fun at Hollywood's big-budget flicks. But now, with the passing of its star, you'll find it replete with metaphors of her life."[85]

In May 2007, the movie was screened at the Cannes Film Festival, where Reuters News Service reported: "Along the glamorous Croisette Boulevard, from the (possibly) sublime—Angelina Jolie in *A Mighty Heart* about the kidnap and murder by Islamic militants of US reporter Daniel Pearl—to the (probably) ridiculous—*Illegal Aliens* starring the now-deceased Anna Nicole Smith—to the (certainly) serious—Leonardo DiCaprio's environmental documentary *The 11th Hour*." And that autumn, it was a huge hit at the Bahamas International Film Festival, where Howard attended, thanked Anna's many fans, and told them how happy she had been in their country.[86]

A month before shooting the film *Illegal Aliens*, Anna, Daniel, Howard, and Larry Birkhead visited friends in Myrtle Beach, South Carolina. At a club called Freaky Tiki, she fortified herself with Red Bulls and vodka, entered a wet T-shirt contest—which she won—and exposed herself, according to an account by MSNBC's *The Scoop* columnist Jeannette Walls. The party girl didn't stop there, apparently. A source told Walls that Anna "got into a loud fight with some guy everyone says is her boyfriend." Anna's own Web site was abuzz with the gossip, with posters writing that Anna was seen "slamming shots," taking pills, and smacking her boyfriend in the face. Soon after, those posts were removed and the forum was closed. "The reason we took down the postings was that we don't want Anna defamed on her own Web site," Stern told *The Scoop*. He said that she did enter the wet T-shirt contest but did not expose herself because she was wearing pasties. He also denied that Smith took any pills or that she had a boyfriend. Stern seemed intent on negating Birkhead's role in Anna's life, even though Larry that night had been wearing a T-shirt that read, "I love my girlfriend." Despite their often chaotic and nonexclusive relationship, there was also genuine affection between Smith and Birkhead. Anna later told his hometown newspaper, the *Louisville Courier Journal*, "Larry keeps me occupied so I don't have to worry about being lonely anymore."[87]

Back at the Myrtle Beach home where they were staying, Anna met a neighbor named "Ben." G. Ben Thompson was a fifty-nine-year-old millionaire real estate developer who fell for the dishy beauty. He liked her free spirit, and she liked his free spending. They began seeing each other and he flew her by private jet to his home in the Florida Keys for a week, and then introduced her to his daughter, Gina Shelley, and her husband, Stancil Ford Shelley, called "Ford." As Gina told FOX News's Greta Van Susteren, "She was a little afraid to meet me because she was dating my father. And my first impression of her was she's not what you see on TV. She's a real person."[88]

While Howard stayed in Los Angeles to get ready for the upcoming US Supreme Court hearing, Anna, Daniel, her assistant

Nathan Collins—who had replaced Kim Walther—and Anna's dogs spent the 2005 Christmas holidays with Thompson and the Shelleys. By the end of that visit, she and Ben had decided they made better friends than lovers. He remained a devoted and protective pal for the rest of her life. Around that time, Anna learned she was pregnant, but she wasn't ready to go public with the news. Stern issued a statement for her Web site that read: "If Anna Nicole is pregnant, she obviously doesn't want anybody to know yet. If she's not pregnant, she's not denying the rumor because she thinks it's funny how much of a stir it's causing. She'll leave it up to you to guess which one it is."[89]

One person who knew about the pregnancy was Larry Birkhead, whom Anna assured was the father of her unborn baby. Larry had accompanied Anna to visits to her gynecologist, saw the ultrasound, and discussed with her what they would name their child, he told my co-author, Kaufmann. Birkhead said that not only had the pregnancy been planned, it was their second pregnancy—the first had ended in a miscarriage some months earlier. Anna told him she had wanted a daughter who had Larry's blue eyes, so she would resemble Marilyn Monroe. "For about two and a half years, our relationship was personal," Birkhead said. "I've been told that I was the father from Anna. She said, 'We're having a baby,' and ever since then, my life has been totally different." During the subsequent paternity action, Birkhead filed legal documents that recounted the two pregnancies and their time together.[90]

In April 2006, Anna went into Los Angeles's Cedars-Sinai for a purported eighteen-day detoxification. Then, the next month, Anna called Ben, and told him she was pregnant and needed to get away from all the press that wouldn't leave her alone. She hadn't been feeling well, she said. Ben and Ford flew to Los Angeles and accompanied her back to Myrtle Beach. They agreed to facilitate her move to the Bahamas, where she could give birth in privacy. Gina told Greta Van Susteren that Anna had admitted to her that Larry Birkhead was the baby's father, but they had split up in November after a fight over a pair of sunglasses. She wanted to have the baby without him, Gina said. The family treated Anna like she was a blood relative, and, in their presence, she could unwind from all the stressors in her life.

Ben came to Anna's rescue by financing a home called Horizons in Nassau, which Anna and Howard moved into. Ford, who was on the FOX News program with his wife, said Anna understood that she would have to pay Thompson back for the property. She was about to get a hefty check from TrimSpa and sent many e-mails to Thompson and the Shelleys stating that she would sign the mortgage and pay back the loan. But then her e-mails changed course—she began claiming that Ben, and not Larry, was the baby's father. Even after Ben explained to her that he had had a vasectomy and couldn't produce sperm, she tried to make him take responsibility for the child. (When Gina visited her in the hospital after Anna gave birth, she introduced the baby as Gina's sister. Gina told Van Susteren that there was never a mention at all of Howard being the father).[91]

On June 1, 2006, a video was posted on Anna's Web site showing her afloat on an inflatable raft in a swimming pool as a small white dog barks in the background. "Let me stop all the rumors," she says. "Yes, I am pregnant. I'm happy, I'm very very happy about it. Everything's goin' really, really good and I'll be checking in and out periodically on the Web and I'll let you see me as I'm growing."[92]

Another friend from Myrtle Beach, Laurie Payne, first met Anna in the summer of 2005, but they became closer during the former Playmate's pregnancy. Debra A. Opri, a top Beverly Hills attorney hired by Birkhead in the paternity battle, filed Payne's sworn statement with the court. In it, Payne attested that a pregnant Anna confessed to her in phone calls and instant messages that Birkhead was the fetus's father. Payne also stated that it was the second pregnancy fathered by the photographer. Payne declared under penalty of perjury that she administered pills to Anna from a bottled marked "methadone" and personally observed Anna taking "a rather high dose of Xanax" during her pregnancy. In an e-mail from Smith to Payne, attached to Payne's declaration, Anna spelled out that she had had sexual relations with two men around the time of conception, but one "cant [*sic*] do what has been done." Payne stated that Anna and Larry had had a "love-hate relationship," and that Smith would refer to Birkhead as "the asshole" in her conversations with Laurie. In other e-mails to Payne, Anna raged that Birkhead won't leave her alone and treats her "like shit in front of his friends," and mentions that she's strapped for cash and counting on the courts to give her the money she needs to start over. [93]

In August, Ford, Gina, and Riley Shelley visited an eight-months pregnant Anna at Horizons. While her family went out, nine-year-old Riley spent time with Anna, who had missed celebrating the girl's recent birthday and had promised her a celebration. Howard Stern's camcorder captured about forty minutes of the occasion, part of which later became hotly debated on TV news shows. In an exclusive for FOX News's *Geraldo at Large*, host Geraldo Rivera interviewed Ford Shelley about the video and played the longest clip that had been broadcast to date—about ten minutes' worth. The tape shows young Riley—her face digitally obscured for her privacy—plastering clown makeup on Anna's face, and the two playing with dolls, when Riley became concerned that Anna seemed to think a doll was her baby. "This is not your baby," Riley tells Anna. "Your baby's still in your tummy." Riley turns to Howard for help, suggesting they get a screwdriver to take out the doll's battery to prove to Anna it wasn't real. "Please, Howard, seriously, help," she begs. Stern, still holding the camera, talks to what seems like a plainly impaired Anna:

> STERN: Anna. Anna. Anna, look at me. Riley thinks you've
>   absolutely lost your mind.
> SMITH: Huh?
> STERN: Riley thinks you've lost your mind.
> SMITH: I didn't lose my mind.
> STERN: She thinks you have.
> SMITH: I didn't.
> STERN: Is this a mushroom trip?

SMITH: Huh?
STERN: Is this a mushroom trip?
SMITH: What?
STERN: Is this a mushroom trip?
SMITH: What do you mean?
STERN: I'm kidding.
SMITH: What does that mean?
STERN: I'm kidding. I bet this footage is worth money.
SMITH: Why? What footage?
STERN: This thing you're looking into?
SMITH: It's a camera.
STERN: Exactly.

Another section of the video shows Anna outside, running on the tennis court, with Howard shouting at her not to fall and hurt herself. Anna is wearing a sarong and her right breast keeps popping out, which she hardly notices until Howard tells her. Riley, by then frantic, can be seen telling Howard that Anna needs help. "She's having brain trouble. I think we need the hospital!" and "Please call the doctor, Howard. Let's call the doctor, Howard, please. Something's wrong!" It would be a while before this video was made public, and when it hit the airwaves, I was as shaken as everyone else who saw it. On the program, Ford Shelley also told Geraldo that his daughter Riley had seen Howard give Anna "something from a white bottle with red stripes."[94]

Also that month, on August 8—almost four weeks before Anna gave birth—a Beverly Hills internist sent a package addressed to Vickie Marshall, in care of a mail drop in Nassau. Inside were vitamins, the sleeping aid Dalmane, and the morphine-like drug Demerol, according to the *New York Post*. The doctor, who later said he had performed some cosmetic surgery on the celebrity, confirmed that prescriptions were sent but weren't written for Anna. He refused to tell reporters for whom the scrips were actually written and did not say why they were sent to Anna, if they were not meant for her.[95]

On August 25, a Los Angeles internist named Dr. Sandeep Kapoor reportedly wrote a prescription for "Michelle Chase," one of many aliases used by Anna. Under California law, it is illegal to prescribe a controlled substance to a false name. The Los Angeles address listed for the patient did not actually exist, and the package was sent to Vicky [*sic*] Marshall in the Bahamas. The medication was liquid methadone, a strong pain reliever that is also used to wean heroin or opiate addicts from their substance abuse, although there has been no suggestion Anna was ever addicted to heroin. Syringes were also ordered through a local pharmacy, which purportedly carried out the doctor's shipping instructions. Alleged copies of both the prescription and the shipping information were posted on the Internet gossip site TMZ.com, along with Dr. Kapoor's statement, issued via his lawyer. Kapoor, a 1996 graduate of the Boston University School of Medicine, explained that prescribing methadone in the late stages of a patient's pregnancy was "medically sound and appropriate." The attorney cited a US Department of Health and Human Services study that the drug will not cause birth defects in a fetus, and also defended Kapoor's use of Smith's alias, saying it was done to protect Anna's privacy.[96]

Anna—under the pseudonym "Jean Smith"—delivered her daughter by cesarean birth on September 7, 2006, at Doctors Hospital in Nassau. Her obstetrician, Dr. Hubert Minnis, who is also the minister of health for the Bahamas, performed the procedure. He described the six-pound, nine-ounce baby's birth as "uncomplicated."[97]

However, Anna apparently felt otherwise. "I actually thought I was dying," she told *Entertainment Tonight* in an exclusive interview that included explicit footage of the surgery, which Stern shot with his camcorder. "They had my arms strapped down, probably so I wouldn't pop anyone," Anna said, and the video shows her in apparent agony as the doctors prepare her. "You sure you want me to film this?" Howard asks, stroking her forehead with his free hand. Anna nods a yes, so he keeps taping. In fact, Howard hadn't originally brought the camera with him. Anna's labor was delayed so that he could drive home and get it. In the interview with the TV show's co-anchor, Mark Steines, Howard sits with his arm around Anna while she recalled why she had the C-section: "They thought the baby was too big, that it was going to bust my womb." Howard said that he was happy he had camera duty so it could keep him "a little distant from the actual surgery." Doctors can be heard saying Anna wants the cut to be "above the tattoo but as low as possible, so she can wear a bikini." And Anna complains that she is not feeling the effects of the anesthetic. "I felt like I was going to die," she informed Steines. "It felt like God and Jesus were like ripping my insides out of my body and like the Devil was yanking my insides from my legs, and they were playing Tug o' War." The video shows the doctor using forceps to pull out the infant, and then Howard is heard saying with a quavering voice, "She's beautiful, she's a beautiful baby." The video ends with the baby, wrapped in a cloth, being put into her crying mother's arms. "The pain went away when I saw her," Anna told Steines. The *Entertainment Tonight* segment was uploaded to YouTube.com.[98]

In watching that video, I had to marvel at the Oscar-caliber acting I saw in that delivery room. Anna's bellows and contortions might make one think she was in obvious distress, unless one realizes that she was likely exaggerating for the video camera. My own daughter, Ingrid, is an obstetrician in Pittsburgh, and I asked her if there was any chance a patient undergoing a cesarean delivery would not be sufficiently anesthetized, and she replied that it was highly unlikely in a modern hospital. I believe it is far more reasonable that these very experienced doctors had performed with utter professionalism, making sure that Anna was in no discomfort. They must have been quite stunned to hear their famous patient complain about pain that was almost certainly nonexistent. *Entertainment Tonight* reportedly paid nearly $1 million for the video and first post-birth interview with Anna and Howard, which ran in November 2006. Would a drama-free, tranquil birth have commanded such a steep price tag?[99]

What should have been a brief hospital stay and the beginning of a joyous family adventure went askew three days later, when Anna's twenty-year-old son, Daniel, died. As you read in the previous chapter, the boy's death set Anna on a disastrous course. Shortly after Daniel's death, I traveled to Nassau to perform his second autopsy, and met Anna, Howard, and their legal team. I continued to consult on a regular basis with them from then on. Stern's name was on the birth certificate for the baby, now called Dannielynn, and while I didn't press him for details, he represented to me that he was the child's father. He announced that he was the "proud father" on a September 26 edition of *Larry King Live*[100]—and two days later Howard and Anna had that non-legally binding commitment ceremony on a friend's boat. Still, I took note of the many TV appearances made by Larry Birkhead as he continued to claim he was the girl's father and that Anna and Howard were keeping him from his daughter. Birkhead told one outlet that he had spoken to Anna the night before she gave birth, and he was hopeful that she'd change her mind at the last minute and let him fly to the Bahamas for the delivery. He seemed bitterly disappointed that he was not allowed to be there. "I've had to look on Anna's own Web site and pay $4.99 a month to get updates about the baby," he said softly. His attorney Opri was pushing for DNA tests, which she felt would prove Birkhead's paternity and help him establish his rights as a father, if there was a scientific match. This simple process would take months to resolve.

On the October 12 edition of Cable Headline News's *The Nancy Grace Show*, Anna's mother, Virgie Arthur, fired the shot that would escalate frictions into a full-fledged war. Stating that she didn't believe that her grandson took drugs, she questioned why he died at such a young age. And after mentioning the possible half-billion-dollar inheritance, she pointed a finger at Howard Stern: "If Howard marries Vickie and Daniel's gone, that leaves Howard and the baby, to inherit whatever money she has." She added, "If Howard Stern marries her and she ends up dead, then who does the money go to?" Then, in a statement directly to the camera, she warned the daughter whose given name she used: "Vickie Lynn, you know I love you, always have. And be very careful about who you hang around with, because you may be next."[101]

This was not some TV talking head expounding theoretically; this was very much an insider whose hurt was palpable and whose feelings had to be considered. News shows picked up the quote, and since I was on many of them during that time while we were waiting for Daniel's toxicology report to come back, I was asked my opinion. I could only urge people to let Daniel's investigation take its course. While Anna was depressed, she was surrounded by loving people helping her to heal. Whenever I called the Horizons home and she would answer the phone, I noticed how lifeless and hopeless she seemed; the mere question of how she was might cause her to start crying. Some of that could also be post-partum depression, I mentioned to Howard, and he assured me that Anna was getting constant medical and psychological treatment. In November Anna went back to the hospital for three days with pneumonia. She was videotaped in her hospital bed, with an oxygen mask over her nose and with a sketch she had drawn of her lungs resting on her chest. As with everything in Anna's life, the clip ended up on TV. There were days when I would flip my remote control from station to station and still catch Anna Nicole news wherever I looked.

A steady parade of friends and employees flooded the Horizons home, to try to lift Anna's spirits and make sure Dannielynn was well cared for. Among the visitors was Dr. Khristine E. Eroshevich—or, as she liked to be called, "Dr. Khris"—Anna's psychiatrist who flew back and forth from California and monitored Anna's intake of prescription medications. Not only were they dear friends, the two women owned homes next to each other in a tony Los Angeles suburb.[102] Anna's frequent bodyguard Maurice Brighthaupt—known as "Big Moe"—and his wife, Tasma—known as "Taz"—were also around. Meanwhile, Howard was occupied quashing Larry Birkhead's paternity claims and finding a way for Anna and him to stay in the Bahamas permanently. Residency could be expedited if a person "of good character" could prove financial means—which Anna could, thanks to her TrimSpa contract—and provided he or she owned a property worth at least

$500,000. The Horizons home qualified for that, as long as Ben Thompson allowed them to continue living there. He kept urging Anna to sign paperwork agreeing to pay him for the estate but, to his dismay, she suddenly insisted he gave her the residence as a gift, in exchange, she said, for "the best sex of your life." Apoplectic, Thompson denied the home was a gift or that there was any deal, stating, "I'm not so wealthy that I can give away a million-dollar home without blinking."[103]

Immigration minister Shane Gibson became a trusted asset to Smith and Stern, fast-tracking their application, a scandal that ended with him resigning from his post after photographs surfaced of him lying on Anna Nicole's bed, with both of them fully clothed, but giving the appearance of inappropriateness. Gibson's family had also befriended Anna. His wife, Jackie, designed the program for Daniel's funeral, and his mother, Gerlene, served as an occasional nanny for Dannielynn.[104] His father, "King" Eric Gibson, a popular singer/musician and boat captain on the island, as well as being Gerlene's ex-husband, performed Anna and Howard's commitment ceremony. King Eric's current companion was Brigitte Neven, who was versed in homeopathy and kept the mood light by singing German songs to baby Dannielynn.[105] It took all of their steady efforts to keep Anna Nicole from plunging into despair, but still it wasn't enough. It didn't help Anna's frame of mind when she and Howard had to travel to California in December for a court appearance in the Marshall inheritance case.

Two Haitian nannies worked round-the-clock shifts, seven days a week, to care for Anna and the baby. Quethlie Alexie, thirty-six, and her sister-in-law Nadine Alexie, thirty-two, were hired in September and fired in December, allegedly after Anna accused Alexie of losing a manual to the new washing machine and Alexie asked too many questions about Anna's medication. Both ladies signed affidavits protesting their terminations, although the paperwork was never filed in court. In her five-page document, Quethlie stated her anxiety over the baby's health, claiming Anna purposely underfed her child to be "sexy." Alexie also declared that Anna had tried to commit suicide twice in her presence—the first time when she downed an entire bottle of a liquid sleeping aid and went into an "unrousable coma" for forty-eight hours. Anna supposedly admitted to her afterward that she "wanted to die. . . . I meant to kill myself."

The second time Anna tried to kill herself, Alexie wrote, was when Stern and Big Moe found her floating face down in the swimming pool—an event that was later corroborated by Dr. Eroshevich. Nadine's affidavit was along the same lines. Both nannies went even further on a Bahamian cable access program, *Controversy TV*, hosted by Lincoln Bain and Utah Taylor, who posted the interviews in multiple parts on YouTube.com. Alexie said Anna instructed her (as with Quethlie) to underfeed the baby so that she would grow up to be a "slim, sexy" movie star. "I used to hide food for the baby because Anna wanted us to give the baby only one and a half ounce of milk and the doctor instructed us to give her more food. So when Anna made the bottle with soy milk I would throw it out and make a proper bottle," Ms. Alexie said. They also claimed that when Dannielynn had colic, Anna overmedicated her to the point where they worried if the infant could be awakened. And they charged that when Anna would fall on the ground, which was "all the time," Howard would not help her up. Alexie, who had studied pharmacology for a year, insisted she complained about the amount of medication—a total of twenty-four different kinds—Anna was being given. And they spoke of the doctor preparing little cups of pills that the nannies allegedly saw Howard give Anna every four hours, even waking her up to take them. Some of the cups would have six pills, some would have ten, they told the talk show hosts.[106]

By the New Year, Howard—nervous that they would lose the Horizons home—was making plans to buy another expensive Nassau house, so he and Anna could maintain residency in the Bahamas. It was being slowly fixed up, including painting its exterior pink. Dannielynn's status wasn't a problem; as a Bahamian-born child of American parentage, she could petition for Bahamian citizenship once she turned eighteen.[107]

On January 2, 2007, a number of medications were supposedly prescribed from Dr. Eroshevich to Howard K. Stern, according to a detailed list posted on an Anna Nicole fan site. These pharmaceuticals purportedly included the muscle relaxants carisoprodol—sold as Soma—and methocarbamol—sold under the name Robaxin—as well as chloral hydrate, a hypnotic, sleep-inducing depressant. On January 6, Anna and Howard made a quick trip to the Seminole Hard Rock Hotel and Casino in Hollywood, Florida, for a World Boxing Championship match, accompanied by Big Moe. News footage showed her hugging promoter Don King and wrestling star Hulk Hogan. And on January 8, more medication scrips were reportedly written from Dr. Khris to Stern for the sedative diazepam—sold as Valium—and the water-retention pill, furosemide—sold as Lasix. Eroshevich allegedly prescribed herself a potassium supplement called Klor-Con M20, which ended up in Anna's possession. On January 26, Eroshevich is said to have written Stern prescriptions for the antiseizure drug Topamax, the antianxiety drug clonazepam, sold as Klonopin, and more carisoprodol.[108] I never heard about these drugs being prescribed for them, much less allegedly in someone else's name, until after Anna's death.

All through January, Larry Birkhead was on the warpath. In midmonth he told my co-author that Anna fled to the Bahamas because she feared her drug habit would give him ammunition to take sole custody of their baby, and that if Anna was brought back to the States, she'd face severe questioning about her ability to care for the child. While Anna insisted Stern was the infant's father, Larry wasn't conceding any ground, and it caused friction between them. Still they communicated with furtive phone calls when Stern wasn't around, or through e-mails and instant messages. Stern caught them talking once and had his lawyer write a letter threatening Birkhead with a charge of harassment, which Larry said he found "ridiculous." And sometimes, Birkhead said, Anna would be so mean, he wondered if he'd ever get through to her. After all that Anna had put him through, Larry didn't want to renew their romance—he just wanted to be part of his daughter's life. He had "baby-proofed" his California apartment and had taken a parenting course and another in children's CPR, the only single father in the classes. It wasn't right, he said, that he missed her birth and important milestones. He had always been Anna's favorite photographer—he should have been taking the girl's pictures, instead of having to buy magazines to see her. Still, when he did, the photos made him swallow hard—Dannielynn had his blue eyes, eyebrows, lips, and crooked smile. For Christmas he shipped the girl stuffed animals, pink dresses, an "I Love Daddy" onesie, and Disney videos— with a video of *How the Grinch Stole Christmas* marked for Anna. He included a handwritten card and a photo of himself so the baby could keep it close until he could finally get to meet her.[109]

Later that month, he told MSNBC's Jeannette Walls that Anna and Howard were making a "cash cow" out of the child. "I'm outraged that they're trying to pimp my daughter. If Anna wants to sell pictures of herself, that's one thing, but to conveniently put my daughter in every single photo to up the ante is sick and disgusting. And what's even more disgusting is that someone would buy them because they are financially assisting someone who's stockpiling money in an attempt to keep my child from me."[110] Larry's attorney began filing motions in various jurisdictions, hoping to find a court that would hear the case and demand the paternity tests. He was being cheered on by Anna's mother, Virgie Arthur, who reportedly wanted the child's father to be almost anyone besides Stern. It was complicated by the fact that Bahamian law favors maternal decisions in matters of family, and since Anna willingly put Stern's name on the birth certificate, the country accepted him as the father. In most paternity disputes, the fight is usually over who is *not* the father—here, there were two claimants both avidly seeking a legal tie to the child.

Birkhead's position was getting a lot of support in the media. If Howard was so certain he was Dannielynn's father, why not take the

DNA test and prove it? His lack of interest in doing so was interpreted by many as stonewalling and not in the best interest of the baby. Frankly, I wondered myself why he wasn't taking this very non-invasive test, which involves wiping a cotton swab on the inside of someone's cheek. I would have liked Howard to explain his reluctance to me, but he never did. He knew I was a lawyer, but my usefulness to him was as a forensic pathologist. He had plenty of other attorneys in his circle to consult with if he had legal questions.

Around the beginning of February, Anna and Howard bought a ten-year-old, forty-foot yacht Anna had christened *The Cracker*. The plan was to fly to Florida, pick up the boat, and sail it back to the Bahamas. King Eric Gibson, who was an experienced captain, his significant other Brigitte Neven, and a small crew planned to be on board. And while in Florida, Smith and Stern would also meet up with the Brighthaupts, Big Moe and Tasma. On Monday morning, February 5, Anna took a dance lesson, and that evening she and Howard flew to Florida, accompanied by Dr. Khristine Eroshevich. The pilot made a mistake and landed in Miami, so the group cleared customs and flew on to Fort Lauderdale. Howard had had the flu for a couple of days and on the plane trip Anna came down with symptoms. She was also complaining of severe pain in her left buttock, stemming from an injection before she left home of human growth hormone, immunoglobulin, or vitamin B12. It's impossible to know which injection caused this problem since Anna was in the habit of self-administering these medications.[111]

The group took a limo to the Hard Rock Hotel and Casino, their favorite spot in decidedly unglamorous Hollywood, Florida, where they were often comped for their stay. Their two-bedroom suite was on the sixth floor—numbers 607 and 609—behind mahogany doors. Anna and Howard were to share 607, while the Brighthaupts were in 609. A living room with an entertainment center connects the master bedrooms, which overlook the swimming pool. Anna's bed was a four-poster canopy, with soft Egyptian cotton sheets and a thick white duvet. Anna's bathroom had a deep whirlpool tub and a glassed-in shower. There's a rock 'n' roll theme throughout the hotel rooms, with *Rolling Stone* magazines in the john and toilet paper rolls sealed by a red concert admission ticket. Gold-wrapped chocolates are on each pillow, a leopard skin ironing board cover is in the closet, and the mini bar holds lubricant and glow-in-the-dark condoms. Normally the suite would cost $1,600 a night; I don't know whether this trip was comped.

Usually Anna would get massages and be seen at the Council Oak Steakhouse downstairs, but on this visit she spent a lot of time in her room, ordering soup from room service.[112] She did go to a shoe store, where she spent $2,000, and early in the trip visited the boat, where she asked for pink interiors and big-screen TVs. She chose the Carver sport yacht because she "liked the fact that there were two separate bedrooms and a forward deck to sunbathe and a salon living area" said Ned Bruck, the general manager of Reel Deal Yachts of Miami Beach that sold her the craft for about $50,000. (Bruck later told Stern he wouldn't hold him to the sale if he wanted to change his mind, but Stern still wanted the boat. Within a few days, *The Cracker*—which would be rechristened *Anna Nicole*—would make its voyage from Fort Lauderdale to Nassau without its mistress. Anna also would not make it to a TrimSpa celebration scheduled for February 19, a video shoot on the twenty-first, her planned wedding to Stern on the twenty-third, or a vacation in Dubai in March.)

That night, Anna's fever spiked to 105 degrees. Howard and Dr. Khris tried to persuade her to go to a hospital, but she refused. Instead, she sat in her bathtub, with ice cubes piled atop her until the fever broke. Khris prescribed for her the antiviral medication Tamiflu, made out to the name of Alex Katz. The next day Anna's fever was down to 100 degrees, and Eroshevich prescribed the strong antibiotic ciprofloxacin HCL, sold as Cipro, also made out to Alex Katz. Anna had trouble urinating that day and her body gave off a "pungent" odor. Khris told Anna she (Khris) had to go back home, which depressed and upset Anna, but the doctor kept in contact by phone over the next couple of days. On Wednesday, Anna tried taking a normal bath, but slipped in the tub and bruised her back. Mostly she stayed in bed, watched TV, ate an egg white and spinach omelet, and drank Pedi-alyte, Fuji water, and chamomile tea. Anna asked for Soma, Klonopin, and Topamax, but it's unknown whether she received or took them. That afternoon, she was found sitting in a dry bathtub, naked and confused. In the evening, she ordered two crab cakes and shrimp, picked at them, and then took another bath.

On Thursday morning, February 8, Tasma and Moe Brighthaupt left the suite to go pick up King Eric Gibson, Brigitte Neven, and a boat crewmember at the airport. Just before noon, the party returned to the hotel. As they waited for the elevator to go up to the suite, Howard came out of the elevator and then went back up with the group. Moe and Taz went into the second bedroom, while Stern stayed in the living room. Moe said he had to go run some errands, and Howard asked Tasma if she and Brigitte could stay behind and watch Anna, who was asleep in her room. Tasma spent some of the time working on the computer in Anna's room. The men rode the elevator to the lobby, and the last time Moe saw him there, Howard was speaking on his cell phone. About 1 p.m., Brigitte Neven looked into Anna's room and found her slumped over, her chin on her chest, mouth open, and not making sounds. She called for Tasma—a registered nurse—to come in, and both women panicked. By now, Howard and King Eric were at the marina, seeing about the boat, and Moe—a certified emergency medical technician and paramedic—was still driving around. Because the ladies had been given instructions to call Howard in the event of a problem, they tried to reach him, but his cell phone went to message mode. Tasma phoned Moe, who told her to try giving Anna cardiopulmonary resuscitation, but the women had trouble getting Anna onto the floor where the hard surface would have the best results for chest compressions. At 1:38 p.m., Tasma called the hotel operator, who called for paramedics to respond. Moe rushed back to the hotel, arriving shortly thereafter.[113]

On *Larry King Live*, Moe described seeing Anna: "I pushed the covers off the bed and I looked at her. Anna has very voluptuous, beautiful lips, and full lips. And when I saw her, her lips didn't look right. They looked kind of pale and blue. So I slapped her on the face and tried to wake her up. And when she didn't wake up, I picked her up off the bed and placed her on the floor." Continuing his story to King, he said, "I thought I felt a pulse but it probably just was my imagination. . . . I was trying to get her back; I figured I did it before. I knew I could do it again." Moe had saved Anna's life in October, when he found her floating lifeless in the pool, so he hoped lightning would strike twice. He disputed that the near drowning was a suicide attempt, insisting that she fell in accidentally. After about fifteen minutes of trying to revive Anna in her hotel room, Big Moe had to admit defeat: "I don't know if it was my arrogance or—I just never thought I lost her, actually . . . deep down I just figured that she was going to see her son Daniel."[114]

By two o'clock, paramedics with the Hollywood Rescue Fire Department had arrived. They noted white towels strewn around the bathroom floor and on the sinks. One sink was caked with yellow-brown vomitus. The white sheet on the bed had a large yellow-brown stain, and to the right of that stain, there appeared to be bloody fluid. The night table held cold medicine, opened and unopened cans of soda, Slim-Fast, empty packets of gum, Nicorette, and an open box of Tamiflu tablets. The table on the right of the bed held a partly covered transparent glass jar containing a brownish liquid. In the closet were men's and women's clothing and shoes, and there was a pearl necklace at the foot of the bed and a Louis Vuitton purse on a chair by the window. Across from the bed was an armoire, with clothes in open drawers and a television set in the top portion. The guest bedroom had three beds, all neatly made. A small table there held numerous medicines, prescribed under different names. There was also a piece of furniture that held a television and a small refrigerator. Police later made a list of all the medications, along with the date prescribed, dosage, and the number of pills remaining in each bottle.[115]

The paramedics bundled Anna onto a gurney and called headquarters: "She's not breathing, she's not responsive. She's, um, actually

Anna Nicole Smith." They rushed her to Hollywood, Florida's, Memorial Regional Hospital, which has a children's wing named for Joe DiMaggio, who, as noted, was once married to Marilyn Monroe.[116]

Anna was pronounced dead at 2:49 p.m. Later that afternoon, Dr. Gertrude M. Juste of the Broward County Medical Examiner's office retrieved the body, which was clad in a light green hospital gown. Cardiomonitoring and defibrillator pads were on the body, and an endotracheal tube with a plastic clamp was in Anna's mouth. The coroner's office photographer, Joseph Anderson, took snapshots of the body—sadly, Anna's last photo session. Juste arranged for the Broward Removal Service to transport the body to her office, where it was logged in at 4:59 p.m., and met by Dr. Perper and others. Anderson took more photos. Juste then took blood and cerebrospinal fluid for testing. No urine was available, even via the suprapubic approach, which is done by inserting a needle into the area by the hairline. Generally these fluid samples are collected at autopsy, and since Perper's team knew there would be one within a day, I'm not sure why they took them at this point. It's remotely possible that because the death scene was on Indian property—which is self-governing—Perper didn't want to lose the fluid samples in the event that the Seminole tribe took possession of the body, for any reason. There have been historical cases where deaths have occurred on a reservation and outside investigators were denied jurisdiction; as it turned out in Smith's case, the Seminole police department was of great assistance to Perper's staff. The corpse was wrapped in a body bag, sealed with evidence tape, and wheeled into a locked cage at the back of the morgue refrigerator. The door of the cage was also sealed with evidence tape, and the cage was draped with a cloth to prevent viewing.[117]

Footage of Anna being loaded into the ambulance, with one EMT pushing on her chest, sold for a reported $500,000, even though Smith's face was covered by an oxygen mask and the video was grainy.[118] Within minutes, the first reports hit the airwaves, the story broken by then-MSNBC anchor Rita Cosby, who would go on to write a best-selling book, *Blonde Ambition: The Untold Story Behind Anna Nicole Smith's Death*, about the case.[119] As soon as I heard the awful news, I called Howard K. Stern but got his answering machine. It would be a few days before he would call me back and ask for my help.

While both Stern and Birkhead dropped out of the media fray for a few days out of respect for the woman they had loved and lost, a new character zoomed into focus: Prince Frédéric Von Anhalt, the sixty-something German-born eighth husband of actress Zsa Zsa Gabor, who is ninety-ish and to whom he had been married for more than two decades. The prince, also known as the Duke of Saxony, had actually inherited his title when the wealthy daughter-in-law of Kaiser Wilhelm II adopted him. Once he had his title, he was free to offer his hand in marriage to the highest bidders. He cheerfully admitted to my co-author that he had married and divorced six women prior to Gabor, in exchange for millions of dollars, so they would be able to claim royal titles.

Von Anhalt first met Anna in the late 1990s at New York's Plaza Hotel when she was still wed to J. Howard Marshall II, he said. She called him when she visited Los Angeles, and what was to be a cup of coffee turned into a secret affair that lasted ten years. "She wanted to be a princess and asked me to divorce my wife, which was out of the question. I asked Zsa Zsa if we could adopt Nicole"—his nickname for her—"but she wouldn't sign the papers." Still he was enamored with the bodacious centerfold's little girl voice and kittenish manner. "She wanted to be protected," he said, adding that they had had relations about thirty or forty times, "always at a private house" in Los Angeles. "She was a woman you just don't kick out of bed," he grinned, explaining, "It wasn't a love affair, it was just sex. Sometimes I'm a bad boy."

According to Von Anhalt, their last physical encounter was around the time her daughter was conceived, which is why, the day after Anna died, he did the gentlemanly thing and held a press conference to suggest he might be the father. The prince was adamant that Anna did not consider either Stern or Birkhead her boyfriend. "Stern was her lawyer, and that was it. She told me she never even saw him naked. As for Birkhead, she called him her 'cheap gigolo' and 'sweet butler,'" he proclaimed. "She didn't love either of them; she only loved her son." Von Anhalt had his DNA tested before the baby's biological dad was finally revealed. "I was prepared to raise the child, if it was proved I was the father," he said, although his wife didn't relish the idea.[120]

The prince wasn't the only possible sperm donor, apparently. Anna's former bodyguard, Alexander Denk, told the TV show *Extra* that he was also a candidate. And Donna Hogan, in her book titled *Train Wreck*, theorized that her half sister might have used the frozen sperm of her late husband, Marshall, for fertilization.[121]

As I watched the network TV coverage about Anna's death, I was reminded of the advice given by Margo Channing, the character famously portrayed by Bette Davis in the 1950 classic *All About Eve*: "Fasten your seatbelts, it's going to be a bumpy night!" (Incidentally, Marilyn Monroe had a minor, but memorable, role in that movie.) In the rush to be first with a scoop, no matter if it was completely inaccurate, *Access Hollywood* gambled and lost with its report that Smith had taken a "children's sedative" and "choked on her own vomit."[122]

Friends, enemies, and family members paid tribute to the fallen beauty. *Playboy* founder Hugh Hefner said of the woman who was one of his magazine's most popular Playmates: "I'm very saddened to learn about Anna Nicole's passing. She was a dear friend who meant a great deal to the *Playboy* family and to me personally."[123] TrimSpa CEO Alex Goen said of his spokesmodel and pal: "Ever since Daniel's passing, it has been a very difficult life. She really was a big-hearted, very caring, very misunderstood human being."[124] And even the family of the late J. Howard Marshall II issued a statement about their courtroom foe: "[We were] shocked by the untimely death of Anna Nicole Smith. We wish to express our sympathies to her family in this difficult time." Understandably, in the vacuum of not having any answers yet, some folks speculated that there might have been foul play or suicide. Part of this was because the people who knew Anna the best and most recently—namely Howard K. Stern, the people from the Horizons home, and those on the trip to Florida—were avoiding the press and very appropriately just talking to investigators. Gail Harrison told *Dateline NBC* of her cousin's demise, "I'm not surprised. She has battled so much lately. . . . I'm not sure if she committed suicide. I don't think we'll know until all the tests are in. But I do know she was so distraught that maybe, at one point, she didn't want to be around."[125]

Less than twenty-four hours after her daughter's death—and before the autopsy had even begun—Anna's mother, Virgie Arthur, appeared on ABC's *Good Morning America*, certain she knew the cause of death: "I think she had too many drugs, just like Danny."[126] Arthur had been suggesting for months that her grandson's death was a criminal act. No doubt she had heard about my second autopsy on the young man—which echoed the Bahamian official's view that Daniel had, indeed, died of an accidental drug overdose. Had Ms. Arthur called me, I would have gladly taken time to go through the evidence with her. On TV, the retired Texas sheriff's deputy was blunt about her estranged daughter's lifestyle: "I tried to warn her about drugs and the people that she hung around with." And she charged that Anna was kept isolated from her family and hadn't allowed Virgie to even see five-month-old Dannielynn. Vowing to travel to Nassau to try to meet the baby, Arthur whispered, "She's the last of the two. I have a dead grandson, I have a dead daughter, and I have a granddaughter that I'm really worried about."

The *Good Morning America* show was not the first, nor last, time Virgie would air her daughter's dirty laundry. The next night she told Deborah Roberts of ABC's *20/20* that "Vickie Lynn never wanted anyone to have anything better than she had." And when Roberts inquired whether Anna shared the wealth with her Texas kin, Arthur replied, "Oh no. She's never helped her family. Her sister had leukemia and we could have used help with the kids, a nanny or something. But nope, she didn't help at all." On that same show Alex

Goen's wife, Monique, spoke of how she once talked to Anna about all of the challenges she faced, asking her if she had it to do all over again, would she do the same thing? Anna said no: "If I had to do it all over again, I'd be back in the chicken place, having lots of babies."[127]

Over the next several weeks, Anna's life—and death—would be explored from all angles. For a woman who craved publicity as she did, it seemed a shame she wasn't around to witness just how much attention she was receiving.

On Friday, February 9, 2007, at 10:36 a.m., Joshua Perper, MD, LLB, MSc, and chief medical examiner for Broward County, Florida, began the autopsy of Anna Nicole Smith. Following the procedure, Perper and Seminole police chief Charlie Tiger held a joint press conference that was covered by the world press and included cameras, tape recorders, and even news helicopters hovering overhead.

Tiger, a former homicide detective, began with an important statement: "No evidence has been revealed to indicate a crime occurred. We found no illegal drugs, only prescription medicines," although he refused to name those medications. The chief said his officers had obtained sworn statements from all pertinent parties, who were cooperating fully. Hotel surveillance tapes were being viewed, he said, but had not as yet produced anything unusual. Then he turned over the spotlight to Dr. Perper.

I first met Joshua Perper back in 1962, when the thirty-year-old had finished his training at the Baltimore medical examiner's office, where I had also received my training. I was then the coroner of Allegheny County in Pittsburgh, Pennsylvania, and brought him to my office where he worked as one of my forensic pathologists. In 1979, when I won the election for county commissioner and served the next few years in politics, Perper took over my job, staying there until he moved to Florida in 1994. (I would later serve another round as Allegheny's coroner from 1996 until 2006; nineteen years, all told.) Born in Romania, Dr. Perper was educated in Israel, before moving to the United States.

Perper addressed the crowd, went through "Mrs. Nicole Smith's [*sic*]" time line, and explained the Florida statute that gives the Broward medical examiner's office jurisdiction over any death that is "sudden, unexpected, and unexplained." He said that he, and his associate, Dr. Juste, had excluded "any kind of physical injury, such as blunt force trauma, gunshot wound, stab wounds, or asphyxia" as contributing to Anna's death. Only one minor bruise to her back was noted, which he attributed to the fall in the bathtub. He said that subtle findings in the heart and gastrointestinal system would be studied microscopically, and that a small amount of blood in the stomach was related to her being in terminal shock just before she died. No determination of cause or manner of death would be announced now, he said, pending a full review of her medical records, witness interviews, and the full array of pathological and toxicological laboratory testing.

Reporters then began lobbing questions, which he fielded with aplomb. The autopsy had lasted about six hours. More information would be forthcoming within three to five weeks. Although he couldn't rule out a drug-related death, no tablets or pills of any kind were found in Smith's stomach. There were no signs that she choked on her own vomit. Neither coroner's officers nor paramedics saw Mr. Stern flushing the toilet—which was a fresh rumor Perper wanted to knock down. And when asked whether Anna might have been dead for hours before being discovered, he stated: "No. And the reason is that according to our information at the time when the medics came to the scene, the body was warm."[128] Finally, Perper revealed that due to the incessant media interest, Anna's body would be held in a VIP area of the morgue, in a vault under twenty-four-hour guard. I knew instantly what that meant—he wanted to make sure no one shot a final photograph of the former *Playboy* centerfold. There were surely many news outlets that would pay a fortune for such a gruesome image.

On February 11 a daunting photo turned up on the Web site TMZ.com. It showed the inside of Anna Nicole's home mini fridge, with a large bottle of methadone, vials of injectible medicine, several cans of flavored Slim-Fast, a nutritional supplement called Miracle 2000, French's Worcestershire sauce, spray butter, and yogurt. An open carton of TrimSpa was on the floor nearby.[129] The photo, it was later learned, was snapped by Ford Shelley, the son-in-law of G. Ben Thompson, who was trying to evict Howard from the Horizons estate. The methadone, in a bottle the size that is usually seen in an addiction treatment clinic, was a reminder that Daniel Smith had died of a combination of methadone and two other drugs—and no one still knows how or from whom he had gotten the methadone.

In an interview on Fox News's *On the Record with Greta Van Susteren*, Shelley said, "Anna was on methadone to help her and we knew that because I transported her from Los Angeles to Myrtle Beach in May and they gave me strict instructions for all the medications in her bag. I wanted to show not that there was methadone there and 'look what she's taking,' [but] if she died of an overdose of methadone, her methadone was at home." He further told Greta, "The name on the methadone was Michelle Chase—that is the name Anna used on her prescriptions," and added: "As long as we've known her, Anna never did illegal drugs."[130] TrimSpa's Alex Goen was curious about whether the refrigerator photo might have been staged to embarrass his company's product. Goen stated that Anna had signed affidavits that she did not use any other diet aid product while she was representing TrimSpa. "I'm not denying that Anna Nicole took methadone; however, from everything that I know Anna never used Slim-Fast," he said, adding, "Dr. Khris, who had been staying at the home, was the one who used Slim-Fast."[131]

Shelley would later testify in court that Anna had given him her computer password, so that "if anything happened" to her, he should take her laptops for safekeeping. Anna seemed convinced that something would happen to her, he claimed, and that the computers might fall into the wrong hands. Shelley made copies of the hard drives of two laptops and an external hard drive, and then turned over the original items to his local sheriff in Horry County, South Carolina, who later forwarded them to Seminole detectives.[132] In order to view the material, a judge would have to issue a search warrant. Since the police were unable to convince the judge that a crime had occurred, the judge wouldn't comply. Broward prosecutors had no choice but to ask Stern for permission to look through the material, which he granted.[133] The hard drives were reviewed by detectives and Dr. Perper's team, and far from being the smoking gun that perhaps some had hoped it would be, the material was useful in proving that Anna was not in fear of her life or suicidal. Her calendar and e-mails showed a woman with a busy schedule and much to live for.

Stern felt betrayed that the home was broken into while he was gone and at his most vulnerable, so his friend Pol' Atteu, who was in Nassau at the time, filed a police report.[134] As of this writing, it is still unknown whether any criminal action will follow for the removal of the property. During the Daniel Smith inquest, Shelley testified that he and another man had witnessed Stern finding two pills in Daniel's jeans, and supposedly flushing them down the toilet.[135] When last I heard, Howard was still living in the Horizons estate, and the Thompson/Shelley family was still fighting to get him out.[136]

Around this time Howard K. Stern returned my condolence call and apologized for the delay in getting back to me. His voice was hoarse and he sounded exhausted. He asked if I could go to Florida as soon as possible to conduct a second autopsy on Anna. He couldn't bear waiting the weeks it might take to find out why Anna died and reasoned that if I performed an independent procedure, I could share the findings with him quicker. I wouldn't mind going, I told him, but it would be unethical to reveal any findings before Dr. Perper showed his hand. Plus, with such a painstakingly comprehensive and top-secret investigation, I might not have access to all of their files until after they declared a result. With the breadth of the ongoing microscopic and toxicological testing, chances were good that even if I did my own testing, the results wouldn't be back until after Perper's office released its findings. Dr. Perper, I assured him, was an experienced forensic pathologist and, knowing the world was watching, would certainly have put together a team of top experts. That didn't mean that I couldn't find some imperfection, were I to delve into it on my own, but it would be advisable to see Perper's work first. If he came back and said the death was "suspicious" or hinted that criminal charges might ensue, then it would make sense for me to go in, conduct a second post-mortem exam, and look for evidence that could challenge him.

Meanwhile, I advised Howard to stay cool and stop viewing those TV programs that seemed to delight in calling him culpable for Anna's death. I knew it was tough for him to maintain his equilibrium, but there was nothing in what he told me of the events surrounding Anna's death that in any way hinted of foul play. Police would have to hand over a real case to prosecutors, and Chief Tiger said from the get-go that there was no evidence a crime had been committed. I asked if Howard had told police everything, and he replied that he absolutely had. I also asked him if he was holding back anything that might surface later and hurt his story, and he said he wasn't. We agreed to wait until Perper's work was completed. I informed him that when I made subsequent TV appearances, I would urge that people stay fair-minded and not assume that because Daniel died of a drug overdose, it necessarily followed that his mother did too, which is exactly what I did.

Anna's will was made public on February 16, and its release led to another round of accusations and countercharges. The seventeen-page boilerplate document, in her married name of "Vickie Lynn Marshall," was prepared on July 30, 2001, with Stern named as executor. The will states that Marshall was unmarried and had one child, Daniel Wayne Smith. But one article caused a lot of flak: "I have intentionally omitted to provide for my spouse and other heirs, including future spouses and children and other descendents now living and those hereafter born or adopted, as well as existing and future stepchildren and foster children." Yet, another section referred to Smith's "children," instructing the executor to manage the estate "such that my children are distributed sufficient sums for their health, education and support."[137] Since the will was drafted before Daniel's death and Dannielynn's birth, why was no codicil ever drafted and filed? Its absence fed a legal firestorm that would soon erupt. Soon after the will hit the press, Anna's mother questioned whether the handwritten signature was that of her daughter. In a *Globe* magazine exclusive, Virgie Arthur stated: "She did not sign that will. I know my daughter's handwriting. I think it was forged."[138] But to date, no legal challenge has been presented over the will's accuracy.

Anna's body was causing a problem for Dr. Perper and his office. Deterioration begins at the moment of death, and embalming and cold storage only slow the process—but Anna's corpse had not even been embalmed yet. If her loved ones wanted to hold an open-casket funeral, they had better move swiftly before her facial color started changing. Perper petitioned the Seventeenth Judicial Circuit Court of Broward County, which assigned Judge Larry Seidlin the task of determining who would get custody of the remains. The judge's first ruling was to allow Perper's staff to proceed with the embalming, which was done on Saturday, February 17. Ordering the funeral was a more complicated matter. Normally the decision of where to bury someone falls to the next of kin, but in this case who, exactly, was that next of kin? Howard K. Stern was executor of Anna's estate and had married the pin-up queen in a non–legally binding ceremony. Dannielynn Hope Marshall Stern was the undisputed next of kin, but she was still very much a minor, and no one was certain of her biological father, who might have some standing in the matter. The closest relative of legal age was Virgie Arthur, but she admitted having been at least partially estranged from her daughter for years. And there were even greater ramifications—not only would someone win the burial argument, but that person would have a leg up in establishing dominion over the J. Howard Marshall II inheritance case.

In an interminable court hearing that became known as the "Fort Lauderdale Follies," Judge Seidlin invited all parties, their attorneys, and the media, into his courtroom. Court TV and other outlets broadcast the live, nonjury proceedings. What viewers saw was more entertaining than many scripted comedy programs. The ratings must have gone through the roof, if my own experience was typical. Although I was working during most of the daytime broadcast and later watched clips on the news, I got numerous cell phone messages from people watching live, gasping: "Oh my God, I can't believe what just happened!" If the proceedings were considered a circus, its ringmaster was fifty-six-year-old Seidlin, a Bronx-born former cabbie who is bald, tan, and a championship tennis player when he's not on the bench.[139]

Seidlin's disarmingly emotional personality had him honking wisecracks at the witnesses, nicknaming lawyers "Texas" or "California," or whatever was their home state, commenting on the good looks of women before him, musing about the need to support our troops in Iraq, taking cell phone calls from his wife, and bursting into tears more than once when the enormity of Anna Nicole's death struck him. At one point during a discussion over what dress Smith might be buried in, Seidlin whined, "This is the one area I always ran away from—the death," causing an attorney to wryly remind him that he was, in fact, a probate judge, referring to the type of court case that involves wills and funerals.[140] At another point when John O'Quinn, the celebrated Houston attorney representing Virgie Arthur, fainted due to a low blood-sugar level, Seidlin handed his own credit card to his bailiff with instructions to buy the attorney some orange juice. When Billy Wayne Smith, Anna's ex-husband and the father of their son, Daniel, testified over the phone from Texas, Seidlin asked how the court might know it was the real Billy Wayne Smith; the judge accepted his testimony after securing the promise that Smith was wearing cowboy boots.[141]

In what should have been a fairly straightforward hearing lasting no more than a day, Seidlin, in either his desire for attention or his honest sense of wanting to hear everyone's two cents, stretched the hearing into a six-day event. I doubt any of the participants can say they were shortchanged in giving their views. Witnesses weren't just asked for testimony germane to the burial issue; they were encouraged to tell their life stories. And Seidlin didn't rely on lawyers to examine and cross-examine witnesses—he took over much of the questioning himself. One of his early duties was appointing Miami attorney Richard Milstein as a guardian ad litem to represent the interests of baby Dannielynn, who was at home in Nassau with her nanny.

Stern was grilled about his relationship with Smith, taking the judge through all of their show business and Marshall case high jinks. Howard admitted he was an attorney with only Anna as a client, and that while she didn't pay for his services, she paid all of his bills and living expenses. He said that while they had had a commitment ceremony, they planned to hold a legitimate wedding in the near future. And Stern argued that Anna wanted to be buried in Nassau, with her casket on top of her son's, in a four-person cemetery plot she had purchased months before she died. Howard, who presented himself as the baby's father, would eventually share that gravesite, as would their daughter, he told the court. He admitted Nassau was not Anna's first choice—originally she wanted to be buried near Marilyn Monroe in Los Angeles, because she always felt she was going to die young, too. But once they moved to the Bahamas and pursued residency, Anna revised her plan. He also spoke of how her son's death affected her: "Daniel was without question the most important person in Anna's life," he said. "From the time I met her, everything that she was doing was for Daniel. From the day Daniel died, Anna honestly was never the same. I would say that physically she died last week but in a lot of ways, emotionally, she died when Daniel died."[142]

Seidlin allowed Stern to play a video from an *Entertainment Tonight* episode where Anna, in her first interview after Daniel's death, lashed out at Virgie Arthur, caustically calling her "Mommie Dearest," and claiming she beat and abused a teen-aged Anna. Dabbing her eyes, Anna snarled: "You wanna hear my child life? You wanna hear all the things she did to me? That's my mother. That's my mom. What do you want to say to her? I want to say to her, how dare you, bitch? How dare you?"[143]

The next day Virgie Arthur responded to the video that had brought her to tears. "She's been on drugs the last ten years," Arthur told the court. "Anything she said during that time isn't that person, is not my daughter." She wanted to bury her daughter with relatives back in Texas and hoped to exhume and move Daniel too—she even got Daniel's father, Billy Smith, to agree in his over-the-phone testimony, even though he hadn't seen his son in twenty years. Virgie also accused Stern of having an ulterior motivation for wanting Anna's remains. "The only one who's ever, ever made any money off of my daughter is that man sitting right over there. I heard that *E.T.*'s buying her death funeral. That's why he wants her body. For a million bucks."[144]

In a more lighthearted moment, the two Larry's—Seidlin and Birkhead—got the courtroom smiling with this exchange:

SEIDLIN: How old are you?
BIRKHEAD: Thirty-four.
SEIDLIN: Any marriages?
BIRKHEAD: No, sir.
SEIDLIN: Any children?
BIRKHEAD: One.
SEIDLIN: How old?
BIRKHEAD: Five months, six months.
SEIDLIN: Ho-ho, okay. That's that little girl we always talk about, Dannielynn. All right, I'm glad you're keeping your sense of humor.

But the testimony turned serious when Birkhead claimed Stern supplied Anna with drugs while she was pregnant in the hospital, trying to kick her addiction:

SEIDLIN: So she's pregnant and now she's taking medications?
BIRKHEAD: She's taking medications before and during the pregnancy.

SEIDLIN: Were you concerned about that?

BIRKHEAD: I was very concerned.

SEIDLIN: Why?

BIRKHEAD: Because we had already had one miscarriage, and every time she put something in her mouth (choking up) I thought that it would . . .

SEIDLIN: . . . that it would affect . . . ?

BIRKHEAD: Yes, sir.

SEIDLIN: . . . the welfare of the child, and her too, as well.[145]

Stern was called back to the stand where the judge pressed him about Smith's drug intake:

SEIDLIN: Did she go into rehab centers after 1996?

STERN: Not into a rehab center, no.

SEIDLIN: Did she need to go into a rehab center?

STERN: I guess that would be open to interpretation.

SEIDLIN: Well, what was your interpretation?

STERN: Anna Nicole took prescription medication, at times for depression. She did.

SEIDLIN: These drugs all came from one doctor?

STERN: Well, at different times, she had different doctors.

SEIDLIN: I'm saying at different times, did she have prescription drugs from different doctors? Where they get multiple drugs from different doctors? A doesn't know doctor B prescribed drugs, so they're sitting there at the pharmacy . . .

STERN: I don't know. You know, she had more than one doctor. I believe her doctors knew about each other.

SEIDLIN: Could you have stopped her from taking these drugs, these prescription drugs? Could you have stopped it?

STERN: Your honor, after her son passed away . . .

SEIDLIN: Prior.

> STERN: I talked to her about it. I mean, I talked to her about
> it. And she did cut down a lot on medication that
> she took. Can anybody stop someone else?

Stern mentioned three medications that he knew Anna had been taking: Topamax, Dilaudid, and methadone. Larry Birkhead's attorney, Debra Opri, still angling for Stern to take a paternity test, used part of her questioning to press the issue. "Mr. Stern," she demanded, "are you or are you not the biological father of Dannielynn?" Opri wanted to ensure that Anna not be buried before the medical examiner's office preserved her DNA. "We do not want a bait and switch of a child," she argued.[146]

Birkhead made a second appearance on the stand, too, when the judge wanted more details about Anna's habit:

> BIRKHEAD: At times I took her medicine and I was told by
> Mr. Stern to give it back because she needed it to live. I
> told her over and over, I said, "Don't. Something's gonna
> happen to you. . . ." (crying) You don't know how many
> times I had to help her and to carry her back and forth to
> make sure she was okay. Sometimes I didn't know if she
> was gonna live and they kept bringing more drugs in the
> house.

Birkhead testified that Smith told him she needed the prescriptions to live and that he witnessed Stern giving her additional drugs into her IV drip when she was in the hospital. When Larry suggested she enter drug rehabilitation, he said she told him: "I'm not a drug addict and quit calling me one."[147]

Ford Shelley testified about the drugs he saw Anna take in Howard's presence and played the clown-face video of the stoned and pregnant Anna, interacting with his nine-year-old daughter, Riley. Shelley said the girl remains traumatized by Anna's death. "I'll never forgive you for that," he said directly to Stern. But Shelley concurred with Stern that Anna would want to be buried with her son, in the Bahamas. Shelley also admitted Anna moved to the Bahamas because that country didn't recognize paternal rights.[148]

Like a maudlin Dr. Phil, Seidlin seemed to work through his thoughts by expressing them out loud. "She stays away from mother, because mama is not gonna like her taking over-medicated drugs." And, "We got Larry who now tells her because she's pregnant and he's concerned about the health and welfare of the baby to be born and Larry tells her not to do drugs." And, about the role of Smith's long-time companion, Stern, the judge pondered: "Is he a bad guy? Or is he a fellow who has some form of a love for her? Whatever relationship he had with her, he would be called maybe an enabler." Seidlin's wrap-up got in a few more pearls of weirdness. "I feel for all parties here," he choked. "I have suffered with this, I have struggled with this. I have shed tears for your little girl." Then, openly sobbing, he blubbered: "There's no shouting, this is not a happy moment. I want her buried with her son in the Bahamas; I want them to be together." To cover Dannielynn, he added: "And I hope to God you guys give the kid the right shot."[149]

Judge Seidlin cited a strikingly parallel legal case about a minor who was the next of kin in a disputed burial case. Then the weepy jurist turned the ball of wax over to Guardian ad Litem Milstein, who made the decision that Anna would be buried in the Bahamas. Attorneys for Virgie Arthur filed an appeal that was rejected. Because of Anna's advanced decomposition, Perper suggested her loved ones visit a special area of his morgue, which he decorated with flowers. So Stern, Arthur, and Birkhead said their farewells at that designated area, and agreed that the actual funeral would have a closed casket. Larry later told a reporter that he wept as he said, "Goodnight, my sweet Anna baby," one last time. It was the phrase she would always make him say before they went to sleep.[150]

The paternity hearing continued in a neighboring courtroom with Judge Lawrence Korda, who threw the case back when he determined he had no jurisdiction. Korda later retired from the bench after being arrested for smoking marijuana in a public park.[151]

Seidlin also retired from the bench after twenty-nine years and moved with his wife, Belinda, and their young daughter to Connecticut. Seidlin was the University of Miami law grad who, in 2004, had ranked near the bottom of Broward judges on knowledge of the law and other categories in a County Bar Association judicial poll and was nicknamed "Lightning Larry" for the way he'd zip through cases on his "Rocket Docket." The *Broward–Palm Beach New Times* published an article on Seidlin, questioning a relationship he and his wife had with an elderly millionaire widow in his building who had rained riches on his family, in exchange for meals and friendship. Then there was the public defender who got regular appointments in Seidlin's courtroom, only to be handed a note by Judge Larry, suggesting the attorney buy Mrs. Seidlin a $1,000-plus Louis Vuitton purse for her birthday. There was a second purse and a man's polo shirt Seidlin asked the attorney to purchase over their years of working together, according to the *New Times* piece. Seidlin also got Belinda a job as an investigator at the public defender's office, but she was fired when staffers found more than three months of untouched work on her desk. In another bizarre instance, Seidlin was criticized in May 2006 after being followed around by a local ABC News team who found him taking three-hour lunch breaks. After fielding some two hundred offers from TV recruiters, he taped a TV pilot for his own *Judge Judy*–type of program that, if it goes forward, could be on the air by the time you're reading this book.[152] He also earned his place in pop culture history when *Saturday Night Live*'s Fred Armisen did a letter-perfect impression of him in a couple comedy sketches.

Access Hollywood, the TV series that reported the bogus story of Anna "choking on her own vomit," reported another exclusive that proved equally wrong. In suggesting that Anna might have had lupus, they contacted a New York physician who had written books on the malady. He said that while the three medications mentioned in the recent testimony—Topamax, Dilaudid, and methadone—were not typically prescribed for the connective tissue disorder, women who had recently given birth can develop painful symptoms of the disease. The TV show found a separate source that cited increased risk of miscarriage in patients with lupus, and since Larry Birkhead testified that Anna had miscarried their first child, and since there were also specious links to breast implants and lupus, it just all made sense.[153] Except it was erroneous, as we would soon learn. Media outlets asked me about the lupus connection, and I refused to comment. Dr. Perper's report had not yet been released, and I preferred not to speculate.

The following weekend the main players arrived in the Bahamas to plan Anna's funeral and to allow Larry Birkhead and Virgie Arthur to finally meet baby Dannielynn. Larry's attorney, Debra Opri, accompanied him and was purportedly disappointed when Larry agreed to a face-to-face meeting with Howard Stern without her, when she was trying to get the Nassau court to arrange for the paternity tests. In time, Stern and Birkhead would form an alleged business alliance, and Opri would withdraw from the case. Birkhead and Opri would take legal action against each other concerning her bill.[154] Those matters are reportedly still unresolved.

On February 24, Howard called me and asked if he could put Dr. Khristine Eroshevich on the line. Of course, I said yes. Like most of America, I had been hearing about this physician and close friend of Anna's who had been on the Florida trip but had left before Anna died. I was eager to get her views and, since the press was pummeling both her and Stern, they were eager to have someone hear their side of things. Khristine Elaine Eroshevich, a 1975 graduate of Ohio State University College of Medicine, is licensed in California as a physician and surgeon.[155] According to public records, she has contributed money to Republican causes, both local and national.[156] Her husband, Wes Irwin, is a noted postproduction manager on many of Hollywood's top TV series and even appeared in several episodes of Anna's E! series.[157]

"Khris," as she told me to call her, represented herself as one of Anna's best friends, who had taken care of this high-maintenance patient for years. Anna, she explained, was always in a great deal of pain, both physically and mentally, especially since Daniel's death. Khris told me that she took on Anna's treatment to ensure that there was one physician who could monitor all of Anna's medications, rather than Smith's getting prescription drugs from numerous sources. Anna's prescriptions were written to other persons to preserve the star's privacy, she said. I later learned that California had recently tightened its laws regarding controlled substances, requiring doctors to use tamper-resistant prescription documents, instead of the old-style pads, for medications that fall under Schedule II to V narcotics. Having other people fill prescriptions intended for Anna might not catch the attention of the state pharmacy board or the Drug Enforcement Administration. That is neither a legal practice nor one that I would recommend, but it may be a way of life for doctors with a celebrity clientele.

Dr. Khris said that Anna had been suffering from a painful and swollen right hand, which she diagnosed as "reflex sympathetic dystrophy," a chronic neurological syndrome that causes extreme sensitivity to touch, excessive sweating, and sometimes pathological changes in the bones and skin. I inquired whether Anna might have had sleep apnea—since I had heard reports of labored breathing—but her doctor said no. Khris and Howard took me through the days leading up to Anna's death, her high fever and flulike symptoms, which included a bad smell, labored breath, and the fall in the bathtub where she bruised her head. Howard said he had had the flu himself and thought Anna had caught his bug. He also said she had felt better the night before she died—so much so that they had had intercourse.

Khris named some of the medications she had prescribed for Anna, which included Tamiflu, Cipro, Klonopin, Soma, Topamax, and chloral hydrate, a syrup used for sedation. I was surprised to learn about that last medication because it is considered a drug that has been superseded by many other, better medicines. Two of my children, who are also physicians, told me that they had never even heard of its being used today, though that doesn't mean that other doctors don't prescribe it. Khris said that the list of medications she prescribed to Anna might seem extensive, but Anna didn't take all of the drugs. Sometimes if she would try something and didn't react well, she would stop taking it, and sample something else—but she might not have tossed out those medications that she had stopped taking. Khris also said that she was personally wounded by the loss of her friend and would never have left her in Florida if she thought she was in any kind of serious trouble. Anna was upset that Khris was leaving, which made the doctor feel all the worse.

Before we three signed off on our conference call, Howard told me that he had granted permission to the Broward authorities to read the contents of the two laptops and one hard drive in their possession. He was angry that the material had been stolen from his home, but assured me that there was nothing in the contents that would suggest foul play or suicide. I commended him for helping the officials and we agreed to continue our dialogue after Dr. Perper's autopsy report was released, should there be a need to address any issues.

On Friday, March 2, Anna Nicole Smith attended her final red carpet event—her funeral. The day began with Anna, in her mahogany casket and accompanied by Dr. Perper, going from the medical examiner's office to Miami International Airport. They boarded a charter jet that took them to Nassau's Million-Air field, where they were met by an escort of limousines and a white hearse.[158] The event, which was televised live in the United States, rivaled the scope of the ceremonies held for President John F. Kennedy, Princess Diana, and President Ronald Reagan. Footage showed the long procession of cars on the way to Nassau's Mount Horeb Baptist Church. But before the casket could be offloaded, there was an hour-long delay while Virgie Arthur's attorneys tried and failed to get an emergency injunction against her daughter's burial. Bystanders in summery clothes lined up behind fences and cheered as people they recognized came into the church.

Larry Birkhead got the biggest eruption of applause; Howard K. Stern and Virgie Arthur both got catcalls.

Dannielynn did not attend the event, but her attorney, Richard Milstein, was there. Doctor Lloyd Smith officiated the ninety-minute service in front of about a hundred mourners, including rock guitarist Slash and country crooner Joe Nichols, who sang "Wings of a Dove." A photo Larry had taken of Anna dressed as Marilyn Monroe was displayed by the altar. Pol' Atteu, who designed Anna's commitment ceremony gown and many costumes, also created her burial dress, made of hand-beaded French lace with Swarovski crystals, as well as the rhinestone-studded coffin cover. Inside the closed casket, she was laid to rest in a tiara, with J. Howard Marshall II's ashes in an urn next to her and notes from those close to her.[159] One letter, faxed to Birkhead, who included it in the coffin, was from nine-year-old Riley Shelley. Riley's mom, Gina, said the young girl stated her love and ended the missive with: "Anna, you know Howard K. Stern is not the father of the baby."[160] The burial was at Lake View Memorial Gardens, in a grave shared with Daniel's casket.

That night's *Larry King Live* program featured several guests who had attended the funeral. Carlos Diaz, a correspondent for TV's *Extra*, complained that he and his camera crew were not allowed to shoot inside the church because *Entertainment Tonight* had paid a "sizable contribution" for the exclusive rights. Harvey Levin, executive editor for TMZ.com, reminded King that the previous week the producer for *Entertainment Tonight* said on Larry's show that "they don't pay" for interviews. But Levin explained that the shows do pay for footage and hinted that this funeral would command a nice paycheck for someone. TMZ later reported that all of the funeral funds went into a trust in Dannielynn's name, which Stern set up, and that he "does not and will not receive any money from it, and is not the trustee." *Entertainment Tonight* and its sister series, *The Insider*, began airing their exclusive footage within days, which seemed more sympathetic to Stern than Arthur.

Levin also told Larry King that an agreement had been struck between Stern and Birkhead. "We are hearing that Howard has all but conceded that Larry is the father and that they are talking about financial arrangements, [and] what kind of presence Howard K. Stern will have in terms of a trust in the estate." Levin also predicted that the Marshall inheritance case would resolve, leaving baby Dannielynn set for life. "I think she's going to have some money, Larry," said Levin, who is also an attorney. "I think there's too much at stake to risk going to trial and losing everything, and usually what happens is there is a settlement. And she could stand to be very, very rich."

On that same broadcast, Carlos Diaz told Larry King that he had spoken to Dr. Perper in Florida and the doctor said everyone would be "very surprised" by the outcome of Anna's toxicology report, but refused to comment further. The report was expected in the next week and it would finally answer which of a plethora of theories—from pneumonia to lupus to a drug overdose—was accurate. Levin added: "Dr. Perper has been very coy about this but if this were as simple as methadone, which is out there right now, that she was taking methadone, if it were as simple as that, I don't think he would be saying that. I think it's got to be something other than drugs. Otherwise, why not say the obvious?"[161]

I had been hearing independently—as had my co-author—that Perper's surprise was that methadone was not a significant factor in Anna's death. Could it be that the painkiller Anna received while pregnant, which had been photographed in her home refrigerator and was also part of the drug cocktail that killed her son, was not to blame for her demise? We would know soon enough.

On the day of Anna's burial, *Access Hollywood* got its own exclusive: an airing of an interview with Larry Birkhead in which he revealed a tattooed cartoon of the departed centerfold and her signature across his back, above the jean line. "It's a picture of Anna, so wherever I go, she goes," he told the show. Birkhead was inked in December 2005, when he and Anna were still hot and heavy. "I really didn't want a tattoo and then we argued about it forever," he said.

"Then finally when I got to the point I wanted to do [it] because I wanted to, then finally she said 'Okay, don't worry about it.' Then I said 'I'll do it.'" She held his hand during the prickly process, and fed him orange juice and candy bars when he nearly fainted. "She's like 'quit being such a baby. Quit being such a sissy,'" he laughed. That night, he removed his bandages before the pair went to bed and discovered the imprint was on the sheet the next morning. "She folded the sheet up and kept it because it had the exact picture of the tattoo, something she wanted to keep," he recalled. She would beam with pride when he showed off the body art at the beach and tease him if his shorts rode too high. "She'd say, 'What are you doing, trying to hide me back there?'" Larry said the duo also wore matching diamond crosses around their necks, which he bought: "She was actually wearing it when she passed away."[162]

Dr. Perper continued making media appearances, if only to say he wouldn't comment until his report's official release. So the nosy press members, having nothing else to talk about, asked him to explain why the left side of his head was oddly misshapen. He joked, "I am definitely not a member of the television's Coneheads. I always used to say that I have extra brains that I could not accommodate in my head." Then he gave the real scoop: An aunt accidentally dropped him on his head when he was young and a blood clot thickened part of his skull.[163]

Perper admitted that, in addition to toxicology screening, which takes weeks, another reason for the delay was the sheer volume of research he and investigators were doing into aspects of Anna Nicole's life. With the help of the Seminole police force, they had been building a psychological profile of Ms. Smith. Besides scouring her computer files looking for threats made against her, they were going through e-mails and correspondence between Anna and her doctors, pharmacists, friends, lawyers, and Stern. If there was any evidence of criminal wrongdoing in her death, it would be uncovered.

A press flurry occurred over a legal declaration filed in the Birkhead paternity matter. Laurie Payne, the Myrtle Beach woman who was a pal of Anna's, swore in her statement that she had been around during Anna's pregnancy. She said: "I asked her why she did not just go into a relationship with Stern, to which (Anna Nicole) responded, 'Ewww, gross! No way! I would never!'" According to the document, during Christmas 2005, Stern began to tease Daniel "about being a nineteen-year-old virgin." Payne asserted that "Daniel looked at Stern and stated, 'I don't know why you're worried about me, you've been around my mother for twelve years and you haven't had any pussy either.'"[164] I have since learned that Daniel's exchange with Stern was made in the presence of a large number of people.

On March 7, *FOX 411* columnist Roger Friedman wrote a scathing article about *Entertainment Tonight*'s coverage of the funeral with "all its tacky preparations." He claimed that sources said the show "paid millions to Howard K. Stern for the right to have a landmark ceiling camera hovering over Smith's casket as it was rolled into the Bahamian church." He saved most of his vitriol for Dr. Khristine Eroshevich, citing a July 7, 2006, firing from the Los Angeles County Employees Retirement Association (LACERA) for "failing to perform her duties properly." According to a memo, the board's legal counsel, James Castranova, recommended terminating her services after Eroshevich, on two occasions, arranged for psychologists to conduct face-to-face examinations of LACERA members, which went against their mutual agreement that stated only board-certified physicians are allowed to do that work. Friedman spoke to Castranova, who explained, "Eroshevich farmed out her duties to other shrinks in violation of her agreement. In other words, she was sending [other] doctors to interview members of LACERA when she was supposed to be doing the work herself." It was not the last of Dr. Khris's problems.[165]

Two days later, Anna's other methadone-prescribing doctor, Sandeep Kapoor, got a press smackdown when reports surfaced that he was refusing to cooperate with Perper's investigation. Kapoor's lawyer, Ellyn Garafalo, issued a statement saying that her client was simply honoring his patient's confidentiality by not discussing why he wrote the scrip to Anna's alias. "The medical examiner's job is to determine the cause of Ms. Smith's death. Dr. Kapoor has no information that will help with that determination," she wrote. "Dr. Kapoor's treatment of Ms. Smith was at all times medically sound and he will continue to cooperate with any formal requests from authorities."[166] Why she didn't consider Perper's request "formal" was not explained.

In lighter news, NBC announced its popular *Law & Order: Criminal Intent* series would do its own version of the Anna Nicole Smith and Howard Stern story, starring actors Kristy Swanson and David Cross; it aired in 2007.[167]

And an independent movie, *Anna Nicole*, starring reality show mainstay Willa Ford in the title role, went into production and was released in 2008.[168]

From what I could see on the TV shows, Howard was getting thumped from every angle. Why hadn't he moved out of the Horizons home? Why was he refusing to concede paternity and reunite Dannielynn with Larry Birkhead, or at least take a DNA test to confirm or eliminate himself as the girl's father? Why was he trying to limit the scope of the inquest into Daniel's death that was supposed to start in Nassau at the end of the month? Not that those weren't good questions, but I think if there had been a way to have worked him onto the Grassy Knoll when JFK was shot, someone would have done so. By staying silent, except for his occasional bits on friendly *Entertainment Tonight*, he was inadvertently fanning the flames.

Jack E. Harding, the California private eye who had met with Daniel before the youth went to Nassau, said on *The Nancy Grace Show*: "[Daniel] contacted me, and he was really concerned about his mother. Someone was taking control over his mother's life, and that was Stern. He told me that he was afraid of Stern and that he was feeding his mother drugs and that he was acting like some kind of Svengali and that his mother was receiving some kind of mind-bending drug. The boy was very concerned, and so I became concerned. And I didn't take the case at that time because he said he was going to get back to me, and I hadn't seen him for a couple of weeks since that time. And he did tell me that he had a nightmare, and this is what spurred him into talking to me, in that nightmare he saw his mother in a coffin."

Harding (who was no relation to the late J. Howard Marshall II's nurse with that last name) described how Bahamian detectives investigating Daniel's death found Harding's business card in the lad's belongings. "They wanted to know why Danny had my card, and did I do an investigation in the Bahamas?" When Anna died in Florida, Harding's suspicions were piqued even more. He said, in essence, that Daniel had blamed Stern for pushing him out of his mother's life. "Danny didn't like him. He was afraid of him." Harding said he hoped to be called to testify at Daniel's inquest and also wished for Florida officials to contact him.[169] He reiterated the same information to my co-author, Dawna Kaufmann. Harding was eventually invited to the Bahamas to give his account to the coroner's magistrate and jury in March 2008, but had to cancel due to illness.

In mid-March 2007, Royal Bahamas police commissioner Paul Farquharson and some of his detectives traveled to Florida and met with Seminole investigators. But the Broward County state attorney's office downplayed the significance of the meeting, saying "no homicide investigation was under way." This was backed by Perper's office, which stated it needed about another week to complete its probe.

FOX News's Roger Friedman was not done with Dr. Eroshevich. On March 16, he published an online bombshell that got picked up worldwide. It was a handwritten fax allegedly from "Khris" to Sandeep Kapoor, the California doctor who prescribed methadone to an eight-months-pregnant Anna using her alias, "Michelle Chase." According to Friedman, Eroshevich, in the Bahamas, was attempting to get Kapoor—a doctor she didn't know—to fill a "laundry list of drugs" to be sent by courier to "M. Chase" in Nassau. Calling the list of different kinds of painkillers "scary and potentially very harmful," Friedman said it included four bottles of 2 mg injectible Dilaudid; two milliliter bottles of Lorazepam (also known as Ativan or Intensol); two bottles of 350 mg Soma, a total of 180 tablets; one bottle each of 30 mg Dalmane and 400 mg Prexige (a British drug); and one bottle of 5 mg methadone tablets (containing three hundred tablets). At the bottom of the fax was written: "You have my local number here. Please call. If half of the amounts can be prepared, I'll have someone take them to a courier to bring to me and he can [illegible] FedEx the rest, except for Intensol, which has to be on ice."[170]

The fax, which included the psychiatrist's medical license number, was dated September 15, 2006, just over a week after Dannielynn's birth and five days after Daniel's death. Kapoor refused to fill the prescription, Friedman wrote, so Eroshevich then sent the request directly to Key Pharmacy in North Hollywood, California—which also refused it. Friedman read the dosages to a pharmacist who told him the amounts were alarmingly high. "All together, these drugs potentially will kill you. I would have refused to fill the order," the pharmacist reportedly told him.

Friedman asserted that all of the drugs carry warnings for pregnant women and caution those who are breast-feeding not to take them. The insert on Prexige reads: "Tell your doctor if you are breast-feeding a baby. Ask your doctor about the risks and benefits of taking Prexige in this case. It is not known if lumiracoxib, the active ingredient of Prexige, passes into the breast milk and could affect your baby." Friedman had a brief conversation with Eroshevich, who acknowledged the existence of the fax but cited "patient confidentiality" when she declined further comment.[171]

Four days later, Friedman blasted her again after Dr. Khris appeared on *The Insider* TV show to defend herself. The program reported that Kapoor received the fax, but failed to mention that it was Eroshevich who wrote and sent it, or that both Kapoor and the pharmacy failed to fill the scrips. Friedman further reported that Key Pharmacy "put Eroshevich in touch with an addiction and pharmacology expert at a prestigious local university" who supposedly scolded her for requesting dosages that were inappropriate and dangerous. Friedman's source told him that the expert told the doctor "she was in way over her head and that Anna Nicole should be hospitalized." The expert allegedly referred Dr. Khris to treatment centers that specialize in helping patients with chronic pain and grief. But, Friedman wrote, Eroshevich would have none of it and ignored the expert. The columnist added that Kapoor was reassured when he heard from Dr. Khris, Smith, and Howard K. Stern that Anna was not breast-feeding her newborn. But Kapoor was apparently horrified when Eroshevich purportedly told him, "I need something to knock her out," Friedman wrote, adding, that Anna had not bonded with her baby girl.

Friedman stated that sister programs *Entertainment Tonight* and *The Insider* had both paid Eroshevich for interviews and were only firing easy-to-answer questions her way. Kapoor, Friedman wrote, inherited Smith as a patient from a doctor who had retired and had been writing scrips for a low dose of methadone for Anna's chronic pain. Friedman reported what Kapoor had said before: that methadone does not affect the placenta of a pregnant woman. Friedman's source claimed that Stern had told Kapoor that Eroshevich was a longtime friend. The source purportedly informed the columnist, "[Stern] said that they hadn't given Anna anything for pain after her C-section. And Eroshevich said she would be with Anna Nicole twenty-four/seven and that she would administer the drugs herself."

In refusing to write the scrips, Kapoor responded that he was particularly concerned about the dose of Dalmane. But Khris told Kapoor in a phone call that Anna was really tolerant of that drug, Friedman reported. Kapoor only heard from Anna Nicole one or two more times—the last time in November—three months before she died, according to Friedman.[172]

I remember seeing that fax and being absolutely stunned. I was surprised that the doctor, if that was her fax, would request such a list of heavy-duty pharmaceuticals from a second doctor she didn't even know. But I was heartened that there was finally one doctor— Kapoor—bold enough to turn down Anna Nicole's endless hunger for drugs. I also wondered who might have been Friedman's source. Obviously it was someone who had access to that fax and knew of the conversations that followed.

The other big news that week was that a Bahamian Supreme Court judge ordered DNA tests to determine paternity of young Dannielynn. Birkhead left the courthouse pumping his fists in the air. If Larry were the dad, the same judge would likely give him expedited custody and an amended birth certificate. Then he would need to get a passport for his daughter before he could bring her to the United States. The next morning, Stern, the baby, and Larry met at a doctor's office where the latter two were swabbed.[173] Stern didn't need the test because the country's law presumed he was the father since his name was on the birth certificate. Should Larry be proved the father, he could then force Stern into taking the test too. The swabs would be sent to a lab in Ohio, and results would come back in a few days. But before the tests were completed, Stern filed an emergency appellate motion, delaying everything until April 3. That hearing took place, but the matter was pushed forward one more week so that Dr. Michael Baird, the scientist who tested the samples, could deliver the news himself. Given so much publicity, Maxfield's, a high-end men's clothing store in West Hollywood, California, celebrated the paternity roulette by dressing its window mannequins in stylish togs, their faces covered by photos of Stern, Birkhead, and Prince von Anhalt, with a caption reading: "Who's Your Daddy?"

The Broward County medical examiner issued the long-awaited autopsy report into the death of Anna Nicole Smith on March 26, 2007, signed by Dr. Joshua Perper; his associate medical examiner, Dr. Gertrude Juste; and his chief toxicologist, Harold E. Scheuler, PhD. Perper and Seminole police chief Charlie Tiger held a joint press conference to announce that Smith had died of an "accidental overdose" from "acute combined drug toxicity." All told there were nine prescription drugs in her system—including antianxiety drugs, muscle relaxants, and antihistamines—but the one that did the most harm was the chloral hydrate, the sleep medication. Verifying the leaks that had been circulating, methadone was only found in trace amounts in her bile, probably from before she left Nassau, and had nothing to do with her passing. The police chief specifically said Howard K. Stern was not going to be charged with any kind of crime, and that his allowing the computers and hard drive to be searched helped confirm that there was no foul play or suicide.

Perper released a forty-page "Investigative Report in the Death of Vickie Lynn Marshall (AKA) Anna Nicole Smith"; an eight-page autopsy report; investigative reports from the scenes; and a well-organized eighty-four-page PowerPoint presentation, all of which can be found online. He listed the names and titles of the full investigative team; the medicolegal findings; the clinical background and circumstances leading up to Anna's death; her autopsy and toxicological results; consultants' opinions; cause, mechanism, and manner of death; contributing factors; summary; and references. Team members traveled to the Bahamas and reviewed medical records from Doctors Hospital, where Anna gave birth and Daniel died; and in Florida, they spoke with the emergency medical technicians who responded to the Hard Rock Hotel and those at Hollywood Memorial Hospital where she was pronounced dead.

Personal interviews were conducted with Howard K. Stern; Dr. Khristine Eroshevich; the physicians who delivered Anna's baby, treated her for pneumonia, and counseled her for grief after Daniel's death; the two Nassau nannies, Quethlie Alexie and Nadine Alexie; family friend Raymond Martino; Moe and Tasma Brighthaupt; Larry Birkhead; and Donald Hogan, Anna's father. I was puzzled by the omission of King Eric Gibson, the boat crewman whose name was never made public, and Brigitte Neven, King Eric's common-law wife—all of whom were in that Hard Rock Hotel room. Neven was the person who first noticed that Anna was not breathing, when she was likely already dead. I also didn't understand the choice not to speak to Anna's mother, Virgie Arthur, who was eager to help anyone probing her daughter's death. Not only might she have had some important information, but excluding her seemed lacking in common courtesy.

I would also have liked there to have been interviews with Jack E. Harding, the California private eye who said that Daniel had told him he was concerned about his mother being isolated by Stern; as well as Gerlene Gibson, the nanny at the home. Gibson's time overlapped with that of the two nannies and was extended after they got fired. And certainly, they should have interviewed the families of G. Ben Thompson, and Ford and Gina Shelley, Anna's friends from South Carolina, who had spent so much time with her at the Horizons home. I would also have included the Shelleys' young daughter, Riley, who was so shattered by Anna's death. Feeling that she contributed something to helping understand the tragedy might have perhaps eased the child's memory over that ghastly clown video.

In the external examination portion of the autopsy report, Anna is described as a "well-developed, well-nourished white woman" of thirty-nine years of age. She was five-foot eleven-inches tall and weighed one hundred seventy-eight pounds. Her scalp hair was blonde, five inches long in the front, and up to nineteen inches long in the back, which included multiple hair extensions and pink strands attached to the natural hair that had brown roots. The irises were hazel. The natural teeth were in good condition (although the report doesn't mention that she had cosmetic veneers), and there were bilateral earlobe piercings, but there was no jewelry on the body. She had piercing above and below the umbilicus—or a belly-button piercing. Her fingernails were long and clean, and her toenails were short and clean. Two reddish and recent contusions were on her upper back, presumably from the fall in the bathtub. Evidence of recent medical treatment by the paramedics was present, including the tube in her mouth, chest pads, and needle puncture marks. A linear half-inch scar was on the anterior right forearm, and two parallel linear scars measuring one inch and two inches were on the anterior surface of the left arm. Were these from the alleged suicide attempt in 1984? No further characterization or explanation of the wounds was given in the report. Other unexplained scars were noted on her thigh, buttocks, and right leg.

While alive, Anna's breasts were her pride and joy. At autopsy, they were an uneasy reminder of what many actresses are willing to do to themselves to attain fame. A 3/4 × 1/2-inch flat scar was on the upper inner aspect of the right breast quadrant. The right inframammary skin—or the crease under the breast—had a linear transverse 3/4-inch remote "chest tube" scar, possibly from her bout with pneumonia. There were bilateral inframammary and transverse linear 3-3/4-inch scars compatible with left and right mammoplasty with breast implants. A 1/2 × 3/8-inch scar was on the medial aspect of the left nipple. I had seen a photo of that breast, taken when she was still in Nassau; the breast looked as big as a pillow, with such scarring on the left areola it was almost unrecognizable as a nipple. When her body was opened with the Y-incision and her implants removed, each contained seven hundred milliliters of clear fluid, which is more than twice the size of typical surgical implants. Thirty milliliters equals a bit more than a fluid ounce, and there are sixteen ounces to a pint. In round numbers, seven hundred milliliters would be nearly a pint and a half of liquid. Next time you pick up a pint of ice cream, think what it would be to constantly have three of those on your chest. Anna's chronic back pain and general physical malaise could well have its root in those breast augmentations. As is routine when autopsying someone with implants, Perper sent them to a laboratory so the fluids could be tested for bacteriological cultures.

Anna also had a number of tattoos on her body: A pair of red lips was on the right lower abdominal quadrant; two red cherries were on the right midpelvis; a *Playboy* bunny was on the left anterior midpelvis; the words "Daniel" and "Papas" were on the midanterior pelvis region; a collage was on the right lower leg and ankle, which included Jesus Christ's head, Our Lady of Guadalupe, the Holy Bible, a woman's naked torso, the smiling face of Marilyn Monroe, a cross, a heart, and shooting flames; and a mermaid on a flower bed with a pair of lips underneath was across her lower back.

Her internal organs were of normal size, color, and consistency, and the procedure ended with Perper taking additional blood and tissue samples for DNA testing, mindful that the paternity matter might require it. Anna's past medical history revealed migraine headaches; insomnia, first treated with Ambien, then with chloral hydrate; muscle strains and back pains; Hashimoto thyroiditis; anxiety and post-traumatic disorder; seizures; pneumonitis, following the near drowning in the swimming pool; self-treatment for longevity and weight control, with repeated neuromuscular injections of vitamin B12, immunoglobulin, and human growth hormones; and alcohol and drug rehabilitation. Her chart cited depression as a result of the deaths of her husband and her son, as well as a number of lawsuits. A forensic examination of her computers outlined her grief and frustration but also showed that she was enjoying life and had plans to have another baby. Additional information gleaned from her medical records, but not having to do with her death investigation, was not included in the public report, due to patient confidentiality.

Perper's autopsy and microscopic analysis found discoloration of the heart muscle and intestinal lining; congestion and enlargement of the liver; a healed cesarean scar; less than an ounce of blood in the stomach, consistent with terminal shock; fibrous adhesions of the right pleural (lung) membrane, and congestion and swelling of the lungs; a small, cystic lesion in the right occipital (rear) lobe of her brain— which might have come from a seizure but had no bearing on her death—recent bruises near her shoulder blade from the previous day's fall in the bathtub; mild dilation of the mitral valve of her heart; a small hemorrhage on her tongue; evidence of the life-saving meas- ures; and remote breast augmentation surgery, but no definite evidence of liposuction scars or recent plastic surgery. Days after the autopsy, following Perper's medical examiner team speaking to Stern and Ero- shevich, the forensic experts went back for an atypical procedure. Both of Anna's buttocks were dissected, revealing extensive scarring with necrosis, or dead tissue, of the fat tissues and formation of cysts. The left buttock contained several abscesses measuring up to one cen-

timeter in diameter and multiple hemorrhagic needle tracks, one per-
forating an abscess. Cultures on the blood were negative, probably
because Anna had been on antibiotics. Tests showed markers of
inflammation but no blood poisoning. Two infectious disease experts
who reviewed the materials were in agreement with Perper and Juste
that the very high fever of 105 degrees was related to the release of
bacteria into the blood from the abscesses of the buttock. Viral
enteritis was probable, given the reports that she had diarrhea, possible
vomiting, and dehydration. But while she had symptoms of the flu that
her companion Howard K. Stern had, tests were negative for Influenza
A or B.

Gross examination and microscopic analysis eliminated acute
myocardial infarct or coronary heart disease (heart attack), pulmonary
thromboembolism (stroke), choking on gastric contents, cirrhosis,
hepatitis, kidney inflammation, pregnancy, diabetes, HIV, lupus,
colitis, gastritis, cancer, leukemia, pneumonia, asthma, large amounts
of pills or capsules in the stomach or duodenum, and needle marks on
the arms. Toxicology readings eliminated the presence of alcohol;
amphetamines or methamphetamine; barbiturates; carbon monoxide;
marijuana; opiates, cocaine or fentanyl; gamma-hydroxybutyric acid;
insulin; salicylates; poisons such as thallium, cyanide, and succinyl-
choline; and heavy metals (lead, mercury, and arsenic). So exhaustive
was the search for substances in her system, a Geiger counter was used
to eliminate radiation toxicity. A few esoteric poisons, such as ricin,
cannot be analyzed by civilian laboratories, but the risk would have
seemed low for the kind of toxin that a secret agent might use on an
enemy.

Anna's infatuation with chloral hydrate, which accumulated in her
system over days, might have caused some of her epigastric distress,
especially if the syrup wasn't properly diluted or was taken on an
empty stomach. Toxic blood levels range from twenty to two hundred
forty milligrams per liter; fatalities are reported at levels greater than
twenty-nine milligrams per liter. Anna's blood level for the drug was

seventy-five milligrams per liter. The lethal drug in her system was the chloral hydrate, without which the others could have coexisted.

Her blood, urine, organs, and ocular fluids were tested and the results showed therapeutic levels of over-the-counter decongestant Benadryl; prescription muscle relaxants/sedatives Klonopin, Ativan, and oxazepam (a metabolite of Valium, meaning its chemical components were starting to break down); and prescription antianxiety drugs Valium and Restoril. Other prescription drugs that had no bearing on her death, but were present in her system, include muscle relaxant Atropine, used in Advanced Cardiac Life Support (ACLS) resuscitative protocols; anticonvulsant and tranquilizer Topamax; antibiotic Cipro; methadone, which was only in her bile; plus over-the-counter Tylenol and an incidental hint of caffeine. Prescription drugs known to have been used recently by Anna, but not present in her system, include the muscle relaxants/sedatives Soma and Robaxin and the antiviral Tamiflu.

According to Perper's findings, homicide could be eliminated because there were no signs of a struggle or force-feeding of medications. Chloral hydrate also has an unpleasant, harsh taste that could not be "slipped" into a drink. The report notes: "One could speculate that Miss Smith was cognitively impaired due to her infections and use of benzodiazepines and that this rendered her susceptible to homicidal poisoning. However, due to the evidence produced by the parallel police and medical examiner investigations, this would represent mere speculation and does not hold up under scientific scrutiny."

Suicide was also eliminated despite signs of chronic depression from her son's death and the painful cesarean section incision. Anna also bought several burial plots and purportedly commissioned a dress for her funeral, but she left no note—not that one is always found in such cases. She told people she "wanted to die" but did not develop a specific plan of action; even her near-drowning episode was not considered suicide by Perper since she thanked the person who revived her. While she had once told someone that she wanted to die as her idol Marilyn Monroe did—and Monroe died of a suicidal overdose of chloral hydrate and barbiturates—it is unknown whether Anna knew which drugs were involved in Marilyn's suicide, even though that information is online. Perper also revealed that some witnesses observed Anna wasn't as infatuated with Marilyn Monroe as she used to be.

Chronic chloral hydrate consumption causes jaundice, which Anna didn't have, and she did not appear to be intoxicated when last seen alive, which would indicate that her last, large ingestion of the drug was in the hours before death. Also a half bottle of chloral hydrate remained near Anna; had she taken it to die, she likely would have downed it all. She may have overmedicated herself with chloral hydrate to alleviate pain from her infection, not understanding that its interaction with the other therapeutic medications in her system was heightening her risk of overdose. She was also known to swig the chloral hydrate from the bottle, making it difficult to determine the exact dosage ingested, and was observed on the Florida trip taking multiple doses of chloral hydrate in combination with her "usual" assortment of pills.[174]

On March 29, 2007, a panel of seven local citizens was seated in the Nassau coronial magistrate's court, waiting to begin the inquest into Daniel Smith's death. Stern's attorney—Bahamian Bar president Wayne Munroe—argued that pretrial publicity, suggesting Stern had culpability in the death, made it impossible for jurors to be open-minded in the case. The judge promised to study the matter while continuing the case another two weeks.[175]

On March 31, Joshua Perper was a guest on FOX News's *On the Record with Greta Van Susteren* and stated that of the eleven prescription medications found in Anna's hotel room when she died, not one was in her name. Eight were written to Stern, two were for Alex Katz—who has still not been indentified—and the last was in the name of Khristine Eroshevich, the psychiatrist who wrote all eleven scrips. He also said the chloral hydrate had been kept in a duffel bag. Van Susteren wondered how someone as weak as Anna could have gotten to the bag and that medicine, and Perper said he asked Stern, Eroshevich, and Big Moe that, but no one had an answer.[176] Perper added that even if someone else gave her the drugs, "It's not wise, for sure, but it's not homicide."[177]

Despite Perper's statement that Anna's death wasn't murder, Howard K. Stern was still concerned that he might be pulled into court and forced to defend himself on criminal charges. In the public mind, both Anna's and Daniel's deaths were entwined, and there were very few talking heads going on the various shows to offer Stern's point of view. On April 3, I got a five-page, single-spaced e-mail from him that outlined "all the egregious falsehoods perpetuated over the last couple months that have poisoned any possible jury pool." He added that the list was by no means exhaustive, and that it would take weeks to make a comprehensive one. Among the media outlets he targeted were: the *Bahamas Tribune*; *Globe*; FOX News's Roger Friedman, *The O'Reilly Factor*, and *On the Record with Greta Van Susteren*; Cable Headline News's *The Nancy Grace Show*; *Star*; TMZ.com; CNN's *Larry King Live*; *People*; *In Touch Weekly*; and *Life & Style Weekly*. My first thought was what a miserable task that must have been to have to go through all that material, finding criticisms, so I was sympathetic to his sense of being picked on.

The stories and reports he found fault with included those suggesting that Daniel's autopsy was faked and his methadone levels were ten to twenty times greater than reported; both Daniel and Anna would be exhumed and new autopsies performed; Stern would be cashing in on insurance policies for $70 million; Stern was paid $3 million for the rights to Daniel's and Anna's funerals; Stern gave Daniel methadone, then flushed more pills down the toilet; Daniel tried to hire a private investigator to free his mother from Stern; Daniel knew Stern controlled his mother with "mind-bending" drugs; Anna blamed Stern for Daniel's death; people heard her scream "You caused this!"; Stern killed Virgie Arthur's daughter and grandson; the two nannies would tell all about the drugs Stern gave Anna; and more.

I went through the items line by line and found a few arguments for his side. It's no one's business but his how much money he makes on selling rights. Also, he's said that the money is going into a trust account for Dannielynn, not that it is required. If there are really seven insurance policies, that will be revealed soon enough; but if Stern is truthful that there are not, he has an absolute right to call that report a lie. The private investigator has told his story many places, as have the nannies, Virgie Arthur, and the two men who supposedly witnessed Stern flushing away the drugs. During Daniel's inquest, I suggested, Howard or his attorney should introduce those topics in open court. You have an advantage of knowing where the minefields are, I told Stern.

As for the escalating levels of purported methadone in Daniel's system and the autopsy being faked, I would be willing at any point to address those stories in the media and bring the official toxicology reports with me. I spent enough time talking with Howard that I believed his grief over losing two people so close to him was real, and it has to be so much worse being viewed as the architect of those deaths. Other parts of his fax had dates wrong and mentions of me that I knew weren't accurate, and when I wrote him back and asked for an explanation, I didn't get one. Perhaps his fax to me was a long stream of consciousness that he needed to expel from his system, and once he hit "Send" on his computer he felt purged. I did manage to assure him that there would be no need to exhume Anna for another autopsy. Perper and his team's work was fine, and they couldn't be more unambiguous, asserting that no murder had taken place.

In early April it was announced that the California medical board was looking into Dr. Khristine Eroshevich's treatment of Anna Nicole Smith. It was also revealed that the board had already begun investigating Dr. Kapoor.[178] But from what I understood, Kapoor was chiefly Daniel's doctor; his prescribing to Anna was limited to the methadone he sent when she was pregnant—albeit to her assumed name—and his refusal to fill the prescriptions Dr. Khris reportedly requested. These probes can take years to complete, with the public not learning the results unless and until the doctor in question is sanctioned or loses his or her license. Generally when a board investigates a physician, it is to see whether the patient in question is actually having physical checkups before a doctor prescribes medicines. In this case, Eroshevich was seeing Anna on a regular basis, even living with her in Nassau and next door to her in California. Maybe the examinations weren't in an office setting, but who's to say they weren't performed when the doctor was at Anna's home? The board also looks for periodic reassessments of medications and accurate record keeping.

Dr. Khris told me that she was always fine-tuning Anna's medication, so that should not be a problem, though I have no knowledge of her record keeping. Another factor is the medical history of the patient; Anna seems to have invested some time with this doctor, which Howard can attest to, as well. So the question is whether this doctor was negligent.

Purportedly more than six hundred pills were prescribed in about thirty-eight days.[179] That certainly seems excessive, but how many pills did Anna take and how many were left in their bottles? Should the doctor have collected the leftover pills? There's no doubt that Anna Nicole was drug addicted, but she was also quite tolerant of medicines and demanding of the people around her. She was the star, the money earner, the domineering queen bee. If someone made her mad, she'd banish them. She had sent Larry Birkhead and her own mother packing. So what does a doctor do with a patient like Anna? Abandon her? That seems more irresponsible than staying aware of the person's treatment.

That said, there are still some issues I would like to address, such as how close a psychiatrist should get with a patient. Anna might have insisted that once a person entered her inner circle, he or she had to ignore boundaries. Anna said on TV that her relationship with Howard K. Stern—her lawyer—bloomed into a sexual affair when she "attacked" him. "I kissed him first," she laughed. Although the American Bar Association codes contain no provision for dealing expressly with a lawyer/client sexual relation, state bars—including California—warn against it.[180] Lawyers are not supposed to sleep with clients because it can lead to a conflict of interest. It's just not a smart, ethical choice. Stern's situation was and is complicated by the fact that he's the executor of Smith's estate. But again, Anna might have insisted upon these kinds of messy situations. Doctors and lawyers with celebrity clients may enjoy a boost to their professional stature in business and social circles. Suddenly they're in the gossip columns and the best restaurants. The celebrity brings attention to the charities and foundations that the professional cares about. So it can be a seductive environment, even if there isn't sex involved or people who are "best friends." It remains to be seen whether the respective state governing boards will take action against Eroshevich—whose offices are now closed[181]—Kapoor, or Stern, but I hope in the future they can comport themselves with more professional distance from their clients.

On April 10, Dr. Michael L. Baird, the laboratory director of DNA Diagnostics Center in Fairfield, Ohio, appeared in a Nassau court, holding an envelope with a name inside. The gentleman whose name he would reveal would not be our next president or win an Academy Award, but would be the only living link between a seven-month-old child and a potential half-billion-dollar fortune. Outside the courthouse, TV and print reporters, who were barred from the closed-door session, were doing live stand-ups, announcing each major player who walked up the path and into the building. Howard K. Stern, Larry Birkhead, and Virgie Arthur all brought relatives, hoping to prove to the magistrate that whomever Dannielynn was going home with would have an extended, loving family. The paternity question would be decided today, but not custody—the magistrate would still hold that card until a hearing later in the week.

After the hearing ended, Larry Birkhead was the first key person out the door. He walked to a microphone in the center of a field of reporters and bystanders and said, "Everyone, I hate to be the one to tell you this, but—I told you so!" A loud cheer ripped through the air, and Birkhead teared up as he thanked his supporters. Dr. Baird told the court there was a 99.99 percent certainty for the DNA test. When asked what's next, Birkhead proclaimed, "I'm going to the toy store!" Disneyland would have to come another day.

Stern walked to the microphone, gave Birkhead a hug, and told the crowd, "My feelings for Dannielynn have not changed. I am not going to fight Larry Birkhead on custody. We're going to do what we can to make sure that the best interests of Dannielynn are carried out. And I'm going to do whatever I can to make sure he gets sole custody."[182] After moving to the Bahamas to ditch Birkhead during the second half of Anna's pregnancy, then denying a simple test to confirm paternity—resulting in keeping the child from her father for more than seven months—his offer seemed a bit weak. Just days before, Stern had asked the appellate court to block the release of the DNA results, citing invasion of Dannielynn's privacy. The judges refused, ordering him to pay $10,000 in court costs for the action.[183] But on this day, Stern told onlookers that Larry could come over to the house and spend as much time with the baby as he'd like. Stern's new spirit of generosity didn't extend to Virgie Arthur, who was the final person to speak. "I'm happy that Dannielynn will know who her real father is, and I look forward to working with Larry, [and] raising my granddaughter," she said. Later that day in Los Angeles, representatives for Prince Frédéric Von Anhalt stated: "We never intended to take Dannielynn from anyone. We were just here in case Prince Von Anhalt was the father. We wish Larry luck in raising Dannielynn and we wish him the best."[184]

Behind the scenes, Arthur's attorney John M. O'Quinn was letting Birkhead know that while the baby's grandma not only looked forward to having an ongoing relationship with the child, she was seeking a written agreement that would ensure her guardianship in the event something happened to Larry. Virgie also wanted a say in how monies in the girl's name would be spent. She gave an example: if Larry wanted to buy his daughter a costly item, "like a Porsche at fourteen, we would have to say, 'No, at fourteen you are not getting a Porsche.'"[185] O'Quinn invoked Section 14 of the Family Act of the Bahamas, which gives a grandparent the right to ask for joint guardianship.[186] O'Quinn, from Houston, is one of the nation's sharpest trial lawyers and a giant in personal injury, corporate, and pharmaceutical litigation. With victories against tobacco companies (a $17.3 billion settlement), Halliburton ($70 million), and a diet pill manufacturer (roughly $1 billion), he could afford to pick up all of the expenses for Virgie, including travel, accommodations, and legal costs, from before the Fort Lauderdale burial case.[187] Equally pugnacious Michigan attorney Geoffrey N. Fieger once said, "O'Quinn's not doing this because he cares about family law—he sees the potential for the J. Howard Marshall II pot of gold, and he wants Virgie Arthur to get her fair share."[188]

But while Larry indicated that he had no qualms with letting "anyone with good intentions" remain in his daughter's life, he balked about any shared custody or financial arrangement. "It would imply that I'm unfit as a parent, which I'm not," he remarked on the *Today Show* the morning after he won the Paternity Bowl. "I'm looking forward to giving Dannielynn everything that she needs and all the love and support."[189] It seemed implausible to think Arthur would prevail in her desire to be named the baby's custodial next of kin. As Dannielynn's sole parent, Larry could draft his own will, granting custody—and all that would come with it—to the person of his choosing. In Louisville, he had a twin brother, a sister, and a half sister who has children, in addition to his mother. (His father, who was divorced from his mother, passed away in December 2007.) Reasonably his designee would come from his own family and not a woman whom he had recently met for the first time and who had had a contentious relationship with her own daughter. Nonetheless, he agreed to a meeting with Arthur, just before he would go back to court to get formal custody.

Within days, Larry and Dannielynn were the cover story for *OK!* magazine. The photos of Daddy and Baby were adorable, and the article revealed that Anna had written him three days before her death, "Don't fall in love again. I'd be a bit jealous." Early in her pregnancy, he told the writer, he and Anna had thought about naming their daughter either Annabella or Marilyn Nicole, or, if it was a boy, Nico. Birkhead said his former foe Stern was helping him learn about the baby's likes and dislikes. "People blame a lot on him, but Anna had her own mind too."[190] On April 25, a Bahamian judge gave Larry the green light to leave the islands with his daughter, subject to at least another custody hearing down the line when he'd have to bring the child back for a look-see. Arthur's attorney filed a last-ditch appeal, trying to block them from leaving Nassau, but the court ruled against her, figuring this family feud should be fought in America. Virgie was also ordered to pay $3,000 in court costs.[191]

Dannielynn's birth certificate was amended to remove "Stern" and add "Birkhead" to her last name, and as soon as her passport came through on April 28, she, Larry, and Howard hopped aboard a plane for the States. The private jet was courtesy of NBC, which brought the trio to a studio for exclusive interviews on the *Today Show*, *Access Hollywood*, and a Bravo channel—an NBC subsidiary—documentary. The reported million-dollar deal went through the network's entertainment division, so that the news operation could continue to say that it doesn't pay for stories.[192] The media spree continued on to Louisville, where Larry's family got to see the girl on their home turf when he attended the annual Barnstable Brown Kentucky Derby eve bash. As he carried his daughter through the airport and past crowds and reporters, he took care to cover Dannielynn's face with his jacket.[193] Was that to protect the child from flashbulbs that might scare her, or so he'd be able to control—and make money from—any photos? Just four months before, he was outraged at Anna's and Howard's attempts to "pimp" his daughter.

In mid-May, Howard Stern's attorney petitioned to file Anna's will into probate in California, seeking to establish a trust naming Dannielynn as Smith's sole beneficiary, although it would be almost a year before the matter was resolved. Larry Birkhead, while not mentioned in the will, was cited as a party with an interest in the estate. A June date was set to hear the petition, as well as one Birkhead filed at the same time for guardianship of his daughter.[194] The earlier will, from 2001, stated that Anna was unmarried and made her son, Daniel, the only beneficiary, purposely excluding any child or spouse that would follow. No codicil was drafted to rectify that after Dannielynn's birth and Daniel's death. If the probate petition were not accepted, the will could fall under the intestacy statute, meaning that the document would cease to exist since there would be no living heir. The state would then administer the estate, taking a large fee off the top.

The probate petition also waived Stern's right to any compensation as executor of the estate, but when the court action was discussed on *On the Record with Greta Van Susteren* that night, attorney Geoffrey Fieger scoffed at the idea that Stern's intentions were strictly altruistic. "He's named as the executor. He'll be the person who pursues all the legal actions, and he's got several pending. The main action is the one against the Marshall estate, in which all those millions are pending," Fieger said. "He reserves the right to name a corporate fiduciary, and I'm certain that he will have a relationship with the corporate fiduciary, and he will get his remuneration that way. So any claim that he's doing this for free and he'll do it for free forever—that's utter nonsense." Lawyer Jeff Brown added: "Larry knows that Howard's going to work with him. Howard knows that he can count on Larry to work with him, as well, to make sure that they go after any assets that are available. So this is clearly a back room deal that we're not privy to that's been cut."[195]

The probate petition listed Anna's assets as personal property of $10,000 and the $1.8 million home in Studio City, which has a $1.1 million mortgage—totaling $720,000. But what about her wardrobe, art, furniture, cars, yacht, bank accounts, and talent guild pensions? Reportedly, she was wearing a six-carat diamond ring when she died, had a pearl necklace in the room, and had another $2 million worth of cash and gems in safety deposit boxes. What happened to the $30,000 gowns she said she bought regularly when she gave testimony during the Marshall case? Where is the money made from the footage and photographs sold after Daniel's death, and her film work and TrimSpa earnings? *In Touch Weekly* estimated her earnings in the last year of her life to be at least $1.3 million[196], and the *National Enquirer*[197] and *Globe*[198] tabloids ranked her net worth as much higher. Could there be off-shore bank accounts hiding some missing assets? "The probate judge should put a freeze on everything until an independent forensic accountant can go through Smith's finances," said Don Clark, the retired Houston FBI chief-turned-investigator for the John O'Quinn law firm.[199]

Also not mentioned are any assets Daniel Smith might have had, which would have reverted to his mother after his death. His grandmother said on *20/20* that J. Howard Marshall II had set up a trust in the boy's name.[200]

Stern's petition asked for the right to represent Anna Nicole's interests in the Horizons home, but while that home's ownership is still in dispute, there was the second home in Nassau they bought together, also unmentioned in the probate petition. TV's Nancy Grace said of the lack of assets: "Something stinks." But a will and probate attorney, Mark Bain, explained to her that another filing could be done later if and when more assets are uncovered.[201] In fact, the California filing adds a page with a box that is checked for filing fee purposes, which estimates the estate value as "at least $1.5 million and less than $2 million," but it is not itemized. And I have since heard that the will has been entered into probate in Florida and the Bahamas, so those documents may list the assets in greater detail. Stern purportedly later filed a claim against the estate, asking for a fee agreement of 6 percent for any monies recovered in the Marshall litigation, which could net him millions, if there is a settlement or victory.[202]

Soon after the California probate action was dissected by TV panels, Howard's sister Bonnie Stern, a Beverly Hills accountant, was invited to write a piece for an online magazine. "I'm proud of my brother, and I know who he really is," she stated, "I want all the

Howard-haters to stop dragging his name through the dirt, so Anna can finally rest in peace." Bonnie spoke from the heart about the toll on their family when Howard was repeatedly called a murderer in the media. He doesn't even kill bugs, she wrote, much less would he harm the woman he was "utterly in love with" and planned to marry. Bonnie also stood up for Anna, saying how charitable she was to groups that helped battered women and AIDS patients. Anna's public persona was extreme, but Bonnie knew the more reflective woman, the one who still mourned her son every day. If Anna didn't have Howard to lean on, she would have committed suicide, Bonnie felt. She also stated that Anna's drug use was nothing Howard, or anyone, could have stopped. "Anna did what Anna wanted to do," she said. "She made her own decisions, and if you went against what she wanted, you were gone."[203]

Howard and Larry attended a court hearing on June 19 before Superior Court commissioner Mitchell L. Beckloff, who announced that Anna's will would, indeed, be admitted to probate, with Larry named as the estate's guardian and Howard its executor. The court would now begin the process of distributing Smith's assets. Beckloff said he would advise Virgie Arthur of his decision, in case she wanted to intervene legally, although Stern's counsel, Bruce Ross, said that he believed Arthur had no standing in the matter. Outside the courthouse, Ross told reporters that he would have the lawyer who drafted the will testify to the commissioner that Anna never meant to disinherit Dannielynn. Ross said Anna told the lawyer, "I probably won't have future children, but if I do, I would want them to be the beneficiaries of the trust." He added that Anna agreed to the clause that specifically left out future children because "she was concerned that someone would pop up out of the woodwork." Howard and Larry were all smiles as they spoke of their plans—Stern would return to Nassau and Birkhead would go to Los Angeles with his daughter, unless the paparazzi attention made that impossible. He joked, "You guys are always taking pictures of me, so I can't take pictures anymore." But he did have an idea for a fallback career: "Maybe I'll go to law school."[204]

On July 6, the California Department of Justice announced it was conducting a criminal investigation into the doctors who prescribed various medicines to Anna Nicole Smith. Agents reviewed more than one hundred thousand computer images and files, analyzed patient files and pharmacy logs, and interviewed Larry Birkhead, Big Moe Brighthaupt, and others, zeroing in on their knowledge of Eroshevich and Kapoor.[205] On October 12, eight search warrants were served on the offices and homes of Eroshevich and Kapoor, although no arrests were made. When Dr. Khris's home was searched, Howard happened to be there, picking up his dogs.

In a press conference, state attorney general Jerry Brown said he launched the investigation on March 30, after learning that Smith had died of a drug overdose and that the prescriptions written for her were from doctors and pharmacies in California. Although he gave few details of what his agents were looking for, he noted, "You don't go to a judge and get a search warrant for somebody's home unless you think some serious crime has been committed." Brown admitted investigators learned "quite a lot" from Bahamian officials, adding, "We do know from the public record that there's someone who's dead and her body, upon investigation, is full of controlled substances and combinations of drugs that turned out to be illegal." Asked whether the probe might include Daniel Smith's death, Brown stated: "We're not setting any limits on this investigation."

Reporters also inquired of Dr. Khris's attorney, Gary Lincenberg, how the medical board probe that began in April was progressing. He stated that it had "nothing to do with whether or not Dr. Eroshevich in any way contributed to Anna Nicole Smith's death," but only concerned whether the doctor's prescriptions followed state law regarding controlled substances. It was also revealed that the medical board had opened an inquiry into whether there was any misconduct by Dr. Kapoor in prescribing methadone to Anna late in her pregnancy and under her pseudonym, Michelle Chase.[206]

The next few months were reasonably quiet. Dannielynn celebrated her first birthday on September 7 with a super lavish party back in Louisville with her daddy, and then they flew to Hawaii for a few days.[207] On September 16, the three-hour-long Fifty-Ninth Annual Emmy Awards celebration was broadcast, honoring primetime's best programming and stars. The Academy of Television Arts & Sciences, which produces the event, ran the standard In Memoriam list of fifty treasured performers and creative people who died in the past year. Anna Nicole Smith was mentioned, along with Merv Griffin, Sidney Sheldon, Luciano Pavarotti, Ed Bradley, Steve Irwin, Tammy Faye Bakker, and Tom Poston.[208] Anna would have loved being in such company.

In mid-October, Moe Brighthaupt gave an interview to *Access Hollywood* to complain that Howard, formerly his good friend, had started a smear campaign against him. Moe pointed to a *Larry King Live* show where Howard insinuated that Moe had released a photo of Anna in which she appeared to have vomit dripping down her chin. Moe said he regretted calling Stern instead of 911 when he learned that Anna couldn't be roused. "I hear some reports that she could have been down since early that morning," Moe said about Anna. But this was negated by Dr. Perper's report, which said that Anna's body was warm when rescue workers got to her. Moe also grumbled about Larry Birkhead's telling Judge Seidlin that he had tried to get Anna off drugs. Moe told the TV show's correspondent that he saw Larry also give Anna "things to make her look or seem very out of it." But he was coy about his allegation, saying, "Let's just say that everything made her tipsy and [it] wasn't always the champagne he was giving her." Birkhead told the program that Moe "has no credibility."[209]

The Bahamian coroner's inquest into Daniel Smith's death finally began in November 2007, then dribbled along, on and off, through the end of March 2008, with about three dozen witnesses testifying before the seven-person jury. At its conclusion, the jury voted that no criminal charges would be filed in the matter. The question of where Daniel got the methadone or Zoloft that were in his system—along with the Lexapro for which he had a prescription—was never answered. Howard told *Us* magazine that the events of the past year had left him drained financially and indebted to his parents for hundreds of thousands of dollars: "There's this impression out there that I am somehow making money off of Anna's death. It couldn't be further from the truth."[210]

Stern put the kibosh on a reported attempt by Anna's Texas doctor, Gerald Johnson, to sell videos of her breast enhancement surgery. Collectibles dealer Tom Riccio was hawking a five-minute presentation of the two-hour surgery, showing Anna, naked and on the operating table, with the *Jaws* theme song and Anna's voice from the TrimSpa ad saying: "Do you like my body?" The FBI looked into the matter, but no charges were filed against the doctor, who claimed that Anna had signed a waiver granting him permission to make use of the surgery tape. Stern argued that was ridiculous and that the videos belong to Anna's estate. A judge agreed, barring Johnson and Riccio from marketing the tape, and all copies were surrendered to Stern. As of 2006, Johnson is no longer practicing medicine.[211]

On November 28, which would have been Anna's fortieth birthday, she was remembered on various TV shows, which recapped her wild life and sordid death. On December 13, Stern, director David Giancola, and executive producer John James presented Anna's last film, *Illegal Aliens*, at the Bahamas International Film Festival. The movie was enthusiastically received, and Howard told reporters that Anna's character used the same baby doll voice as she used in the notorious clown-face video, suggesting she was only goofing around on the tape and not really under the influence.[212]

Birkhead is awaiting his day in court against his former lawyer Debra Opri for allegedly overbilling him, and Opri has filed a lawsuit against him for purportedly slandering her on *Larry King Live*.[213] Anna's estate has been hit with a number of lawsuits: Dannielynn's former guardian ad litem, Richard Milstein, also filed for monies owed for his work on the case;[214] Anna's former California law firm, now retained by Birkhead, sued her estate for $163,000 in unpaid legal fees;[215] and a Texas law firm she used in the 1990s wants payment for services they rendered on the Marshall case.[216] Howard Stern is suing Virgie Arthur's lawyer John O'Quinn for implying on various television programs that Stern killed Anna and Daniel. But Stern was dealt a serious blow when the Seminole police department, citing tribal immunity, refused his request to furnish documents about their research into Anna's death. However, Seminole cops have decided to help California authorities with their ongoing investigation into the doctors who furnished Anna with drugs.[217] And, of course, the J. Howard Marshall II case is still wending its way through the court system and will eventually give Howard K. Stern another shot to feather the nest of Anna's estate with a piece of her late husband's billion-dollar fortune.

The E! Entertainment Channel—the network that aired Anna Nicole's reality series—is considering doing a reality series about Birkhead, showing the doting dad and his darling daughter in their normal daily lives.[218] The paparazzi hang out in front of Tinseltown's popular stores and restaurants, waiting to take snapshots of Larry when he's in the vicinity. When Dannielynn is with him, they circle like vultures. The toddler who looks more like her gorgeous mother each day seems to bask in the attention—maybe it's in her DNA.

In January 2008, Larry and Dannielynn were on *Entertainment Tonight* and *The Insider* so that he could discuss the eye patch that the sixteen-month-old girl had been sporting in recent photos. His daughter, he said, suffered from strabismus, or the crossing of one eye, a condition that affects 5 percent of people. It is a genetic malady and not at all related to Anna Nicole's drug usage. Anna had noticed it early on and had already begun talking to pediatricians in Nassau before she died, Birkhead explained. The child's California doctor recommended the eye patch over her stronger eye to build up the weaker one's muscle—and Larry said that he wore one too, so they could play "pirates" together.[219] But the eye needed surgery, and in February, Dannielynn had the simple procedure done. A second operation may be necessary in the future, which is not unheard of.

To commemorate the first year since Anna Nicole died, the same two television programs produced a several-days-long exclusive where cameras followed Larry and Dannielynn as they flew to Nassau and visited Anna's grave. It was the baby's first trip back to the Bahamas. One part of the interview showed Dannielynn dropping a pink toy turtle on her mother's grave and saying, "Mama," while Larry set down a spray of flowers. He explained to correspondent Jann Carl that Anna's and Daniel's graves were still unmarked because he had commissioned an elaborate headstone that would cover both mother and son, but it wasn't finished yet. Larry also said it was "weird" having the two plots in a different country from where he and Dannielynn live, but that he'd wait until she turns eighteen to see if she wants to exhume her relatives and re-bury them in the states.[220]

For his part, Howard K. Stern had a more modest way of honoring Anna. He spoke at a private gathering at the Lake View Memorial Gardens, saying about his former lady love and client: "I worshipped her and I still do." He mourned the loss of his friend who was much smarter than people thought she was, and who, if she were alive, would be bragging to everyone about her baby girl. Wistfully, he told the crowd that he couldn't stop thinking, "Why are things the way they are instead of the way they should be?"[221]

The official Anna Nicole Smith Web site has been redesigned to promote the newly formed Anna Nicole Smith and Daniel Wayne Smith Charitable Foundation. The organization will benefit causes that Anna felt close to in her life, such as underprivileged youth, AIDS patients, and the elderly. Another page announces Larry Birkhead's sponsorship of "Dannielynn's House," for the construction of a new Habitat for Humanity home in Louisville, Kentucky. A single mother and three daughters, two of whom have spinal bifida, will be able to purchase the home at a low cost when it is completed. "This entire project is about the strength it takes to be a single parent, the difficulties you have to face. I can relate to that now, raising Dannielynn on my own," Birkhead stated. "Anna Nicole's struggle as a single parent with her son, Daniel, was another reason that inspired my sponsorship of Dannielynn's House," he said.[222]

On March 4, 2008, a judge in Los Angeles named Dannielynn Hope Birkhead the sole heir to her mother's fortune. A trust was also set up in the child's name, with Larry Birkhead and estate executor Howard K. Stern as cotrustees.[223] Regardless of whether Stern is able to prevail in court against, or in a settlement with, the Marshall estate, Anna's little girl will be able to derive income from the merchandising of her mother's name and likeness. As we've seen with other deceased celebrities—from Elvis Presley, to John Lennon, to Marilyn Monroe—that can be a lucrative enterprise.[224]

Anna Nicole Smith, who wanted to be like her idol Marilyn Monroe, got her wish in life and death. Their similarities were chilling. From their blonde bombshell looks to the public's adoration, first in *Playboy*, then on screen, and from their exhilarating achievements to the soul-crushing depression that made them want to stop living. Marilyn orchestrated her own exit, helped with pills and chloral hydrate. Anna died accidentally also due to pills and chloral hydrate, a syrup sedative that was popular back in Monroe's day but is almost never used today. Information about Monroe's death is easily found online. Did Anna embrace the syrup because she knew—even subconsciously—it was what Marilyn took in her final hours? Perhaps her psychiatrist will weigh in on this someday, or maybe we'll never find out.

As interesting as their deaths are to me, I would have preferred seeing Anna and Marilyn live to a ripe old age. Instead, they will both be given permanent status as two of the most remarkable pop culture queens of our time.

STEPHANIE CROWE

Could there be anything worse for a family than to go to bed safe and sound and then wake up to learn that someone had entered their home and stabbed one of their children to death? For the parents of Stephanie Ann Crowe, the answer is yes. Not only did their young daughter die tragically in this way, but the Escondido, California, police department and the San Diego district attorney's office failed to latch onto evidence of the real killer and instead blamed the vicious crime on their teenage son and two of his friends.

This roller coaster of a case is appropriately studied in criminal justice classes because it illustrates important issues such as coerced confessions, the collection and analysis of forensic evidence, and how we as a society treat violent offenders with mental disorders.

I was brought into the case by Milton J. Silverman, the Crowe family attorney, during the civil rights lawsuit that he filed four years after the murder, against the City of Escondido, et al. Silverman felt the more I knew, the more I could be of help, so he sent me a mountain of information to review. In addition to the expected numerous crime scene, autopsy, and other photographs, I also had access to the actual clothing and bedding, along with depositions and expert witness reports from both the side of the plaintiff and the side of the accused.

My extensive written notes provide the factual background here, with additional sources, as indicated.

On Tuesday evening, January 20, 1998, police in the town of Escondido received complaints that a brown-haired, bearded bum who "looked like Jesus" was bothering people and peering into windows. Several residents phoned that this stranger was walking onto properties and saying he was looking for a woman named Tracy, who used to live there. He even walked into a home, said he was looking for his girlfriend, and stared at a woman and her teenage daughter. Another person saw him talking to himself, shouting, "I'll kill you, you fucking bitch," and demanding that someone appear and talk to him, even though nobody else was there.

Officer Scott Walters was dispatched to the scene and used his floodlight to search the areas where the man was seen. At the north end of a common driveway on Valley Center Road was the Crowe home. Walters hit the building with his spotlight but saw no motion around the home. The double garage door was closed, but to its left, the laundry room door stood wide open and a light emanated from inside. As his squad car pulled closer, a security light activated and lit up the area. Then, the door closed. However, Walters would later say he had no idea whether the door closed on its own or someone closed it. He turned his car around and slowly left the area, typing into his dashboard computer that the mysterious man was "GOA" or gone on arrival. The time was 9:56 p.m. He drove to a nearby Spires restaurant, signed off, and then went inside for a hot meal.

Ramblewood Ranch is a semirural area some thirty miles northeast of San Diego and was a wonderful and safe place for the Crowe family to raise their kids and care for their two cats and a dog. The Crowes had rented the one-story ranch-style home with a swimming pool at 24940 Valley Center Road for five years. Stephen "Steve" Crowe, thirty-five, worked as a painter at an auto body shop, and his wife Cheryl, thirty-three, was a data entry operator at a magazine distribution office. Their three children were Michael, an academically gifted fourteen-year-old high school freshman with a flair for mathematics; Stephanie, twelve, a popular student and volunteer of the year at the local library; and ten-year-old Shannon, a sensitive girl who did well at her elementary school. Cheryl's fifty-seven-year-old mother, Judith Kennedy, visiting from Florida, was staying with the Crowes while receiving treatment for breast cancer.[1]

For dinner, Grandma Kennedy had made a hamburger dish, which all three kids protested. Michael and Shannon, nursing the flu, didn't feel like eating much anyway, and Stephanie helped herself to a ready-made salad with ranch dressing in the refrigerator at around 7:45 p.m. Steve and Cheryl took their dinners into their bedroom to watch television. While her parents were eating, Stephanie walked into their room with a goofy grin and two half-pencils sticking out of her ears. "That's real cute," Steve laughed. "Now get them out of your ears before you get hurt." He asked if she had finished her homework, and she said she had, that Michael had helped her.[2]

Stephanie walked into the living room where she and her brother spread out on the sofa to watch the sitcom *Home Improvement* and then another comedy called *Soul Man*, starring Dan Aykroyd, which the siblings found "lame." They were razzing it so loudly, Judith and Shannon decided to retire to the bedroom they shared to watch the show themselves. Michael soon after went to his room, watched a few minutes of *World's Scariest Police Chases*, then turned off the TV and fell asleep. Around 9:25 p.m., Stephanie knocked on her grandmother and sister's door to say goodnight, then went to say goodnight to her parents. Both Steve and Cheryl were asleep, but Cheryl woke up enough to share an "I love you" with Stephanie, before falling back to slumber. Cheryl would later tell police that sometime that night she heard a pounding on a door or wall and also heard her bedroom door opening and closing, but figured it was one of the cats and did not get up.

Stephanie went off to her room, eager to talk to a girlfriend on the private phone her parents had gotten her for Christmas. There was much to catch up on, from news of her church, United Methodist, to their favorite movie, *Titanic*, with its teen idol star, Leonardo DiCaprio, to their male friend's birthday. Stephanie and her girlfriend chatted until 10:00 p.m., when the friend's mom came on the line to tell the girls it was time to wrap up the call. After hanging up the phone, Stephanie went into the bathroom, brushed her teeth, washed her face, and put her long, brunette hair into a ponytail. Then, still wearing her street clothes, she crawled under the covers of her bed. Sometimes, when it was cold—and the outside temperature that night was 45 degrees—she would change into her nightgown while under her covers. She was likely about to do that when someone walked into her bedroom and murdered her.

Stephanie was either under her comforter or had it thrown over her when she was stabbed nine times in the head, neck, and adjacent upper trunk. If she screamed or cried out, nobody in her family heard her. Based on the amount of blood in her bed, it appears that she stayed there for a short time, then went to the foot of her bed and crawled to the door. There is some debate as to what happened next. It appears that she remained inside the door of her room and brushed up against the inside of the door and the adjacent wall. Her brother, Michael, awoke around 4:30 a.m. with a headache. He turned on his TV with its sound down. The television's glow provided a nightlight as he made his way down the hallway and into the kitchen where he grabbed some Tylenol and a glass of milk. He thought the door to Stephanie's room was closed when he walked past it.

At 6:30 a.m., Judith awoke to hear her granddaughter's alarm buzzing. She went down the hall to see why Stephanie did not turn it off and found the door either closed or slightly ajar. Upon opening it, she found Stephanie on the floor just inside the door. She called to the girl's parents, saying that Stephanie was covered in mud. Steve and Cheryl entered the room and saw their daughter, with her big brown eyes open and still.[3] It wasn't mud that covered her, but blood. Steve's first thought was that something happened with those pencils in her ears.[4]

Finding no vital signs on his daughter, Steve turned to his wife and whispered, "She's gone." Panicked and sobbing, he moved the child from her original position inside the room to more into the hallway, and away from the bare cement slab near the doorjamb. He wasn't thinking about compromising a crime scene; he just didn't want his girl to be cold. Then he jumped into Stephanie's room to search for her phone. He pulled back the comforter on the bed and saw a pool of blood; then he grabbed the phone, called 911, and ran outside to wave down the rescue squad. When Steve reached the laundry room door, it didn't open. The deadbolt was locked and, in his haste, he unlocked the deadbolt and locked the doorknob—an odd fumble, as he would later tell police. Cheryl laid upon her daughter, trying to keep her warm and begging her to come back to life. Paramedics, who responded, pulled Cheryl off the girl; they found that Stephanie was not breathing and had no heartbeat. Their notes indicate that her jaw was in full rigor mortis.

The Escondido police began their investigation as soon as they saw Stephanie. Detectives Mark Wrisley, Ralph Claytor, and Barry Sweeney went inside the home while Officer John Johnson held an outside post. Within ten minutes of his arrival, Johnson was approached by a neighbor who told him about the transient who had frightened people the night before and suggested that the officer talk to other residents. A few hours later, another neighbor came by and told Johnson a strange man had pounded on her door the night before. Two other officers arrived, and Sweeney handed them an eight-year-old photo of an individual named Richard Tuite and told them to create a photo lineup and show it to people in the neighborhood.

Of the ten witnesses who told police they had seen the transient, two positively identified Tuite and one tentatively did. Of the remaining seven, four were not shown any lineup photos, two failed to identify Tuite, and one discounted all of the photos out of hand, saying the drifter she saw had longer hair than was on any of the faces in the photos. While some of the witnesses referenced hearing the stranger say the names "Tracy" or "Richard," officers never spoke to one resident who told someone else that the man who had banged on her door, looking for Tracy, was probably looking for a woman named Tracy Nelson, who used to live in the community and had a boyfriend named Richard Tuite.[5] A door-to-door canvass would have gotten this witness's comments on the record.

Richard Raymond Tuite, pronounced TOO-it, was a twenty-eight-year-old drifter, well known to police in the vicinity. He had served time recently for methamphetamine possession and vandalism, and while in lockup had been diagnosed with paranoid schizophrenia.[6]

One resident looked at the photo lineup, said he hadn't seen anyone the night before but recognized one face as someone he had seen five minutes earlier at the laundromat. The man he pointed to was Richard Tuite. Two officers were dispatched to the laundromat, where they detained Tuite and called Detective Sweeney. Sweeney spoke briefly to Tuite and then took him to the police station.

It's unclear whether Sweeney checked Tuite's criminal record at this point, but Tuite had amassed a great many charges over the past ten years. There were six arrests on drug charges, one for possession of a loaded firearm, five for auto theft, two for car chases and attempts to evade police, one for possession of burglary tools, one for trespass, one for vandalism, three for prowling, one for burglary, and two for annoying or molesting a child under the age of eighteen.

There were also episodes of random violence. According to a briefing I received, in 1993, at a homeless camp in Oceanside, a man had just exchanged jackets with his girlfriend and suddenly felt someone pull the coat over his head. Unable to react, he felt a "bam, bam, bam" to his head and shoulders. He had been stabbed three times before he was able to turn and grab the blade of the steak knife. Witnesses said the assault began with Tuite jumping out of some bushes and attacking from behind the victim. A bunch of men tackled Tuite and began beating him. He promised them money if they would stop. Police arrived and arrested Tuite, who denied having anything to do with the stabbing. As the victim was being wheeled away to the ambulance on a gurney, he looked at Tuite and asked why he did it. Tuite shrugged and said it was a mistake. The victim's girlfriend felt Tuite had probably wanted to target her and jumped on the jacket she had been wearing. When the victim did not show up in court, the prosecutor did not pursue the case. Later the man would say Tuite's friends threatened him with a shotgun to keep his mouth shut.

In 1986, Tuite was involved in a robbery murder, when he and two pals decided to rip off a marijuana dealer. While Tuite was digging up some pot plants, someone was shot and killed. Tuite fled and later, for reasons unknown, the district attorney chose not to file charges against him. During Sweeney's investigation, he interviewed an inmate who told him of this crime, adding that Tuite had said he fantasized about stabbing someone in the head. Sweeney wrote the information into a report but never signed or filed it. When Tuite was behind bars, he attacked at least one inmate and took a swing at a social worker. He spent a year at Patton State Psychiatric Hospital, admitted with a diagnosis of methamphetamine abuse and schizophrenia.

Tracy Nelson, also known as Tracy Ann Chaffin, would later tell investigators that while her old friend Richard Tuite was never violent with her, she knew he had stabbed a man and had been to prison. But she didn't know about his year at Patton or his mental diagnosis. She and Tuite were high school chums, who liked to do drugs together. Tracy, a pretty brunette, thought Richard was "laid back" except for when he would do speed—then he would "get weird" and imagine people were following him. Her former neighbors at Ramblewood Ranch told her he'd come around, looking for her, and each time he seemed more disheveled. Her relatives would encounter him and run him off, saying Tracy wasn't there; one time someone even found him in their living room.

Dr. Brian D. Blackbourne, the chief medical examiner for the county of San Diego, arrived at the scene that Wednesday afternoon at 12:45 p.m. He was able to examine the body at 3:30 and noted Stephanie to be in full rigor, or stiffness, and to have lividity—or discoloration from the blood settling—present in the position in which the body lay.

The autopsy of Stephanie Crowe was performed by Dr. Blackbourne the next day, on January 22. The report describes her as a white female weighing one and hundred and ten pounds and measuring five feet tall. External examination revealed evidence of six stab wounds and three incised wounds. All but two were shallow and hit no vital structures; those two, however, were deep and deadly. One entered her left armpit above Stephanie's left breast and penetrated her chest; the other struck her high on the back on the right side between her neck and shoulder and penetrated down into her chest. Both wounds transversely severed a major vessel—one an artery, the other a large vein.

Wound A was described as a 9/16-inch stab wound of the midleft cheek that penetrated upward and backward for a distance of 1/2 inch. Wound B was a jab of the left ear of unstated length; it cut into the outer ear cartilage and penetrated to a depth of 1-1/4-inches. Wound C was an incised cut of the upper right ear lobe of unstated length, and a separate 3/16-inch-long superficial cut just about the anterior margin of the incised wound. No major structure was injured by any of these wounds of the head.

Wound D was a 1-7/16-inch oblique stabbing of the midportion of the left side of the neck. The wound included a perforation of the left sternomastoid muscle, which connects the top of the breastbone to the area behind the ear. This wound cut the small veins beneath that muscle before cutting crosswise into the fifth cervical vertebra, just above the bony protuberance at the base of the neck. The trajectory was one inch deep and went rightward and backward, and the spinal cord was not injured. Wound E was a 2-3/4-inch slightly curved, very superficial incised wound of the neck from the posterior midline to beneath the right earlobe. No vital structure was injured. Wound F was a 2-1/2-inch oblique incised cut of the right shoulder, which penetrated up to 3/4 inch deep without injuring any vital structure.

Wound G was a 15/16-inch jab of the lateral right shoulder. The stab wound penetrated backward into the underlying soft tissues and left clavicle, or collarbone, for one inch, creating a 1/4-inch slice in the lateral end of the clavicle. Wound H was of the posterior right shoulder, approximately one inch below its superior aspect, or the crest of the shoulder. While this wound had an overall length of 1-1/4 inches, Blackbourne thought it might represent two separate stab-bings. This 5-5/8-inch wound went forward, leftward, and downward, through the muscles of the top of the right shoulder and perforated the right subclavian artery, below the collarbone, laterally with an exten-sive blood clot along the wound tract. Wound I was in the left anterior axillary fold, or under the armpit, and its length was unstated. It went rightward and slightly upward through the muscles of the anterior right shoulder and the pectoral muscle, and then perforated the left subclavian vein and apical pleura, or top of the lung, of the left chest cavity for a total depth of 5-1/8 inches. Associated with this wound was a left hemothorax of 375 ml, or blood in the chest cavity. Dr. Blackbourne also noted a 1/4-inch-long superficial laceration of the radial, or outward, aspect of the back of the middle segment, or phalange, of the right index finger. No other trauma was noted.

Examination of the stomach revealed 250 ml of thick tan semifluid material with partially digested portions of lettuce and intact portions of carrot shavings. No other significant findings were noted. Cause of death was noted as stab wounds and manner as homicide.

In his deposition of October 17, 2002, for the civil suit the Crowes filed against the city, Dr. Blackbourne stated that Stephanie was in full rigor mortis at 6:30 a.m. when she was found. He said she had been dead about six hours—making her time of death no later than 12:30 a.m. When asked about lividity, he said that it was fixed at the time he saw her body at the scene. The stomach contents he noted were discussed and deemed consistent with the salad she was known to have eaten. He added that he would have expected the contents to be there for two and a half to three hours. On discussing wound I, he agreed that whatever knife produced this wound went in 5-1/8 inches deep. He stated that the wound had a "little mark on the top of it, which might be a hilt mark, which would indicate it was in as far as the blade would go." At no time did Blackbourne state that he was certain that the mark was a hilt mark, although when questioned if that was the most likely explanation, he replied he thought it was.

Blackbourne was asked about a one-page report prepared by a witness for the city, Dr. Werner U. Spitz, regarding a knife detectives believed was used in the attack. Dr. Spitz had said that that knife, or one just like it, was used to kill Stephanie, and Blackbourne responded in general agreement. In a report by Jon Bedinguette, crime lab investigator for the Escondido police department, dated March 31, 1998, he discussed Dr. Blackbourne's examination of the knife in police custody and noted the doctor could not rule out that it was the murder weapon. But both reports were not scientifically precise enough to include or eliminate the police knife as having been used in the crime.

Escondido investigators never recovered a knife from Richard Tuite. The knife they insisted was used in the attack—a Best Defense brand knife—came from another source and had been in police lockup since shortly after the crime. More about that knife later.

The autopsy photographs showed the stab and incised wounds described by Dr. Blackbourne. In his autopsy report he noted that wound H was 5-5/8 inches deep and he made no comment about any contusions or abrasions around the wound. I looked at these photographs, too, and didn't see any associated trauma. Based on the autopsy description, the angle of the blade would not have prevented the noncutting side of the hilt, which was only 4.53 inches from the tip of the blade, from impacting the skin if this were the knife. But the photos show no associated hilt mark. As far as I was concerned, this eliminated the knife in police custody as the weapon used on Stephanie.

In Blackbourne's autopsy report he noted that wound I was 5-1/8 inches deep and made no comment about any contusions or abrasions around the wound. In his deposition four years later, he said that it did have a "little mark on the top of it which might be a hilt mark, which would indicate it was in as far as the blade would go." But on reviewing the photographs, I saw a small incision or abrasion that was very thin; it was only one to two millimeters from the stab wound. It was present above the wound, near but not at the lateral end. As the mark was not at the lateral end of the stab wound and the wound had no curve to it to suggest that the blade was turned, it was further proof that the Best Defense knife was not used in the attack. If the Best Defense knife's hilt had hit the skin, it would have made a much wider mark than the thin, fine mark that was present. Additionally, the mark was too close to the stab wound for it to be considered a hilt mark as the ends of the hilt were 1/4 to 1/2 inch away from the edges of the blade.

Finally, neither of these wounds—H or I—showed evidence of small tears on one edge of the wound, which could happen if the blade were pushed to its complete depth, based on clay models that were made. Photographs of the Best Defense knife did show it to have a distinctive notch on the cutting side near the hilt. The hilt was oblique with the side opposite the cutting edge almost at the same level as the end of the cutting portion of the blade, in other words, just at the start of the notch.

The afternoon before Stephanie's death, an officer responded to a 911 call at an apartment complex and found citizens restraining a man identified as Richard Tuite. He had scared two kids by following them into the courtyard and he punched a woman at random. The police report reflected that Tuite was wearing black jeans, a white T-shirt, and a red sweatshirt, but he was not taken into custody. And on the morning of the day that Stephanie's body was discovered, January 21, a woman at another apartment building near the center of town encountered a frightening-looking man with a wild look in his eyes. She hurried to her car and sped away from him. An hour later, another woman outside the complex said the stranger had followed her down the street until they were both running. She dived into her apartment, shut the door, and the man began pounding on it and ringing the doorbell. She called 911, and police found Tuite in a small, detached laundry room.

Police searched his pockets and found nothing but toilet paper—no knife, no money, no candy or cough drops, and no matchbooks. According to police statements I reviewed, although the man was evasive about his identity, officers determined it was Tuite and said he rambled on about a woman he needed to find. One investigator said that Tuite was shabby and wearing jeans and a red sweatshirt. Knowing that a local girl had been found stabbed less than an hour before, the officer eyeballed Tuite's clothing for blood but saw none. The policeman filled out a Field Interrogation form and then told Tuite to leave the premises.

Back at the police station with Detective Barry Sweeney, Tuite was asked if he knew anything of the murder that had happened the night before at Ramblewood Ranch. Sweeney assured him that he wasn't being arrested and didn't give him a Miranda warning, regarding custodial interrogation, nor did he video- or audio-tape the conversation. Tuite stated he knew nothing about the murder but had been in the area looking for his friend, Tracy. He admitted he knocked on doors but said he had not gone into any homes. Even though other officers had informed Sweeney that Tuite had walked inside, uninvited, into one neighbor's home, the topic wasn't pursued. Sweeney also didn't ask Tuite what he had been doing at the laundromat, what he had been wearing the night before, or where he slept. He didn't inquire of Tuite which homes he had visited or anything to do with Tracy. Sweeney never searched the laundromat for bloody clothes, nor did he get the laundromat's surveillance tape. And there wasn't a single question posed by Sweeney regarding the Crowe home or family. For reasons unknown, he simply concluded the interview, apparently convinced that Tuite was too mentally ill to have committed the Crowe murder.

Sweeney did collect Tuite's clothing, in a swap for a new pair of blue sweatpants, a black sweatshirt, and new tennis shoes. Tuite was photographed clothed and unclothed, and the contents of his pockets were photographed—there were three dollar bills, loose change, two matchbooks, and assorted debris. Just hours before, the officers who had stopped the transient and searched his pockets found only toilet paper. To me that denotes Tuite had a secret stash somewhere where he picked up those items—perhaps where he also left his knife.

The currency and matchbooks were not sprayed with ninhydrin, nor was the metal dusted with black powder to check for fingerprints—and none of it was checked for DNA. Sweeney gave back the items to Tuite and offered to give him a ride anywhere in the city, which Tuite declined. No samples of bodily fluids were requested or collected from Tuite, and he was released before anyone fingerprinted him—although he was found the next day, brought back, fingerprinted, and released again.

There really wasn't much reason for the police to harass Tuite. As was apparent in the police statements I reviewed, Sweeney believed that Stephanie's killer was a member of her family, and he communicated that to Detectives Ralph Claytor and Mark Wrisley. There was no forced entry at the home, so it had to have been an "inside job." The entire family was brought to the police station, separated, and forced to pose naked for photographs. Steve Crowe argued strenuously that a female officer should photograph the women, and officers finally relented.

Steve was the investigators' first suspect; they seemed to be building a case of sexual molestation and murder. Ten-year-old Shannon was the first person interviewed, and many of her questions had to do with "good touching" versus "bad touching." Only after the results from Stephanie's autopsy showed her genitalia were consistent with that of a girl who was sexually inactive did they turn their attention to their next suspect—Stephanie's brother, Michael. Over the next several days, Michael and Shannon would be housed at the Polinsky Children's Center, while the adults were taken to a motel and kept under constant police scrutiny.

The detectives felt Michael wasn't grieving in an appropriate way. He was playing a handheld video game instead of seeming miserable like everyone else in the family. When they learned the youth was into Dungeons & Dragons, a fantasy role-playing game that involved swords, the cops felt sure they had the case cracked. In particular, they doubted Michael's story about not seeing his sister's body extended from her bedroom into the hallway when he went into the kitchen for Tylenol and milk. Police didn't make the connection that Steve had moved his daughter's body into the hallway.

Detective Mark Wrisley advised Michael of his Miranda rights; he was the only Crowe family member to be Mirandized. Wrisley and Detective Ralph Claytor took turns interviewing the lad. Michael didn't think Stephanie had enemies, he stated, and didn't know anyone who would want to hurt her. He woke up that morning to the sounds of his parents shouting; he had thought Stephanie might be dead, but no one confirmed it for him. Michael told the authorities all of his actions on the night in question and mentioned hearing someone "really pounding" on the garage door, which woke him. When it stopped he figured one of his parents had dealt with it. He estimated this was before midnight. During a break, Michael called his best friend, Joshua Treadway, to tell him the bad news. Soon Joshua and another friend, Aaron Houser—both age fifteen—would find themselves suspects in the crime.

I also reviewed the statements of sociologist Richard Ofshe, a Stanford University PhD and professor at the University of California at Berkeley. Dr. Ofshe had viewed sixteen hours of the videotaped questioning of the three teen boys, even though that was just a portion of the amount taped. Ofshe, a nationally recognized expert on false confessions, called the footage the "most brutal" psychologically coercive tactics he had ever witnessed. The police theory became that Michael and his two pals conspired to kill Stephanie. Detectives isolated the boys from each other and their families and pummeled away verbally, without the boys having access to attorneys. Over days, with the kind of questioning that might be more appropriate for terror suspects at Guantanamo Bay, the police lied about evidence—which is permissible—stating that Stephanie's blood was found in Michael's room and that his hairs were found in her hand. Almost anything goes in these kinds of sessions except that, by law, police cannot promise leniency in exchange for a confession or threaten harsh treatment if the suspect fails to talk.

I recall seeing the videotapes and being flabbergasted by the way the Escondido detectives interviewed the boys, destroying, dismantling, and undermining confidence in each one's own memory. And despite the law against such tactics, the cops used explicit or implicit threats on one hand and promises of leniency on the other. They also suggested that the boys might be raped in prison if they didn't cooperate—but if they did cooperate, police would put them in protective custody where they would be safe.

Finally, Detective Chris McDonough used a Computerized Voice Stress Analyzer on all three boys, separately, telling them they failed the test. McDonough told them the machine's accuracy was above dispute, when it is nothing of the sort. Much later, the detective would call in to a radio talk show and say it was "completely irrelevant" whether the equipment actually worked.

Wrisley persuaded the Crowe boy that there were "two Michaels," one compassionate toward his sister and the other resentful and jealous of her. The detective even got Michael to claim that he had moved his dead sister, by giving her one last hug. And Wrisley asked whether a person who was stabbed in the neck, chest, or head would bleed a lot, thus searing the wound sites into Michael's consciousness.

Detective Claytor then asked Michael to write his sister a letter, asking for forgiveness. He left the room while Michael penned the following [errors intact]:

Dear Stephanie,
I'm so sorry that I can't even remember what I did to you. I feel that it is almost like I am more being convinced of this than really knowing it. I will always love you and can still remember you in life.

You have always given so much that [you] likely must be an angel. I tried to be as loving as possible to you. I'm still crying for you and I pray to God that you forgive me for what they say I did.

Sometimes I think it would be better if I could remember but I don't really want to try. The fact that I can't remember is a blessing from God. I only want to remember the way you were when you were with us. I hope that you love me forever and that I never forget what you were, a truly loving person.

They are putting me through hell and I think this is what I [UNCLEAR].

I will always hold you dear to my heart. If I did do this then I am insane, I hope both you and God will forgive me for this. We all miss you and I feel that I am being ripped from everything I know.

I never meant to hurt you and the only way I know I did it is because they told me I did. I hope you understand that I don't know what I was thinking when I did this. I hope I never remember because I don't think I could ever forgive myself if I know what I did.

I want you to know that I was not myself when I did this they want me to help them but I can't I feel because of that that I am letting you down. I should help you but I simply can't.

If you don't forgive me then I can understand. You showed me what God could do for you and now I have excepted him myself. I shall one day see you in heaven and I hope that I shall have an eternity to serve you for this.

Never forget that I always loved you.

Love, Michael

At the end of a relentless eleven-hour interrogation, Joshua Treadway capitulated and confessed his role in the murder. Only Aaron Houser firmly resisted every effort to involve him in any part of what happened to Stephanie. The police investigation revealed that Aaron collected swords and knives, and one of his knives was missing. Joshua was questioned on January 27, 1998, and said he took the knife on January 16. He just wanted to draw it and was planning to give it back, he said. A search warrant was served at the Treadway residence, and Aaron's knife was recovered under Joshua's mattress. This was the Best Defense knife that I mentioned earlier.

Joshua changed his story of how he obtained the knife, finally stating that Aaron had given him the knife five days after Stephanie was stabbed. Aaron had done the stabbing and then washed the knife off in the Crowe's kitchen sink, Joshua said. A report dated April 16, 1998, revealed that the examination of the Best Defense knife was negative for the presence of blood. This is critical because in a crime as messy as this one, blood would have gotten into the nooks and crannies of the weapon. While invisible to the naked eye, by taking apart the knife and doing chemical testing, the blood would have easily been detected. When the lab took apart the Best Defense knife, there was no trace of blood.

Michael and Joshua told police that Aaron had stabbed Stephanie while Michael held down the comforter and Joshua stayed outside the house to act as a look-out. Since it was cold outside, Joshua ultimately came into the kitchen, where he supposedly saw Aaron washing the knife.

No time was given by the boys for when they allegedly killed Stephanie. Joshua's parents heard him talking with his brother until at least 11:45 p.m., and his brother says he fell asleep around midnight, so Joshua could not have left until then. He would have had to walk to the Crowe residence, which is over four miles from his house. This would have taken him at least forty minutes, or more likely, one hour. Therefore, if he helped to kill Stephanie, it would have been some time after 1 a.m. Interestingly, Joshua had a final exam the next morning, which he had been studying for that night, and he apparently "aced" the exam, as did Aaron on the exam he took. Michael did not take the test that day due to his sister's death.

No blood, fingerprints, or other forensic evidence tied any of the teens to the crime. But several days after police had taken over the home, someone found the words "kill, kill" penciled in small letters outside of Stephanie's bedroom window. Who put it there, and when, remain unknown. The prosecutor who suspected the kids of the crime hired a handwriting expert who favorably compared the writing to that of Michael, but the expert never testified before a jury.[7]

Because Tuite's shirts and jeans were in custody, they were sent to the crime lab and tested, even though police didn't believe he had anything to do with the crime. This was standard procedure, so detectives could eliminate him as a suspect and instead concentrate on the three boys as the killers.

George Durgin, then head of the Escondido crime lab, tested Tuite's red sweatshirt with a blood-detection method known as fluorescein, which was not widely used in law enforcement, nor had it been subjected to peer-review validation studies, according to John F. Fischer, a former crime lab analyst and co-author of *Crime Science: Methods of Forensic Detection*. In fact, fluorescein sprayed on various surfaces reacted to blood in the same way it reacted to urine, soil, copper, beet juice, and knife cleaner—making it a less than reliable means of detecting blood evidence than more traditional chemicals. The fluorescein detected no blood on Tuite's red sweatshirt, even though there were blood droplets on it. Visible bloodstains discovered on Tuite's white undershirt were found to be his own.[8]

Eventually the three boys were arrested and charged with murder. Each boy had a different lawyer. Joshua Treadway had a court-appointed attorney, Mary Ellen Attridge, who led the defense in this case. She slogged through the police files and was puzzled that no real attention had been paid to the menacing transient who had admittedly been near the scene at the time of the murder and whose clothes the police had collected. Attridge asked to examine the clothing that had been recovered from Richard Tuite and had Dr. Edward T. Blake, a serologist with Forensic Science Associates, examine the sweatshirt. He identified blood spatter on a sleeve and, using DNA analysis, identified it as Stephanie's blood. This finding led to the dismissal of charges against the three boys on February 25, 1999. However, detectives and members of the district attorney's office still maintained that the three boys had killed Stephanie. Their view of the case was so rigid, they refused to consider this new information.

In January 2000, the case was turned over to the sheriff department's cold case team, under the supervision of Detective Vic Caloca. This team straightforwardly concluded that Richard Tuite killed Stephanie Crowe. Because the district attorney still did not want to pursue charges against Tuite, the state attorney general took over, and on May 14, 2002, Tuite was charged with the murder of Stephanie

Crowe. Michael Crowe, Joshua Treadway, and Aaron Houser were at last officially exonerated of involvement in the crime.

In 1998, Dr. Werner Spitz, then chief medical examiner of Macomb County, Michigan, and author of numerous textbooks about death and its causes, was asked to examine the Crowe case. Spitz's assignment was to determine whether Houser's Best Defense knife—designated as number 265—was the knife that killed Stephanie Crowe. He issued a report dated October 13, 1998, stating that the cuts in the clothing and comforter and wounds of the body were consistent with the knife. Dr. Spitz wrote that wound D, which injured the left side of the girl's neck, had dimensions consistent with that knife. Spitz also felt that wound I, which injured Stephanie's left armpit, had the same characteristics as the knife, including the dimensions of the blade and those of its hilt. Overall, he stated: "Based on the above, it is my opinion that the knife designated as number 265, or an identical knife, was the weapon used in this murder."

Mary Ellen Attridge requested Dr. John L. Thornton, a retired forensic science professor from the University of California at Berkeley, to examine the knife, plus the clavicle and vertebra that had been preserved. He issued a report dated November 29, 1998. The knife had a blade 5-1/4 inches long and up to 1-1/4 inches wide. San Diego medical examiner Brian Blackbourne had stated that the knife was 4.53 inches to the end of the hilt on the noncutting side and 5.51 inches to the end of the hilt on the cutting side, with the portion of the blade that has an edge 5.08 inches long, in other words, to the start of the notch.

Thornton measured the blade to the midpoint of the hilt in giving his length for the blade. He found that the clavicle and vertebra had no aspect that "in any way suggest[ed] the dimensions of the cutting tool used on these body parts." He made replicas of the stab wounds using Sculpey modeling/casting material, which had been baked to make it solid. He noted: "A conspicuous and wide hilt mark is seen, which is more pronounced on the upper side of the blade than on the bottom (cutting) side." This was due to the hilt being oblique and not perpendicular to the blade. The hilt side away from the cutting edge was the lower one. Also, on the cutting side, he found a notch between the cutting surface and the hilt. When he pushed the blade in to the hilt, the notch interfered with the blade's withdrawal. He stated: "When the knife is then withdrawn, the blade is unable to follow the same path it took upon entry. Stated differently, when the knife is withdrawn, it hangs up and pulls and tears the substrate rather than cuts it. The appearance of the one side of the mark is therefore not a clean cut, but a cut with a component of tear."[9]

Finally, someone was getting specific about why Aaron Houser's knife did not fit Stephanie's wounds. Detectives had had his report for quite a while—why did they choose to overlook it?

Later, when Tuite was finally put on trial for Stephanie's murder, microscopic drops of her blood were found on the hem of his white undershirt. His lawyers suggested that Stephanie's blood on Tuite's shirts had to be planted by someone or was the result of accidental transfer in the lab. They even floated the idea that a tripod used in the photographing of the crime scene might have been inadvertently planted in a pool of blood, causing dry blood to later fly onto the shirt when it was photographed back at the police lab. After an expert stated that the blood flecks would have to be in liquid form to accomplish that goal, a defense attorney stated the drops must have become rehydrated but never explained how that might happen. Dr. Thornton also characterized the tripod and flying blood theory as "preposterous."[10]

Assistant district attorney Summer Stephan requested that A. C. "Sam" Bove of Forensic Arts and Investigations examine the knife. He made test cuts into pork ribs and balsa wood using the Best Defense knife, a similar Compass knife, and a scalpel. He also looked at the right clavicle and vertebra. He concluded, based on examining only those three blades, that the Best Defense knife "is the only one that could have made the wounds to the victim's clavicle and vertebrae." It is unclear why he added a scalpel to the mix or never thought to test any other type of knife. He also looked at a faint impression on the blue top sheet from Stephanie's bed. He could not rule out that the

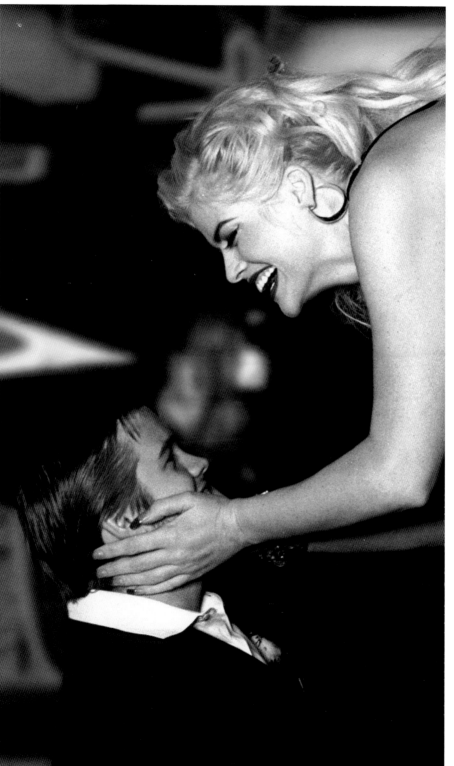

Anna Nicole Smith reaching out to her son, Daniel (*TrimSpa, Goen Technologies Corp. Photographer, Antoine Verglas*)

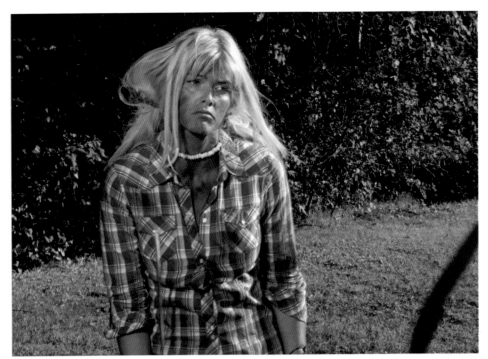

Actor/producer Anna Nicole Smith in character on the set of her 2005 cult hit spoof, David Giancola's *Illegal Aliens*. (2007, EdgewoodStudios.com)

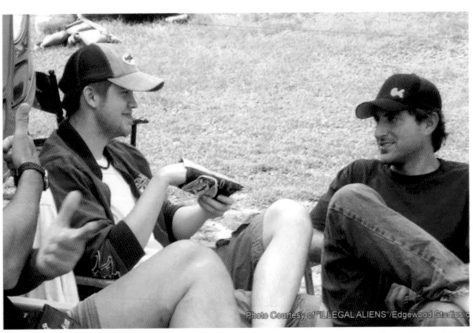

Daniel Smith and Howard K. Stern share a light moment between shots on *Illegal Aliens*. (2007, EdgewoodStudios.com. Illegal Aliens' *production photography used with permission provided by Edgewood Studios Ltd., and in the property and copyright 2007 of EdgewoodStudios.com. All rights reserved I. A. Film Profiteers LLC*)

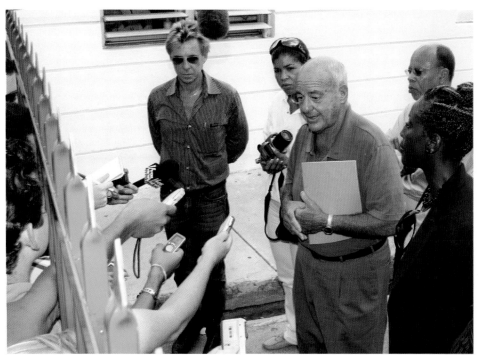

Dr. Cyril H. Wecht answers reporters' questions after performing Daniel Smith's second autopsy on September 17, 2006, in Nassau, the Bahamas. *(AP/Wide World Photos/Tim Aylen)*

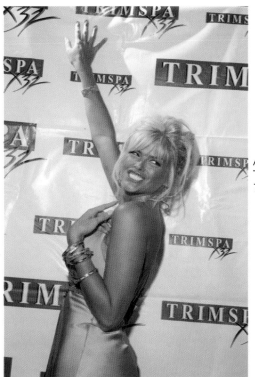

Anna Nicole, as spokesperson for TrimSpa diet plan. *(TrimSpa, Goen Technologies Corp.)*

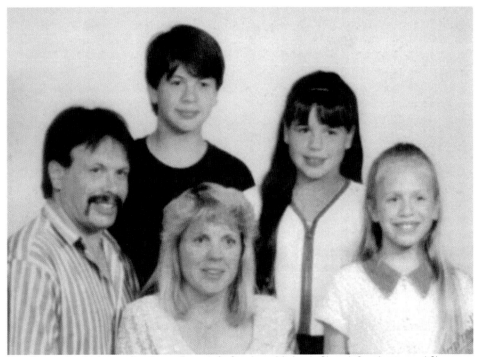

The Crowe family, in happier times. From left: Stephen, Michael, Cheryl, Stephanie, and Shannon. *(Olan Mills Photography, Inc.)*

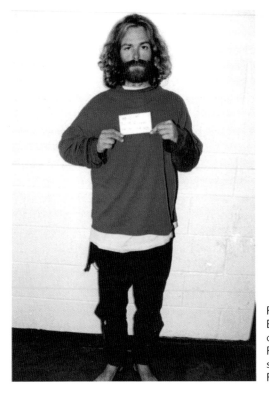

Richard Raymond Tuite, photographed by an Escondido police detective on January 21, 1998, one day after Stephanie Crowe was killed. Police missed seeing bloodstains on his red sweatshirt. *(Court exhibit, The People v. Richard Raymond Tuite)*

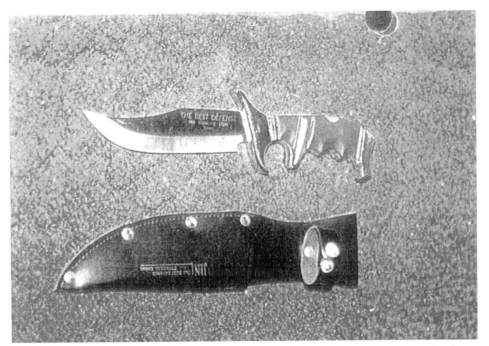

Aaron Houser's Best Defense knife, found under Joshua Treadway's mattress, had no blood on it when scientists took it apart. Richard Tuite's knife was never recovered. *(Court exhibit,* The People v. Richard Raymond Tuite)

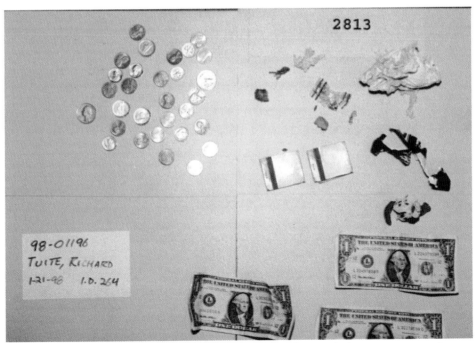

The contents of Tuite's pockets included money, matchbooks, cough drop wrappers, and a torn Snickers bar wrapper, all items that likely came from from the Crowe home and patio. *(Court exhibit,* The People v. Richard Raymond Tuite)

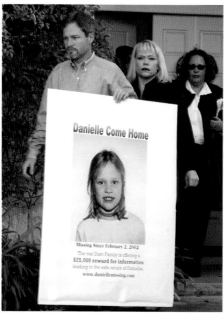

Followed by his wife, Brenda, Damon van Dam carries a poster of their young daughter, Danielle, who vanished on February 2, 2002. Note the child's distinctive necklace. (AP/Wide World Photos/J. T. Lovette)

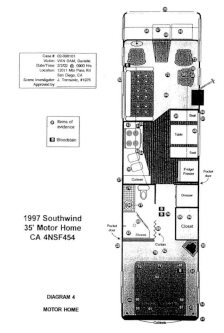

Floor plan of David Westerfield's RV where Danielle's blood, hair, and fingerprints were found. (Credit: Court exhibit, The People v. David Westerfield)

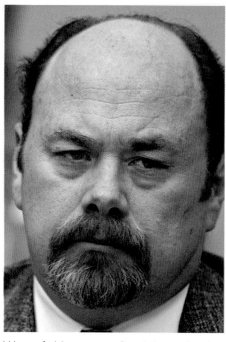

Westerfield sat stone-faced during his San Diego trial for the murder of Danielle van Dam. (AP/Wide World Photos/Denis Poroy)

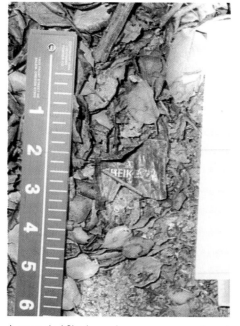

A crumpled Sheik condom wrapper was found under Danielle van Dam's body but was never linked to the case. (Court exhibit, The People v. David Westerfield)

V.I.C. Carville, LA

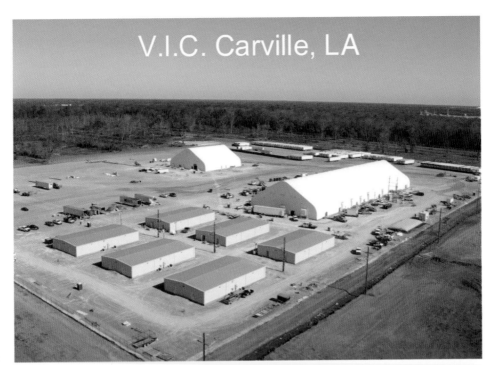

Victims Identification Center, near Carville, LA,—the "forensic Taj Mahal" for autopsying Hurricane Katrina victims. *(Dr. Frank Minyard, Coroner of Orleans Parish, LA)*

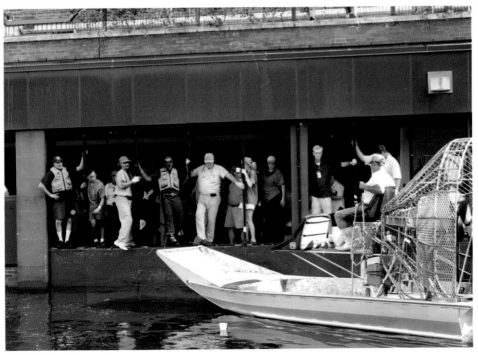

An airboat helps to evacuate patients and staffers in New Orleans, following Hurricane Katrina in 2005. *(AP/Wide World Photos/Bill Haber)*

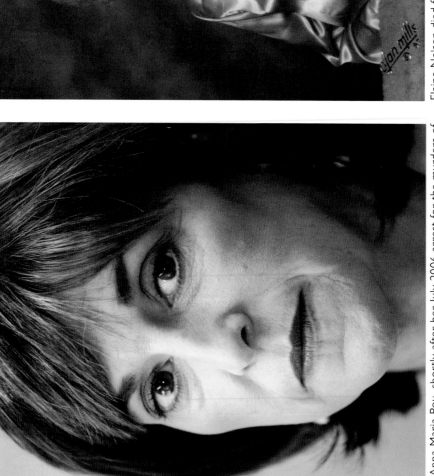

Dr. Anna Maria Pou, shortly after her July 2006 arrest for the murders of patients at New Orleans' Memorial Medical Center. (AP/Wide World Photos/Alex Brandon)

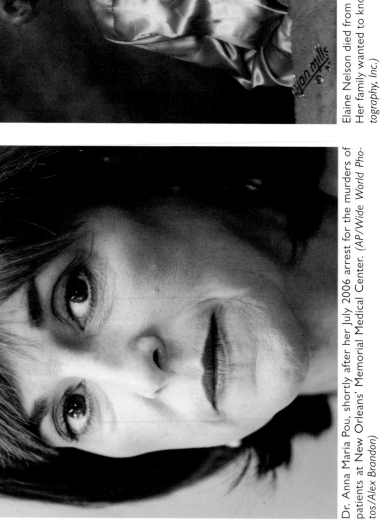

Elaine Nelson died from an overdose of morphine, fentanyl, and Demerol. Her family wanted to know why she was given those drugs. (Olan Mills Photography, Inc.)

blade of the Best Defense knife could have made the stain. He also said it could simply have been a transfer mark from her clothing or another sheet.

Brian E. Kennedy, senior crime scene analyst of the Escondido police force, examined the bedspread that covered Stephanie Crowe when she was stabbed. He, along with several other people, used another bedspread in an experiment to reproduce the wounds in the actual case. He concluded that "a single assailant is unable to hold the bedspread stable enough to focus all the stabbing in a ten-by-nine-inch area, while the victim rolled under the bedspread." Furthermore, he said only two individuals could be involved with the actual stabbing, stating there was "insufficient room" for a third person to take an active part in the restraining and stabbing of Stephanie Crowe. I believe that only reinforced prosecutor Stephan's resolve to see Michael and Aaron on the inside, committing the murder, and Joshua as the lookout outside. She apparently did not want to believe that a slovenly, mentally ill individual acting on his own could have accomplished the crime.

Kennedy reported that after being stabbed, Stephanie eventually moved off the bed, crawled across the floor to the door, "brushed her head against the wall next to the door, dripped and transferred clots to the baseboard, and left her fingerprints on the leading edge at the base of the door. After getting the door open, Stephanie crawled into the doorway and succumbed to her injuries, hemorrhaging from the major wounds of her torso and through the carpet at the doorway." He did not take into account Stephanie's father's statement that he had moved his daughter into the hallway.

Milt Silverman and his associates who were representing the Crowe family, and the lawyers for Treadway and Houser, realized that just getting the boys off the hook wasn't enough—the attorneys would have to actually solve the murder. So Milt put together a team of forensic experts who would be up to the task at hand, no matter what court venue might follow. In September of 2002, he prepared a legal brief entitled *Crowe, et al. v. The City of Escondido, et al.* to serve notice that

the family was fighting back. The first order of business was for Silverman to file a federal court claim, stating that the Crowes' civil rights
had been violated. That's when I joined the team and immersed myself
in all of the photographs, written scene reports, witness statements or
summaries of them, and other details. I reported my findings to Silverman in November 2002 and again in January 2003.

In examining the pictures, I pointed out that a qualified crime
scene criminalist would be the best person to give a detailed recon-
struction or any description of the comforter or other bedding. I
offered, however, my experience in forensic pathology and the
numerous murder scenes I have visited and examined to comment on
Stephanie's final body position and to discuss whether there was any
post-mortem moving of the body by some other party.

In the Crowe scene photographs, Stephanie was lying on the floor,
on her right side, in her doorway. Her head, neck, shoulders, and upper
chest were outside her room, in the recessed area that leads off the
hallway into her room. Her door opened into her room. There are pictures of two partial bloody prints, identified as Stephanie Crowe's left
ring and middle finger, on the hallway side of the bedroom door, as
well as a smear on the side of the door—in other words, the portion
that goes next to the door frame. This established that the door had
been opened after Stephanie was stabbed. However, there was also a
distinctive continuous smear on the bedroom side of the door and
molding, showing that the door had also been closed after the stabbing. Because of the absence of any blood near the door handle, or for
that matter, a few inches off the floor, and the absence of blood in general—except that which seeped under the door from the puddle
inside—my conclusion was and is that Stephanie attempted to get out
of the door and, in her struggle to do so, closed it.

On examining the photographs of the carpeted floor after her body
was moved, I noticed that an exposed portion of concrete was mini-
mally bloodstained—described as a fabric contact pattern in the
bloodstain pattern interpretation report by the San Diego Sheriff's
Crime Lab. The stains were at the right side—when inside the room—

of the door frame that was partially inside and outside the door frame/room. Just to the left of it was a circular area of blood, which would be more inside the room than outside it. Its circular area looked like it would have soaked through the rug. Other photos showed labels on the floor to indicate sites of blood staining. First, there was the previously described circular bloodstain. Second was a small area of superficial blood staining of the rug near the midportion of the door, which was fully opened. Finally, there was a large stain in the rug—which appeared to have soaked through in other pictures—just to the left of the foot of the bed, when looking inside the room from the doorway. There were no obvious stains in the carpet just outside her room, nor were there any described in the bloodstain pattern interpretation report. If she had died in the position she was in, then the photographs would have demonstrated a large stain under her head—but there was none. Rather, the type of stain I would expect was the one seen at the door. In my opinion, that was where her head was, and the blood then spread to seep under the door.

Below are the various medicolegal questions that were posed to me, along with my answers and opinions.

Was the Best Defense knife, or one identical to it, the only knife that could have caused Stephanie's wounds?

One cannot make such a statement with scientific validity. A forensic pathologist might be shown a knife and asked if it could have caused a specific stab wound. Typically, the only answers one can give are yes or no. By yes, one means that the dimensions of the knife make it possible that it caused the wound. The same would be true if the knife went through clothing or some other material. If the wound is too small for the dimensions of the knife, then it can be ruled out as the weapon. This means that one could be given a large number of different knives, and each in turn would be examined to rule it in or out as a possibility. If one finds a tip of the knife, then one can match it to a specific knife exactly. If one sees evidence of trauma that is consistent with a serrated knife, then one could rule out other nonserrated knives. If the knife perforates, or cuts through, something that retains its exact shape and/or dimension, such as bone or cartilage, then one may draw a stronger inference for a specific knife. If the blade only partially cuts into the edge of the bone or cartilage, it is very unlikely to give sufficient unique characteristics to say that knife is the only one that could have made the defects, unless a small amount of metal flaked off and is tested along with the knife in question to show they are identical. Finally, if blood is found on the knife that matches the victim's, then one may infer that was the knife that cut or stabbed the decedent. In this case, Dr. Spitz said that the knife, or an identical one, was the only knife that could have caused the wound without giving any scientific basis for that statement. Elsewhere in his short report he said the knife had dimensions consistent with the various wounds.

In Mr. Bove's report, after making the cuts into pork ribs and balsa wood, he tested three different blades and concluded that one of them—the Best Defense knife—had to be the murder weapon. He cited that unique cuts had been made into Stephanie's clavicle. But there were no unique features to those cuts to have enabled him to make such an assumption. Indeed, there are several arguments against the Best Defense knife being the one used on Stephanie. First, no blood was found on the knife. Second, to have impacted the skin, there was no hilt mark present. That small mark adjacent to stab wound I could not have been a hilt mark from the Best Defense knife due to its size, shape, and proximity to the stab wound. Finally, as Dr. Thornton's model(s) showed, the knife should have made a small tear if it was inserted to the notch. Again, two wounds were present, but no skin tearing was noted. My opinion was that the Best Defense knife did not create the wounds identified during Stephanie Crowe's autopsy.

Was Stephanie inside or outside her door when she was found?

Based upon the photographs, it is my opinion that she was inside the room when she died.

What was the time of death?

In determining the time of death, a number of factors must be examined and considered in arriving at a reasonable estimate. These factors include livor mortis (lividity), algor mortis (temperature), rigor mortis (rigidity), decomposition changes (if present), stomach contents with history of last known meal, and information regarding the last time the deceased was seen or spoken to.

The first four factors are all influenced by the surrounding environment. All are increased by warm temperatures and decreased by cold temperatures. However, in average temperate conditions, development of these factors is fairly standard, allowing for a more reproducible estimation of time of death.

Livor mortis is usually a purple to pink discoloration of the skin that comes from the gravitational settling of the blood. Livor is usually evident within one-half to two hours after death; it becomes fixed by eight to twelve hours, under normal temperatures. When a body is cooled, fixation may be delayed up to twenty-four to thirty-six hours. Prior to fixation, if the body is moved to a new position, some of this blood will redistribute to the new dependent areas. The sooner the body is moved after death, the more blood will redistribute. However, if movement is delayed until almost the time of fixation, then little will redistribute. For the most part, livor is not a good measurement of determining time of death but, rather, better for determining if a body has been moved after death. In this case she was found at 6:30 a.m., but Dr. Blackbourne didn't examine her until 3:30 p.m. At that time he found fixed lividity, which only indicates that she had to have been dead at least eight to twelve hours before—in other words, she died between 3:30 and 7:30 a.m. Since she was found at 6:30 a.m., it obviously had to be before then.

Rigor mortis is the stiffening of the body due to permanent complexing of actin and myosin in muscle, which is secondary to depletion of the energy source required to make them move. That energy source is ATP (adenosine triphospate). Rigor begins in all muscles at the same time and is evident first in the muscles of smaller mass, specifically those of the face around the jaw. Rigor usually begins at two to four hours after death and can be fully developed, or fixed, by six to twelve hours. There's a wide variable for this. Generally though, as long as rigor is present, even if it becomes broken (if the individual is moved), the decedent has been dead less than thirty-six hours. In this case Stephanie Crowe was found to be in full rigor at 6:30 a.m.— she would have been dead no later than 12:30 a.m. that same day.

Was algor mortis a factor in this case?

No decomposition was present on Ms. Crowe's body. Dr. Blackbourne found stomach contents consistent with the salad Stephanie was noted to have eaten around 7:45 p.m. There is no indication that she ate more at a later time. The average emptying time for digestion and movement of this kind and quantity of food from the stomach is two to three hours, which Blackbourne also mentioned. Different foods can have different emptying times, and the time it would take a garden salad to leave the stomach of a young, healthy individual would likely match Dr. Blackbourne's estimate, which placed her death somewhere between 9:30 and 11:00 p.m.

What other time line issues are there?

Stephanie was on the phone with her schoolmate until around 10:00 p.m., when the friend's mother had them finish their conversation. Based on all of the above facts, Stephanie had to be dead after 10:00 p.m. and no later than 12:30 a.m. When the stomach contents are considered, I would move her time of death to somewhere between 10:00 and 11:00 p.m. I think this was a blitzkrieg attack, with the assailant getting in, stabbing the girl nine times, and exiting the home in something that may be best measured in seconds, rather than minutes.

Based upon a reasonable degree of medical certainty, Stephanie Crowe's cause of death was multiple stab wounds of the trunk.

As the deepest stab wounds had fairly smooth edges and no evidence of hilt marks around them, I found it unlikely that the weapon that caused them was the Best Defense knife. The lack of blood on that knife also argued against it.

Based on the photographs and other case information, my opinion was that the door to Stephanie Crowe's room was closed when she died.

My opinion on the cause and manner of, and other particulars about, this death closely hewed to that of Dr. Blackbourne, who performed Stephanie's post-mortem examination.

I was impressed with the report by Gregg McCrary, the former profiler with the Federal Bureau of Investigation at Quantico, Virginia, and now head of a consultancy firm called Behavioral Criminology International. His assignment was to study the analysis written by Mary Ellen O'Toole, PhD, a supervisory special agent with the FBI's National Center for the Analysis of Violent Crime. Dr. O'Toole stated that she had reviewed various items, but she didn't identify any reports or evidence.

McCrary assessed a very low risk factor for a girl like Stephanie to get murdered in her home. She wasn't in a gang; her family was stable with no history of domestic violence or abuse. A small amount of methamphetamine was discovered in a space most controlled by Cheryl Crowe, but McCrary deemed it an artifact and unrelated to Stephanie's murder. Paul Pfingst, San Diego's district attorney in 1999, said he would not prosecute anyone for the drug, out of sympathy for the Crowes' loss of their daughter.

McCrary stated that the only variable that elevated Stephanie's risk potential for becoming the victim of violence was having Richard Tuite, a mentally disordered violent offender with a long criminal history, prowling through her neighborhood, knocking on doors, and attempting to enter or entering the homes of strangers. He outlined Tuite's criminal history and known behavior in the hours leading up to the murder and after the crime. He also reported Officer Walters's drive through the area and his sighting of the Crowe laundry room door closing. He pointed out that Stephanie was the last person in her family to go to bed that night, and she was on a phone in her bedroom that did not have a long tether. Coupled with the banging on the door that Cheryl and Michael heard, and the reports of Tuite banging on neighbors' doors that night and Tuite's entering at least one other domain, McCrary inferred that it might be reasonable to believe that Tuite was the person who closed the Crowe's laundry room door, after finding that door unlocked. Each member of the Crowe family was in his or her bedroom when Officer Walters observed the outside laundry room door closing. The logical question was who was closing the door. Walters had been responding to a 911 call from the Crowes' neighbor, whom Tuite had been harassing. Not finding Tuite at the caller's residence, Walters drove next door to the Crowes' and saw that door closing.

Dr. O'Toole stated that the sliding glass door in the Crowe parents' bedroom was noisy and any entrance or egress would likely wake up Steve and Cheryl. In fact, Steve Crowe had recently repaired the glass door to be silent. When Steve and Cheryl noticed the door the next morning, they saw that it had been opened overnight and that a vertical flap, which would often get stuck when people would exit through that door, was indeed stuck.

O'Toole estimated the time of death to be sometime after midnight and into the early hours, not recognizing the time line that Stephanie's gastric system provided when medical experts pointed more to 10:00 to 11:00 p.m.

O'Toole noted that no other criminal activity, such as robbery, seemed apparent, thus eliminating someone like Tuite—but, in reality, the photographed contents of his pockets told a different story. He had matchbooks that resembled the kind on the Crowe family patio table, and Tuite's three dollar bills and loose change was a similar amount to what Steve Crowe had put on a dresser and was missing; also, the TV on that dresser had been moved.

O'Toole also theorized that the offender was probably someone with familiarity with the home interior, but McCrary parried that with five people and a dog in the home—it was high-risk behavior, whether or not he knew where he was going once he got inside. Besides, the home was small, at only eighteen hundred square feet, and pieces of twigs found inside the next day were further clues that an outsider had been in the residence.

O'Toole believed that the attack was organized and well planned—but McCrary only spotted organization with the comforter over the slain girl's head, which might have muffled any cries and, serendipitously, minimized the amount of blood spatter or blood transfer from the girl to her attacker. Tuite had also previously stabbed a random man, after pulling the man's jacket over his head.

Post-offense behavior was also a tip-off to McCrary. Aaron Houser's teacher affirmed that his high grade on the test he took on Wednesday had to mean he stayed home and studied Tuesday night, instead of traipsing miles back and forth to commit a terrible crime. Tuite, on the other hand, was found that morning in a laundromat, after bothering at least two women. McCrary had also learned that someone fitting Tuite's description and wearing clothes similar to what the police gave him was present at Stephanie Crowe's cemetery service. And four days after cops caught and released him, Tuite was found in a Best Western Hotel parking lot, where he told a witness that this was where the "family of the kid who got killed" may have been staying. Days later, on February 12, he was arrested for telling two preteen girls, "Come here, I want to have sex with you" and calling one Tracy. He was transferred to a mental health center after saying he was suicidal, but soon after, he was on the streets again, testing door knobs, pounding on doors, and yelling for Tracy, as he had on the night of the murder. Over the next several days, he was questioned for window peeping, vagrancy, and numerous attempts to enter locations without permission.

O'Toole, one might conclude, had not revised her work to factor in that Tuite was now the target, instead of the boys. She later issued a supplemental report after reading McCrary's; she stuck to her former opinion and ignored the evidence of Stephanie's blood on Tuite's clothing. She was a defense witness for Tuite in his criminal trial and testified that the fact the victim's blood was found spattered on Tuite's sweatshirt and undershirt was irrelevant to her expert analysis.[11]

Over the next several months, Court TV produced and aired a TV movie called *The Interrogation of Michael Crowe*, starring Ally Sheedy as Cheryl Crowe, and various news magazine programs aired clips of the actual interrogation footage of the boys. Perhaps more egregiously, shortly before the start of the Supreme Court trial of Richard Tuite, a book was released in the San Diego area. Titled *Who Killed Stephanie Crowe?* it was written and self-published by Paul E. Tracy, PhD, a criminalist and University of Texas professor specializing in juvenile justice. His two collaborators on the book were Detectives Ralph Clayton and Chris McDonough, both of whom were involved in questioning the boys—McDonough operated the voice stress test. Tracy told a reporter that "I listed the detectives as collaborators . . . but they in no way influenced my judgment in the case." Tracy said there was too much reasonable doubt to convict anyone, but added: "I believe the weight of the evidence suggests it's more likely the boys committed the murder than Richard Tuite."

Milt Silverman had a ready reply, saying the book was "full of lies, half-baked truths and innuendo," in an interview with a local reporter. "These people have no shame," he blasted. "You see here Richard Claytor and Chris McDonough, the two cops in the case. I do not know of any case in the history of the United States where the two detectives who were the lead detectives on a case are writing a book to exonerate the killer of a little girl. It's sickening."[12] Causing more pain for the Crowes was the recent death of Judith Kennedy, Cheryl Crowe's mother, and Cheryl's own diagnosis of cancer.[13]

On the eve of Tuite's preliminary hearing, prosecutors also had a surprise. New eyes reviewing old crime scene photos and the photos of Tuite's pocket contents noticed that an open bag of Smith Brothers cough drops was on the Crowe kitchen counter and that a crumpled Smith Brothers wrapper was in the suspect's pocket. Additionally, he also had part of a Snickers candy bar wrapper, and Cheryl Crowe had told investigators that she would cut Snickers bars for family members to share. Along with Tuite's matchbooks that seemed to resemble those on the Crowe patio and Steve's remark about missing money from his bedroom, it would make for tantalizing testimony. It would have been preferable had the items been confiscated and forensically analyzed, but it was more than they had before.

Tuite's attorney, Brad Patton, wouldn't comment except to promise that he and his partner Bill Fletcher would point to the three youths as Stephanie's killer, rather than their client. In this most upside-down case, Tuite's defense would be using the San Diego district attorney's former strategy. Senior assistant attorney general Gary Schons, who was heading the case, along with his team of Assistant A. G. David Druliner and Deputy A. G. Jim Dutton, pledged they'd fight to get before the jury all evidence of Tuite's criminal history, mental illness, and drug abuse.[14]

In January 2004, Judge Frederic Link ruled that more sophisticated DNA testing that found Stephanie's blood drops on Tuite's white T-shirt would be allowed in as evidence. Patton's protest that prosecutors had not made it clear to him that the shirt was being tested fell on deaf ears when it was disclosed that a defense expert had been present for the testing.[15]

A month later, as the case was seating a jury, Link ruled that the fantasy writing of Michael Crowe would be admissible. Five weeks before the slaying, Brad Patton said Michael wrote a story about a brother killing his sister, utilizing mythical characters; Michael later said the story was a school assignment. Also, the judge ruled that most, but not all, of the three youths' videotaped "confessions" would be seen by the jury.

But that wasn't the real bombshell of the day's proceedings—Richard Tuite had escaped from custody.[16]

In a jaw-dropping scenario, Tuite, now spiffed up with a haircut, a clean shave, and tidy clothes, had spent the lunch hour with other detainees and bailiffs in an empty third-floor courtroom. Tuite was handcuffed to a horizontal steel pole next to a bench, while eating a bologna sandwich. He asked a bailiff to switch the handcuff from one hand to the other so he could more easily feed himself. A moment later he had vanished from the room, the floor, and the building. The bailiff was unclear why the lock failed, and no one saw Tuite leave, although surveillance footage showed him sauntering out to the street. Sheriff's deputies passed around a photo of him, asking bystanders if they saw which way he went, but the photo was from a previous court appearance when he had a goatee. News hit the airwaves and sent the town into overdrive with tips of sightings pouring in.

Before being caught, some three and a half hours later, Tuite would ride a bus across town. A woman on the vehicle desperately phoned her friend with a "You won't believe it, but that guy is on my bus" call, and the friend phoned 911. Two stops later, Tuite got off the bus and began strolling down the street. A man and his family were with a travel agent in the Auto Club office, planning a vacation, when people started whispering Tuite's name and pointing. The man, who worked as a high school security guard, announced to the crowd, "Come on, guys, we can take him." He ran outside to confront Tuite, only to realize everyone else had stayed behind in the office. He dialed 911, but the call didn't go through, so he tried flagging down a passing police cruiser, but it didn't stop. The security guard decided to follow Tuite from a safe distance. Luckily, two police officers showed up with guns drawn and one shouted: "Drop to your knees!" As Tuite complied, the man told the cops, "He's harmless. He's not going anywhere. He looks like he doesn't know if he's coming or going." One of the officers pulled a San Diego Jail T-shirt from the back of Tuite's slacks.

Sheriff's Detective Vic Caloca called to tell Cheryl of the aborted escape, and she called home to talk to Michael and Shannon. Once she could catch her breath again, she thought of Tuite and told a reporter: "This shows his stealthiness, how he sure could have sneaked into our house and killed my daughter. It takes forever to get into the courthouse. How did he get out?" Under the circumstances, Michael just had to laugh at the bizarre episode: "I was shackled to that same kind of bench and there were never fewer than two people watching me. I can't imagine how he got away—he had to be pretty wily."[17]

As the trial proceeded, defense witness Ralph Claytor—who had already resigned as an Escondido cop and moved to Oklahoma—took the stand to explain his detective work He admitted to tricking the three boys in their questioning, which he said was permissible, and he complained of making "nothing" from the book, for which he and the other detective were to split 20 percent of any profit.[18]

The next day he testified that when he had told the grand jury that the knife recovered at Joshua Treadway's home had blood on it, he might have been mistaken. "It's possible I was wrong," he said. He stated that he wasn't sure whether the misinformation about the blood being on the knife came from a forensic lab report or from George Durgin, the crime lab boss who had been touting fluorescein.[19]

On May 27, 2004, after a three-month-long trial, Richard Raymond Tuite was found guilty of the voluntary manslaughter of Stephanie Ann Crowe. Six and a half years after her senseless death, her family would finally get some closure. After watching about forty hours of interrogation tapes, the jury of eight women and four men deliberated for eight days and then found that the detectives had abused the three boys and that their incriminating statements were coerced. But jurors also found that Tuite had committed the crime without malice—what could have been a twenty-seven-year sentence for murder ended up as thirteen years behind bars on the lesser charge.

For a long while, jurors had hung at ten–to–two, in favor of conviction, until one of those who were acquittal minded inadvertently gave the defense team hope for a new trial. He spied in the jury room a poster that had not been approved for evidence, showing text suggesting that Tuite's hair might have been found in Stephanie's hand. "That turned it around it for me," said the juror, who switched his vote and caused the other holdout to give up. This accidental exposure to a theoretical piece of evidence that was never presented at trial—bolstered by the admission of the juror that he had changed his mind after seeing it and influenced another juror—would be later argued in appellate court as proof of "reversible error." If an appellate panel agreed, Tuite could be granted a new trial.

"I'm disappointed in the verdict," defense counsel Brad Patton said of his client's conviction. "It continues to be my belief that there is substantial reasonable doubt in this case." Tuite also received an additional four years and four months for his courthouse escape.[20]

Later that year, US district judge John S. Rhoades dismissed the Treadway and Houser family complaints and in March 2005, he scrapped much of Milt Silverman's civil rights lawsuit on behalf of the Crowes. Gone was the claim that police violated their Fourth Amendment rights against unreasonable search and seizure, and the family cannot sue over Michael's lengthy police interrogation or that he was wrongly arrested. While Rhoades stated that the police detectives' conduct in the interrogation was "not laudable," he felt it did not rise to a level of violating Michael's constitutional rights. Michael's statements, even if they were coerced, did not get used against him because he was never put on trial. The judge stated that the youth's arrest, and subsequent seizure of blood and hair samples, was due to a "reasonable suspicion" of guilt. Cops had no such right to demand and take blood samples from Steve and Cheryl, Rhoades said, and he allowed the parents to sue on the basis that the police wrongly took their two children away from them early on. Rhoades also found no justification for the strip searches for Steve, Cheryl, and Shannon Crowe.[21]

The following month, in more housekeeping on the case, Judge Rhoades allowed the Crowes to sue the National Institute for Truth

Verification, which manufactures the Computerized Voice Stress Analyzer; he said a jury should decide what value to place on that possible infringement.[22] A trial was scheduled but before it could go forward, an out-of-court confidential settlement was arrived at in May of 2005. Although the Crowe attorney, Silverman, referred to the device as "a fraud and a sham," the West Palm Beach, Florida, based company insisted the settlement was not an "admission of liability."[23] The updated version of the CVSA continues to be in wide usage today among law enforcement, military, and governmental agencies as an alternative to a polygraph machine.[24]

In December of 2006, the state appellate court handed down a sixty-eight-page decision upholding Richard Tuite's conviction. While the defendant's lawyer, Jerome Wallingford, argued a half-dozen reasons why his client deserved a new trial—including the glimpse of the poster in the jury room and issues regarding the DNA testing of Tuite's shirt—the judicial panel disagreed. Wallingford stated his dismay and vowed to take his case to a higher court, even though the odds were against him prevailing there. The California State Supreme Court only accepts about 3 percent of the approximately fifty-five hundred cases petitioned before it annually.[25] So it was no surprise when, three months later, the high court rejected hearing the matter. Tuite's sister, Kerri, who adamantly believes in her brother's innocence, is urging Wallingford to pursue the case in federal court. "We will take it as far as we can for Richard. He deserves it," she told a reporter.[26] In an eerie coincidence, Kerri Tuite was also touched by a random crime—in 1994, her fifteen-year-old daughter Brooke was slain while riding in a car. Police never caught the unknown shooter, but they don't believe the teenager was the intended target.[27]

Milt Silverman wasn't content to let Michael Crowe's civil rights suit be decimated without a fight. With his panoramic knowledge of the case and ability to construct powerful arguments, Silverman went to the Ninth Circuit Court of Appeals for a hearing in June of 2008. A three-judge panel heard him suggest grounds for why the case should be reinstated, including that the police interrogations of the three boys "crossed the line." One of the sticking points was that federal Judge Rhoades, now deceased, had improperly ruled that Fifth Amendment protection from self-incrimination in a coerced confession only applied during a criminal trial and not during police questioning or pretrial hearings. A decision is not expected for several months, after this book is completed. If the case is reinstated—and I hope it will be—it will head to a jury trial.[28] It's unlikely that I would be called to testify, since the issues pending litigation don't require the expert opinion of a forensic pathologist.

While I'm certain that a judgment in a civil lawsuit would be welcome to the Crowe family, no amount of money can compensate them for the loss of the lovely young girl with the radiant smile and the sweet sense of humor.

Michael Crowe is married now, has a job, and is soon to graduate from Palomar College. His family has moved to another home in the area. The California Commission on the Fair Administration of Justice recommended that police questioning for serious crimes be tape-recorded. Chris Boscia of the commission offices said: "The Crowe case is a major California case. That [video-taped] interrogation kept Michael Crowe from being convicted. They were able to see how coercive the methods were on a child." Governor Arnold Schwarzenegger has twice been asked to approve legislation to have officers videotape interrogations, but in 2006 and 2007 he vetoed both bills. San Diego district attorney Paul Pfingst lost his job when the Crowe family campaigned for his opponent. The new district attorney, Bonnie Dumanis, has Stephanie's photo on her desk—it represents all crime victims and reminds Dumanis of her responsibility to monitor police investigations.

On the tenth-year marker of Stephanie's death, her family visited her grave and spoke of the young girl who never got to become the teacher she aspired to be but whose death has taught so much to so many. "Anybody who ever said time heals didn't go through what we did," Steve Crowe remarked. "All time does is make it easier to deal with."[29]

I still look back on this case and all of its facets: How could Tuite come in through an unlocked laundry room door, lock it behind him, go down a hallway into the room where Stephanie was sleeping, commit a bloody murder, leave through the parents' bedroom—first stopping to grab some change, candy, and cough drops on the dresser and move the TV ever so slightly—and then exit from their sliding glass door, grabbing some matches from the patio table? How could a mentally ill, babbling, hairy, sloppy guy, prone to violent outbursts not be heard or seen, or leave fingerprints, shoe prints, hair, skin cells, saliva, or any trace of himself, except for a few twigs that may have come in with him or from anyone else in the household? The answer is that it was a busy household, where those who lived there came into contact with Stephanie's body and room, from the moment her alarm clock kept buzzing to when her dad moved her and her mom threw her own body on top of her daughter's. Plus there were paramedics on the scene. These individuals unwittingly covered over any traces of Tuite that might have been present—but the fact remains that Tuite, and Tuite alone, was responsible for Stephanie's death. Scores of fingerprints were taken to the lab for analysis, along with bags of trace evidence, but none of them linked back to Tuite. His fingerprints were not on the doors, so perhaps he pulled down the sleeves of his red sweatshirt to cover his fingers. Remember, this is an individual capable of canny self-survival. He didn't start shrieking and announce to the world when he slipped out of his handcuffs. No, he just quietly walked out of the courthouse, got on a bus, and kept his focus until he was out of harm's way.

I would certainly like to know who wrote those words "kill, kill" on the windowsill and when they were written. But there was never any link between that message and any of the suspects—or to the investigators, for that matter.

For all the unknowns of this case, there are many more issues that were explored and resolved—and I'm proud to have been a part of that process.

DANIELLE VAN DAM

What are the odds that two cases, very near in time and location, could both involve young girls who were murdered by assailants who boldly came into a family home while everyone slept, committed a horrific crime, and walked out, leaving behind virtually no forensic proof of having been there? While the Danielle van Dam case has distinct similarities to the Stephanie Crowe chapter we just visited, there were vast differences in the ensuing investigations and trials regarding these two girls' deaths.

Danielle van Dam was the middle child and only daughter of Damon, a software engineer for Qualcomm Corporation, and his wife of thirteen years, Brenda, a stay-at-home mom who was very involved in her children's lives. Their bustling household was in the upscale community of Sabre Springs, about nineteen miles northeast of San Diego. It was an area designed for families, with beige $800,000 tract homes, good schools, plentiful playgrounds, and, on Mountain Pass Road, friendly neighbors who barbequed together and treated each other's kids as their own.

Seven-year-old Texas-born Danielle liked dolls, spicy food, and drawing colorful pictures; she was also learning to play the piano and taking ballet lessons. She enjoyed getting her nails done with her mom and had recently gone with her father to a Dad-and-Daughter's dance at her school. On Friday, February 1, 2002, she went to bed about 10:30 p.m. Her brothers—Derek, nine, and Dylan, five—hit the sack around the same time, in their separate bedroom. All of the family's sleeping quarters were on the home's second floor. Damon, having babysitting duty that night, had played video games with the boys while Danielle read a book. At about 9 p.m., Brenda had gone out with some lady friends, one of whom was moving away soon. Brenda, the two women, and two male pals returned around 2 a.m., woke up Damon, warmed up some pizza, and then the friends left. Before Damon and Brenda retired, they noticed that their burglar alarm panel's red light was blinking, but there was no sound. They found the sliding glass door at the back of the house and the side garage door were open—not uncommon in an environment where people were coming and going all the time—so they closed the doors and went to bed. To their eternal regret, they did not look into the children's rooms.

At 9 a.m., as the boys chased each other around and Brenda fixed breakfast, a little girl from the neighborhood dropped by to play with Danielle. When Brenda went to wake up her sleeping daughter, she instead found an empty room. She yelled for Damon and they began scouring the home and yard, in vain. The boys also had no idea where Danielle was.[1]

Brenda placed this call to 911 at 9:39 a.m.:

DISPATCHER: . . . Emergency, Diane. San Diego Emergency, Diane.

BRENDA: Yes, ma'am, I have an emergency.

DISPATCHER: What's your emergency?

BRENDA: My daughter's not in her bed this morning. She's only seven.

DISPATCHER: OK.

BRENDA: Um.

DISPATCHER: How, when did you find her? Just now?

BRENDA: Just now. I thought she was in there sleeping and I went in there because someone came over I was baby-sitting and she's not there.

DISPATCHER: What's your name, ma'am?

BRENDA: Brenda van Dam.

DISPATCHER: She doesn't have any history of running away or anything, right?

BRENDA: No, no, not at all and, and. . . . Oh, my gosh.

DISPATCHER: All right, take a deep breath, OK?

BRENDA (talking away from phone): Did you find her? Is she anywhere?

DISPATCHER: What's your daughter's name?

BRENDA: Danielle.

DISPATCHER: And her last name is the same?

BRENDA: Van Dam.

DISPATCHER: That's V-A-N-D-A-M, right?

BRENDA: Yes.

DISPATCHER: OK. And how old—you said she's seven. What's her date of birth?

BRENDA: 9/22/94.

DISPATCHER: How tall is she?

BRENDA: Um, I don't really know. . . . She has brown short hair, we just had it cut, it's right to her shoulders. . . .Um, she's probably about sixty pounds. And um, um, I don't know how tall. I don't, I just can't. . . .

DISPATCHER: How tall are you?

BRENDA (talking away from phone): How tall is she? How tall is she, Damon? I don't know where she could be (children's voices in background).

DISPATCHER: OK, how tall are you, ma'am?

BRENDA: I'm five four.

DISPATCHER: OK, and, and, and is she how much shorter than you, do you think?

BRENDA: Oh, about . . .

DISPATCHER: Picture a ruler in your mind.

BRENDA: She comes up to my chest.

DISPATCHER: She comes up to your chest?

BRENDA: Yes.

DISPATCHER: So she's probably about four- . . . four-foot-, probably about, what, eight?

BRENDA: Yeah.

DISPATCHER: OK.

BRENDA: Yeah. Yeah. Maybe a little shorter.

DISPATCHER: Probably about sixty pounds, right?

BRENDA: Yeah.

DISPATCHER: And she's got brown short hair to the shoulder? And then what color eyes?

BRENDA: Um, they're green (children's voices in background). Oh, my gosh.

DISPATCHER: It doesn't look like anybody broke through the house or anything?

BRENDA: Well, last night when I came home, 'cause I went out with my friends . . .

DISPATCHER: Uh huh.

BRENDA: . . . there was a door open on the house and I couldn't figure out which one it was and it was our side garage door. But, but, um, I didn't check the bed and um, I came up . . .

DISPATCHER (interrupting): About what time did you come home?

BRENDA: I came home about two. And my husband was home with them. He was home. And he said goodnight to them and I guess he went to sleep. The back door was cracked, he said. The back door and the side garage door, he found the back door cracked. (long silence during which you can hear the dispatcher typing) Oh, my gosh.

DISPATCHER: And have you checked with any of her friends to see if she's possibly with them?

BRENDA (speaking over the dispatcher): Not yet. Not yet. I haven't.

DISPATCHER: OK.

BRENDA (talking away from phone): Damon?

DISPATCHER: OK, ma'am, we have an officer coming there.

BRENDA: OK.

DISPATCHER: If you think of anything else or if you call her friends and find out anything, give us a call right back, OK?

BRENDA: OK.

DISPATCHER: OK.

BRENDA: Thank you.

DISPATCHER: Take a deep breath and calm down. It sounds like you have other kids there.

BRENDA: I have my husband and two other children and, and my neighbor just brought her kids over. I need to call her so she can come back and get them.

DISPATCHER: OK. Think, think positive thoughts and every thing will be OK, OK?

BRENDA: Thank you. Thank you. Bye.

DISPATCHER: Bye.

(Tape ends)[2]

There was no way that Danielle walked off on her own. With each passing hour, investigators and the family had to accept that this was an abduction. But what kind of abduction? There was no ransom note left behind and no communication from any kidnapper. Damon and Brenda were the girl's natural parents, so there was no disputed custody issue. And there was no individual the van Dams knew of who could do such a thing as come into their home during the night, grab their baby, and take her away. Ridiculous. All the bedroom doors were shut—how did this monster know which one was Danielle's? Had someone been targeting her? Who? Why? Department of Justice studies show that stranger abductions make up less than 1 percent of the nation's eight hundred thousand missing children cases each year. In San Diego County, in the year 2000, of the 6,342 children who vanished, only 2 were abducted by strangers.[3] Yet a stranger abduction had to be the explanation here.

San Diego detectives arrived and jumped into action, and soon after FBI personnel joined them. Neighbors organized search parties, and as word spread on the local news stations, people arrived from all over to distribute Missing Person fliers or bring snacks and water to the command post. Friends set up Web sites with Danielle's information, and Damon and Brenda stared into TV cameras, begging whoever took their daughter to please return her. The story spread like wildfire around the nation, as reports were carried on cable news, which is how I first became aware of the case. A missing child case always grips me, being the father of four adult children and the grandfather of eleven youngsters. I've met many parents who have lost a child and I know their pain is endless. On a professional basis, the news reports reminded me of the JonBenét Ramsey case, where a blonde moppet, just a year younger than Danielle, had gone missing in her family home and hours later was found murdered in the basement. That Boulder, Colorado, case was a botched investigation from the start, which is why there have been no real arrests in the matter. As an author of a book on that case, I am frequently consulted by television hosts who want my opinion when there is news on the case, and often where there are elements of that case that appear in other crimes. So I knew to pay close attention to the unfolding van Dam investigation, because it might be one I would be asked to speak about. Weeks later, when an individual was arrested in the van Dam case and faced trial, I would become a member of his defense team.

As the investigation proceeded, Danielle's second-grade teacher at Creekside Elementary School showed police a journal that the girl kept in class, but it offered no leads. Teachers and parents fretted about how much to tell their young charges. The TV trucks and helicopters couldn't be ignored, and the kids were picking up on the panic. With Danielle still missing and her abductor unknown, how could any child feel safe? The thirteen registered sex offenders (RSOs) living within the zip code were grilled by police officers, as were the thirty-one RSOs in nearby Poway. Sightings of Danielle were called in and checked out, to no avail. In all, some nine hundred tips would be analyzed before the search was over. On one TV interview, Brenda held up a pair of flowered blue pajamas, identical to the ones Danielle wore when she was last seen, and asked people to be on the lookout for them. When I saw that, I wondered if she was subconsciously admitting to herself that the live recovery of her daughter was unlikely—as if telling people to start looking for discarded pajamas that might be separate from Danielle's body. What a terrible thought process for a mother to go through.

Search dogs from the police department and sheriff's office and their trainers went door-to-door to each of the 184 residences in the housing tract in hopes of finding Danielle. A civil rights advocate protested the move as invasive, but all the families involved eagerly volunteered for their homes to be scouted. Had anyone balked, the San Diego district attorney's office would have quickly served up a search warrant. One of the first homes searched—two doors away from the van Dams—belonged to a forty-nine-year-old neighbor named David Westerfield. A self-employed design engineer and inventor, Westerfield was a divorced father of two young adult children and lived by himself. He told a reporter, "Police asked me if they could check out my house and I agreed, of course." Two sheriff's dogs went through his home and yard but didn't "hit" on anything. Westerfield also mentioned that while he didn't know the van Dams well, he spoke to Brenda and her two girlfriends that Friday night when they all happened to be at Dad's Cafe and Steakhouse.[4] In fact, he claimed he had danced with Brenda that night and bought drinks for all three women.

On Wednesday night, the van Dams were guests on *Larry King Live*, along with John Walsh, host of *America's Most Wanted*, which would be featuring the case on its next program. Walsh had special empathy for Damon and Brenda, given that he and his wife Revé lost their first-born child—six-year-old Adam—to a predatory kidnapper in 1981. The murderer has never been found. Walsh turned his grief into activism, fought for tougher legislation against pedophiles and violent criminals, wrote books, gave lectures, and in 1988, became the star of the FOX TV network program that has captured more than a thousand fugitives to date. Walsh announced that the van Dams had taken police polygraph exams without protest and complimented the couple for opening their lives to investigators. He also urged them to never give up hope if there's a shred of a chance for a recovery. But he cited bleak Justice Department statistics that said most children snatched in stranger abductions are dead in the first four hours. Brenda told Larry King of the need to hold things together in front of her sons, but that when she hits her bedroom, "I just scream and cry into my pillow." Damon choked up when he described his last night with his daughter: "She liked to read to her brother before she went to bed. She read to him, and she was tucked in and I gave her a good-night kiss."

The family was planning a trip to Italy, Damon said, and Danielle, on the day that she went missing, had had her photo taken for her passport, showing off her new haircut. The van Dams held up the photo, which was now being used on the Missing Child poster. It showed the girl's gap-toothed grin and said she was four feet tall and weighed fifty-eight pounds. Brenda pointed out the brown, plastic looped necklace and pierced Mickey Mouse earrings with blue stones, which Danielle had gotten the month before at Disney World and hadn't taken off since. Larry asked about the neighbor whom police seemed to be questioning and, without mentioning his name, the van Dams affirmed that he had not been arrested, adding that they only knew him slightly.[5]

From Monday morning, February 4 on, police had focused on Westerfield and put him under round-the-clock surveillance. They got a judge's okay to tap his phone and took a sample of his DNA and sent it to the FBI lab in Washington, DC, for testing. Westerfield was also polygraphed, but unlike the van Dams and the many other people who were tested, Westerfield failed the exam. He flunked so badly, in fact, that the interrogation specialist said there was a "greater than 99 percent probability" that Westerfield was lying.[6] Polygraphs aren't admissible as evidence, but they were helpful here to the police in assembling the case.

Westerfield had been talking to police without a lawyer present, but that changed on February 5, when Detectives Michael Ott and Mark Keyser really leaned on him. Conflicts had been showing up in Westerfield's time line. He said that after leaving Dad's restaurant, he went home and then drove out eight miles to where he kept his 1997 thirty-five-foot Southwind recreational vehicle. He spent the next day or so racking up five hundred fifty random miles in the RV, driving around the desert of neighboring Imperial County. He was by himself the whole time, he told them. When he arrived back at Sabre Springs, he found the law enforcement and media frenzy, insisting that he only then learned that his neighbor's daughter was missing.

Witness interviews and lab results had been coming into the command center and, although detectives were careful not to publicly proclaim the balding and profusely sweating engineer a "suspect," he was deemed a "person of interest." Cops with warrants returned to Westerfield's home for another search and took thirteen bags of goods back to the crime lab. They also seized his Toyota 4Runner and RV. But when Ott and Keyser suggested they go on a friendly ride in the police cruiser—right then and there—so they could retrace the route of his desert jaunt, he had no good reason to resist and he climbed into the backseat.[7]

That evening, back at their San Diego police station, the two detectives interviewed Westerfield on videotape for forty-five minutes. The tapes were never discussed publicly until January 2003, when the *San Diego Union-Tribune* prevailed in getting a judge to order the district attorney to unseal the tapes, along with numerous transcripts, documents, and pieces of evidence. The videotape shows a small interrogation room, with Westerfield slumped in his chair across the table from Detectives Ott and Keyser.

> DETECTIVE MICHAEL OTT: Things are falling apart around you.
>
> DAVID WESTERFIELD: They've already fallen apart. . . . As far as I'm concerned, my life is over. The life that I had, the life that I was living is over.
>
> OTT: But you can't blame anybody for that but yourself, Dave.
>
> WESTERFIELD: And I have no problem with that.

Minutes later, the defeated Westerfield, who had been discussing his failures in his personal life and business, suggested that the cops leave him alone in the room for a few minutes with one of the detectives' guns.

DETECTIVE MARK KEYSER: That's silly.
WESTERFIELD: Why is that silly?

When the police asked about child pornography that had been found on his computers, Westerfield said it must have been downloaded without his permission when he was legally downloading adult porn. He wasn't sexually attracted to children, he claimed. He liked "women with boobs." And when the duo asked about his ex-wife's claim that he had used binoculars to snoop on neighbors, Westerfield just said he was "checking on suspicious activities." Cops knew that a pair of binoculars was kept in his personal bathroom, with its unobstructed view right into the backyard of the van Dam home.

At one point, Ott leveled with Westerfield that, after twelve years as a homicide detective, he knew instinctively that Westerfield had something to do with Danielle's disappearance. Ott wanted her body—and he used every possible argument about why Westerfield should reveal where he left it. The van Dam family deserves to have its child back. Let them give her a proper burial, Ott said. But when the detective brought up Westerfield's own kids—teenagers, living with their mother and estranged from their father for months—the man in the hot seat had finally had enough. Westerfield stood, called an end to the questioning, and announced that he was hiring an attorney. "I have a mind-set as to what I want to accomplish and get taken care of and allow him to do that interface for me because that's what a lawyer does," he explained.[8]

As of Wednesday, Westerfield hired Steven E. Feldman, one of San Diego's leading criminal defense attorneys, who is known to be combative and seldom misses a legal trick. When Westerfield made his first trip to visit Feldman's office, he was followed by a dozen under-cover police officers in unmarked cars and several news vans.

The saturation of media coverage brought out one witness who would help narrow the police search. Dan Conklin was a tow truck driver who specialized in assisting recreational vehicles that were stuck in the desert sand, and he told police he had spent two hours on Saturday, getting Westerfield's RV out of a rut. After the vehicle was freed, Westerfield was in such a hurry to get out of there, he left behind his motor home's leveling ramps, Conklin said. Soon law enforcement helicopters and more than three hundred volunteers began doing grid searches of the area.[9] Conklin would later amend his encounter with Westerfield as happening on Sunday, not Saturday.

On the home front, the van Dams were responding to whispers over their lifestyle after callers to a local radio program stated they were pot smokers who also indulged in promiscuous sex acts. At a news conference on her front lawn, Brenda begged reporters not to concentrate on "distractions," such as rumors about their private life. "We are here today to focus on finding Danielle."[10] If she thought that would stop the wagging tongues, she was mistaken. Soon the names of other women alleged to be the van Dams's sex partners were bandied about.

To try to stem the avalanche, Damon and Brenda appeared again on *Larry King Live* on Monday, February 11. After announcing that there was now a $25,000 reward for the safe return of Danielle, King asked about the "spousal swapping" rumors that had been swirling in the local media and on the Internet. The van Dams both refused to talk about the situation, so Larry pressed on. "Personal life is nobody's business, but when people come in the spotlight as you two have, you know how reporters are," King said. "If you're not denying the story, do people who live this lifestyle—does that mean you might be less attentive to children, since most people don't have that lifestyle?" Again, Damon and Brenda refused to answer the question.[11]

It was an uncomfortable spot for them, but also for their supporters who might have hoped to hear a resounding denial. As the press macerated this over the next several days, making the Sabre Springs community sound like *Peyton Place*, a hearty debate ensued over how the rumors, if true, might impact the investigation. Did the van Dams allow someone with an unsavory, high-risk sexual appetite into their home? Were they holding back information that could solve the crime because it reflected poorly on them as parents or people? Were their three children aware of any sexual high jinks or drug usage? Should the two boys be removed from the family home and put in protective custody? And how well did they actually know David Westerfield, their neighbor who said he danced with Brenda at Dad's but she maintained she hardly knew? Was he a fall guy? Was there some other scenario in play?

As I watched the coverage, I felt that the rumor alone would be helpful for any defense case, and that if it were substantiated, the van Dams could lose sympathy in the court of public opinion. But the nagging thought remained: If consenting adults engaged in private sexual behavior, and even marijuana use, outside of their children's view, could they still be considered good and loving parents? I had to say yes. I didn't think the van Dams owed the world press any explanation for their personal lives, but I strongly hoped they were sharing any and all details with investigators.

Over the next several days, the reward for Danielle's safe return zoomed to $175,000, and her pink and purple bedroom was searched even more carefully. A bloodhound was brought in to try to detect Westerfield's scent in the van Dam home, and a more proficient chemical method was used to try to pull up foreign fingerprints in the room. Homicide detectives refused to share their findings, saying only that they were not ready to make an arrest in the case.[12] Searches continued in dumpsters, sewers, riverbeds, and any place handy for disposing a body. Despite the gossip surrounding them, the van Dams wisely stayed in the media spotlight because their daughter's plight outweighed their own embarrassment.

To a local reporter, Brenda theorized that since Danielle was such a heavy sleeper, she probably didn't wake up when her abductor lifted her from her canopy bed, brought her downstairs, and left the house with her. If she cracked her eyes open at all, she probably thought she was safe in her daddy's arms. Brenda also explained that while they had a sleek, gray Weimaraner named Layla, it never barked—it had been raised in a kennel where other dogs of that breed had had their larynx surgically removed, so Layla didn't "learn" to bark.

Brenda also elaborated more on David Westerfield, telling the reporter that he had never been invited into the van Dam home but that she, Danielle, and Dylan had been in his home the week before when they were going door-to-door, selling Girl Scout cookies.[13] When he asked them in and bought four boxes of cookies, it was the first time she ever learned his name, although they had recognized each other from a January 25 outing at Dad's. That night he had bought her a cranberry juice and vodka cocktail and flirted with her female friends. While the kids ran around his backyard swimming pool, Westerfield told Brenda he wanted to meet her pals. Tell them you have a rich neighbor to introduce them to, he chuckled. She replied that they might all be at Dad's on Friday night, if she could get a babysitter— her husband was going to be out of town, she recalled telling him. As she and the kids left, Westerfield jotted down her phone number and mentioned that he "had adult parties and barbecues." Brenda would later say she wasn't sure what he meant by "adult parties." She was so unsettled by the remark that she called Damon at work when she got home and told him about it.[14]

Brenda also wanted to clarify to the reporter that she never danced with Westerfield at the bar, despite his telling that to the *San Diego Union-Tribune*. She introduced him to one of her friends that night and saw them drinking together. Brenda danced and played pool, but not with Westerfield. When she and her friends left the bar, he had already gone. The three women ran into two other friends, both males, and all five went to the van Dam home for pizza with Damon.[15]

On February 22, after lab results found Danielle's blood on Wester-field's jacket and in his motor home, he was arrested for burglary and the kidnapping of Danielle van Dam. He was jailed without bond and, on February 25, spent his fiftieth birthday behind bars, isolated from other prisoners for his own protection. Would all of his birthdays from now on also be spent in lockup?

Born in Southern California, Westerfield moved to Maine for a while, and then returned to the San Diego area where he got a job as a draftsman. An early marriage when he was twenty-one lasted six years and produced no children, but he wed again in 1979. A son, Neal, and daughter, Lisa, were born before that marriage ended in divorce. In 1996, Westerfield was arrested for drunk driving—he pleaded guilty, paid a $1,325 fine, and received five years probation. The next year he moved into his four-bedroom home in Sabre Springs. A woman he was dating and her teenage daughter, also named Danielle, lived with him for some of 2000, but the mother found photos of her bikini-clad daughter on his computer, including shots with the girl's legs spread apart.

He bragged of being a Mensa member, but the local branch didn't show him on its roster when police asked them to check. Through his company, Spectrum Design, Westerfield holds patents on three medical inventions: a pulley device to help people undergoing rehabilitation for injured bone joints, a surgically implanted prosthesis to replace joints, and a device that aids in joint rehabilitation—the last two inventions share creative credit.[16]

Under California law, kidnapping someone under fourteen years of age carries a maximum sentence of eleven years in prison. However, kidnapping with intent to sexually assault carries a potential life term. Presumably this was a sexually motivated crime, but without Danielle's body—and probably even with it—there might not be proof of a sex crime. Was there enough proof that a murder occurred? So far the only charges were burglary—for the illegal entry into the van Dam home—and kidnapping.[17]

That answer came on February 25—Westerfield's birthday—when

San Diego district attorney Paul Pfingst added a murder charge to the list. "After consulting with Police Chief David Bejarano, my prosecutors, and the van Dam family, I must conclude that Danielle is no longer living and was killed by her abductor," he told reporters. "Today I am announcing my office will file one count of murder against David Westerfield for the abduction and killing of seven-year-old Danielle van Dam." A murder charge with special circumstances, such as kidnapping, could bring the death penalty for the defendant, if convicted—but Pfingst wouldn't say whether he would seek it. The district attorney did say that the reason for filing the murder charge now, the day before the arraignment, was to avoid a possible legal minefield. If Westerfield were to plead guilty immediately to the kidnapping and burglary charges, his attorney might be able to argue double jeopardy if a murder charge was to be brought later. It's not an issue they would want to test, Pfingst explained.[18]

A misdemeanor count of possessing child pornography would be added after evidence technicians waded through Westerfield's multitudinous computer files, CD-ROMS, DVDs, and videos. Of the approximately sixty-four thousand pornographic images and twenty-two hundred MPEG-format videos, including scenes of bestiality and bondage, many featured females who seemed to be underage, but it was impossible to know whether they were minors. Fewer than one hundred images and videos featured children who were indisputably under age, and they were logged on zip drives under titles such as "youngones," "tooyoung2," "Lolita.com," and "youngvirgins.nu." Some of the most offensive of these were Japanese animes, or animated videos, usually featuring sexual situations and maybe a bit of edgy behavior. But these examples Westerfield had were extreme, with some showing little girls crying as they were being held down by adult males and raped. One cartoon's victim was a young blonde girl in pigtails, similar in appearance to Danielle van Dam.[19]

All of the pressures were mounting for Westerfield, who was in the downtown San Diego jail. Feldman, and his co-counsel Robert Boyce, had advised him that the game was over—he needed to tell authorities where Danielle's body was, in exchange for prosecutors dropping the death penalty and letting him serve a life sentence in prison without the possibility of parole. On February 27, the two lawyers had their client's permission to nail down the deal with the prosecutors. But when the attorneys got to the Hall of Justice, members of the media were gathering, and someone told them that a searcher in the desert had found a body that was very likely that of Danielle van Dam. The prosecutors gave the defense counsel a map of a rural area east of El Cajon, marking a spot off Dehesa Road, between Sloane Canyon Road and Willow Glen Road. The plea bargain evaporated and would never be mentioned to the jury during the trial.[20]

Dr. Brian Blackbourne—the chief medical examiner for San Diego county, who performed the autopsy on Stephanie Crowe—was called to the scene, along with local entomologist Dr. David Faulkner, from the San Diego Natural History Museum. While the nude body was partially mummified and decomposed, and parts were missing due to animal activity, there could be little doubt that it was Danielle. Her face, even in its leathery and blackened condition, with its eyes missing, resembled the little girl, and her light brown hair was still attached to her scalp. Around her neck was the brown, plastic looped necklace she loved so much, and the cartilage of her ears still sported the Mickey Mouse pierced earrings, with one of the backings missing. She was found on a brushy hillside, under an oak tree. No clothing was found at the scene. A Sheik condom wrapper was under the body, but it was never linked to the case.

In his official report—which I received, along with all other pertinent documentation and photos when I joined the defense team—Detective James Tomsovic noted that the body "seemed posed." She was on her back, with her head turned to the side and resting on her right hand, with her left arm extended straight out. The left foot was missing at the ankle, and both ankles were about eight inches apart. Both thighs and the upper torso were stripped of flesh, and the odor of putrefaction was evident but relatively mild. The torso and head were infested with maggots and tiny flies, and black beetles were present in the abdomen. Dr. Faulkner collected the insect evidence, and other investigators processed the scene for trace evidence. Then paper bags were placed over the head, hands, and feet, and the body was wrapped in a white sheet, put into a vinyl body bag, and taken to Blackbourne's morgue. Investigators noticed tire and motorcycle tracks in the vicinity, but none appeared suitable for casting. Soil samples, underbrush, and trash were all collected and sent to the lab.

The next day, Dr. Blackbourne performed the autopsy on the body. The deceased was fifty-one inches tall and weighed thirty-six pounds. Through dental records and DNA taken from one of the victim's ribs, a positive identification would be made to Danielle van Dam. Tape lifts and trace evidence from the body were collected by forensic specialist Dorie Savage and criminalist Tanya DuLaney and sent to the lab. The mummified hands were given to fingerprint specialist Jeffrey Graham Jr., who rehydrated them until he could make prints, which he would later link to one palmprint and one fingerprint found in Westerfield's RV, on the wall near the bed. Forensic odontologist Dr. Norman Sperber—who had worked on many high-profile trials across the nation, from Ted Bundy's to Jeffrey Dahmer's—was also at the van Dam autopsy. He noted that Danielle's mouth was missing four upper front teeth, only one of which was found in her oral cavity. Dr. Sperber would testify that there were no signs of fracture or trauma to the mouth and that it was possible that decomposition could have loosened the teeth from the alveolar bone. Neither the missing three teeth nor Danielle's left foot were ever recovered.

Dr. Blackbourne's autopsy report and subsequent testimony reflected that while Danielle's skin and muscles were missing from her chest, her organs were intact. He collected fluid samples from each pleural cavity for toxicological testing. The heart and lungs were decomposed, but the valves and arteries seemed normal, and the lungs had some edema. Below the rib cage, organs were missing because of animal activity. The liver and right kidney were partially present but decomposed, and the bowel was intact but extruded. The genitalia were all missing, due to scavengers, and the pelvic organs and tissues were decomposed. He identified a portion of the rectum and swabbed it and gave the swabs to the criminalist. Later he looked at the rectal piece microscopically but found only bacteria and no mucosal cellular lining, which might have been tested for signs of sexual activity. He looked for any tubular structure that could be a vagina and found what was probably the bladder, so he swabbed it, but it, too, lacked mucosa when seen under the microscope. He also swabbed Danielle's mouth, seeking evidence of sexual involvement, even though he admitted that the longest he had ever seen sperm last in a dead body was five days. Without some evidence of sexual trauma, Westerfield could not be charged with rape, even though that was certainly the prosecution's theory behind what motivated Westerfield to kidnap and kill the girl.

While Blackbourne was able to assert that Danielle's case was homicide, he could not determine the cause of death. There were no bullet or stab wounds, no ligature marks, and there was no damage to the hyoid or thyroid cartilage, which can happen when someone is strangled. Blackbourne admitted the one method of death that might have been employed was asphyxiation, that something was placed over her mouth and nose until she stopped breathing. Often, fingernail marks or abrasions will show up on a smothering victim, but with the mummification, no subtle marks could be observed on Danielle. A pillow or plastic bag over her head could result in her death without leaving telltale signs, he said.

Perhaps most important, Blackbourne was not able to pinpoint the exact time of the girl's death, except to say the decomposition and other factors were consistent with occurring during the three and a half weeks she had been missing. This was a critical question because Westerfield had been under 24/7 surveillance from the time he returned to Sabre Springs after his trip to the desert. If he killed Danielle, he had to have disposed of her before February 4. Any suggestion that she was placed in the dumpsite after that would exclude him as a suspect. I was brought in as a defense expert in May to determine whether my review of the materials would provide an alternative opinion from Blackbourne's.[21]

In the past, I've made jokes about California murder trials being stretched to absurd lengths. While the murder trials of O. J. Simpson, Scott Peterson, Robert Blake, and Phil Spector meandered for months before getting a verdict—with Simpson and Spector getting subsequent trials—*The People v. David Westerfield* was a model of efficiency. From the preliminary hearing, through the eight-week trial, to the sentencing phase, it was presented well and packed with interesting testimony from a broad variety of forensic disciplines.

Presiding over the proceedings was the Honorable William D. Mudd, a fourteen-year veteran of the San Diego Superior Court and formerly a civil attorney. Known for his dry wit and even hand, Mudd made headlines in a previous trial of a man who killed a neighborhood bully by reducing the murder conviction to manslaughter. The prosecution team was led by Jeff Dusek, a former pitcher for the Chicago White Sox's minor-league team, who had been a prosecutor for the past twenty-five years. A low-key yet meticulous advocate, Dusek was the office's most experienced prosecutor of capital cases; he had previously sent three men and a woman to California's death row. His chief associate was George "Woody" Clarke, one of the nation's leading DNA experts, who lent support to Los Angeles prosecutors during the Simpson criminal case. They would be well matched against Westerfield's attorneys, Feldman and Boyce, both of whom earned rave reviews for their creative defense tactics in earlier cases. Feldman, known for his energetic gesticulations to connect with a jury, was awarded a public service honor from the local defense bar after winning acquittal for a murder defendant who had spent five years in jail awaiting trial. In another murder trial, Feldman's client was found not guilty after the jury only deliberated for twenty-five minutes.[22]

The public, which had invested so much time and interest in the disappearance of this young child, would be able to watch her get justice when Judge Mudd allowed Court TV to broadcast the trial, gavel to gavel. The channel's ace reporter, Beth Karas—a former Manhattan assistant district attorney—would provide her usual outstanding color commentary outside the courthouse. The trial would bring a ratings bonanza to the cable channel, as it was preparing to promote its upcoming made-for-TV movie, *The Interrogation of Michael Crowe*, which was in production during the Westerfield trial.[23] While I spent most days in my office and missed the live trial coverage, sometimes I would see a report on one of the nighttime cable shows when I got home—but at this time I only had a general sense of what was going on in the case, not an up-close view.

Opening statements began on June 4, 2002, before a jury of six men and six women, with six alternate jurors. A preliminary hearing before a different judge in March—also televised—had outlined the prosecution's case against Westerfield, and Dusek's opening revisited those points and added new information. Thanks to excellent legwork, police got to a dry cleaner where Westerfield had dropped off his green sports jacket, two comforters, and two pillow covers, recovering the items before they had been cleaned, which would have lost valuable forensic evidence. Instead, lab technicians found Danielle's blood on Westerfield's jacket and hairs from the van Dam dog on the comforter, likely a result of secondary transfer from Danielle. And there would be more forensic bombshells, Dusek promised.[24]

Among the first witnesses were Brenda and Damon van Dam, who recounted their life with their daughter and the agony of discovering her missing. Judge Mudd had not allowed them to sit in the courtroom prior to their testimony, but after they finished on the witness stand, they sat in the front row for the rest of the trial, except for a brief banishment of Damon when he was caught grimacing at Westerfield. The van Dams had to remove buttons with Danielle's face, which they had worn on their lapels, when the judge agreed with a defense argument that the buttons might be prejudicial.

Both parents confessed to smoking pot on the night Danielle went missing, saying that on occasions when they would indulge in a few puffs from a marijuana cigarette, it would be in the locked garage and away from the children. While Feldman seemed to mock the parents here by pantomiming taking a drag off a joint, he ironically was an advocate for legalizing marijuana use, as one of the members of the state legal committee for NORML, the National Organization for the Reform of Marijuana Laws. As such, he would defend people charged with marijuana use, sometimes for no fee.[25]

Asked about their sex lives, the van Dams told the courtroom under oath what they wouldn't divulge on *Larry King Live*. They didn't think of themselves as "swingers," because they did not go to clubs to engage in extramarital sexual activities. They had, a few times, invited various female friends to join them in their bedroom—again, away from the children—or at someone else's home. One of the women who went to Dad's that night with Brenda and came back to the van Dam home was someone they had been intimate with. At Dad's she dirty-danced with the other female friend and tried to grab Brenda's breasts. But later, as the pal went into Damon's room to wake him, he only kissed her and rubbed her back before they both went down for pizza. Nothing else happened of a sexual nature that night.[26] Some of the jurors would later say that the sex and drug testimony had no detrimental impact on how they viewed the van Dams.

Damon told the court that he was supposed to be on a business trip on February 1, but it had been postponed. That supported a statement from one of the detectives who testified that Westerfield had mentioned he thought Danielle's father had been out of town when he saw Brenda at Dad's restaurant.

Other prosecution witnesses included the following: a neighbor of Westerfield who noticed that all of his shades were drawn on the morning of Danielle's disappearance, something she said was unusual; numerous people who saw Westerfield's motor home during his trip, including some who said the RV had not been in the Sabre Springs area for weeks; a first-time visitor to the van Dams who was not barked at by the dog; various campers at Silver Strand State Beach who noticed the RV's shades pulled down; the tow truck driver who said he heard voices inside Westerfield's RV when he helped him get out of the sand, although he couldn't hear what they were saying; a detective who saw Westerfield's shopping list, with the word "bleach" at the top; an FBI lab expert who said bleach is often used to diffuse DNA; forensic specialist Karen LeAlcala, who seized clothes from Westerfield's home clothes dryer and found hairs in the sink trap of his RV; a second fingerprint examiner who confirmed Danielle's prints in the RV; blood analysts who found Danielle's blood on Westerfield's jacket, as well as a spot of her blood on the floor of his RV; DNA experts who affirmed the matches; and another San Diego police criminalist, Jennifer Shen, who said orange acrylic fibers entwined in Danielle's necklace matched those found on a blanket on Westerfield's bed.[27]

In July, as Feldman and Boyce were into their defense case, I flew to San Diego and drove with them to the Dehesa recovery site. Later we went to where Westerfield's motor home was being held and did a walk-through of it. Being one of the few Americans who hadn't been watching any of the televised trial, I had to be brought up to date on what witnesses had said. The attorneys advised me that they would like to call me to the stand that next day, although I told them I had nothing to add that would differ from Dr. Blackbourne's opinion. This was unquestionably a homicide, but from a forensic pathologist's viewpoint, with the severely impaired condition of the body, there was no way to give an exact cause or time of death. Instead, I argued that while their examination of me might net them some points, in terms of my years of experience, on cross-examination I would have to answer questions that could harm the defense. If Dusek asked me about whether Danielle was smothered with a pillow—something I, like Blackbourne, thought probable—why reinforce that image with jurors? Even my stating that there was no way of proving a rape had occurred would remind jurors that there were all of these other reasons, such as the violent animated porn and Danielle's palmprint and fingerprint near Westerfield's bed, that would point to rape as almost surely a motivating force. I encouraged Feldman and Boyce to hammer away on the forensic entomologist front, where there are often more divergent opinions. Sure, if I testified, I could charge the attorneys a lot more money, but I wasn't comfortable with that, ethically. They asked if I would stay that night in a local hotel and be available to come to court if they decided to call me, which I agreed to do. The next morning, I got a call that they concurred that my testimony wasn't necessary, so I wished them well and flew home to Pittsburgh. I never met David Westerfield.[28]

Defense witnesses included the following: a neighbor who saw Westerfield's RV unlocked on their street at least once, giving credence to a suggestion by Feldman that Danielle might have gone into the RV at some previous time and cut herself or had a bloody nose, which could account for her blood and prints there; a computer security expert who testified that Westerfield's eighteen-year-old son might have downloaded the child porn onto his dad's computer; various people who saw Brenda and her girlfriends at Dad's, partying hard, and some who said they saw Westerfield and Brenda dance together provocatively; friends of the defendant who attested to his spur-of-the-moment camping trips; and an ex-girlfriend who still cared for Westerfield but said he "changes" when he drinks.

Some witnesses created confusion or fireworks. The trainer of the cadaver dog, who allegedly hit on an outside compartment of the RV, would later admit to not reporting the dog's reaction to police for weeks. Also, an e-mail was found on the day of Westerfield's arrest, in which the trainer wrote that perhaps the dog's cadaver alert was done to please the trainer, and Detective Tomsovic testified that he didn't see the dog react to the compartment. The founder of Quest-Gen Forensics in Davis, California, which specializes in animal DNA, stated that Layla's dog hairs were found in the RV, but the expert also made a mathematical error in her computations and stated that she had a "spiritual" connection with her DNA sequencing duties. One of the detectives disputed a defense photo that allegedly showed her wearing an orange shirt at Westerfield's home, which Feldman suggested was the source of the orange fibers on Danielle's necklace. She stated that her shirt was actually red in color, and criminalist Tanya DuLaney microscopically compared the fibers and said the red one was not a match. And Westerfield's teenage son, Neal, was called as a reluctant prosecution witness to clarify his connection with the pornography. A college student, he said he liked to use his dad's computer because it had Internet capacity, unlike his own. He admitted downloading material from adult sites, using his password "Bob Dole"—the name of the conservative former US senator got quite a laugh from the folks in the courtroom—but that while he saw nude females on his dad's hard drive, the women were all adults. He said he never saw any of the zip drives with the child porn.[29]

The biggest controversy came as a result of the dueling entomology experts who tried to ascertain when the body was left in the desert. Making insect testimony interesting to a jury is always a challenge—there's always the chance of boring them with statistics or just plain repelling them. Generally, scientists can narrow the time of death of a body from the age of the insects, usually flies, scavenging it. While a medical examiner depends on rigor mortis, body temperature changes, and level of decomposition to set a time of death, after a couple of days those windows of opportunity pass and, with that, the chance of narrowing the timeframe. But a forensic entomologist will assess each insect's life cycle to get a more accurate reading, a discipline that is being used more frequently in courts these days. Some of the insects taken from a body are kept alive in a container with a piece of liver, so they can complete their life cycle, and others are preserved with alcohol and studied microscopically. Insects can also be liquefied in a blender to determine whether the deceased had alcohol or drugs in his or her system, if the human's body is unable to provide samples for toxicology testing. A fly can smell a dead corpse from a mile to a mile and a half away, get to it within hours, and begin laying its eggs; a day or so later, larvae, or maggots, evolve. The prepupal stage takes another five to twelve days for the maggots to feed on the flesh. In the next, or pupal, stage, the maggots migrate from the body, shrink in size, and get a protective cocoon. The adult fly then grows inside that shell, or pupae. On average, it takes about fourteen to twenty-four days for an egg to reach an adult fly stage, but weather and humidity are key factors in its development. In warm weather, a fly can survive about three weeks, but a cold climate can extend its life to six months. Wrapped bodies or those buried in a shallow grave will slow down the flies' efficacy.

Prosecution rebuttal witness Dr. William Rodriguez, a forensic anthropologist, testified that Danielle's diminutive size might have caused her body to mummify more quickly than an adult's body would and that the process might have begun within twenty-four hours after her death. He also stated that the condition of Danielle's body might have delayed the flies from entering it and that fly larvae might have been carried away by ants. Based on the gross physical condition of the body, he estimated that the date of death was between four and six weeks of discovery. The body was found on February 27, so his earliest estimate was an impossible January 23, since Danielle was safe in her home until the night of February 1. Dr. M. Lee Goff, chairman of the forensic sciences department of Honolulu's Chaminade University, said he understood Rodriguez's four-to-six-weeks estimate but thought that the body was more likely disposed of between February 2 and 12. On cross-examination Feldman found five mathematical errors in Goff's assessment of the post-mortem interval. The lawyer also cited that one of Goff's comments about Danielle's time line contradicted a similar situation the professor had mentioned in a textbook he co-authored.

In a surprise move, Dr. David Faulkner, the entomologist who went to the dumpsite, witnessed the autopsy, and collected and analyzed insects from both locations, testified for the defense, rather than for the prosecution. His "very confident" estimate of when Danielle died was between February 16 and 18, long after Westerfield was in custody. Indiana-based Dr. Neal Haskell, one of the nation's most sought-after forensic entomologists, estimated that the flies only found the remains after February 12 and probably more likely the fourteenth. Defense rebuttal witness Robert D. Hall, whose father authored a classic textbook on forensic entomology, testified that flies are resistant to drought and that his time of death estimate was between February 12 and 23, but there was some evidence that set the date back to February 1. He admitted the wide variance in dates among all the experts was "unusual."[30] So how did jurors react to all of the insect testimony? According to statements made after the trial, they ignored it. David Westerfield never took the stand in his defense, not that it was required of him.

On August 21, 2002, jurors convicted David Westerfield for the kidnapping and murder of Danielle van Dam. They deliberated for forty hours over ten days, asking for readbacks of testimony from Drs. Blackbourne and Faulkner and the criminalist who matched the orange fibers in Danielle's necklace to Westerfield's blanket. They also reviewed the pornographic imagery and the defendant's February 4 police questioning.[31]

The next week, during the penalty phase, the prosecution called several individuals: Westerfield's nineteen-year-old niece testified about a time when she slept over at his home. She was seven years old at the time, Danielle's same age, and became aware of someone fondling her. At first she pretended to be asleep, but when he stuck his finger in her mouth, she bit down on it. She opened her eyes to see him walk away, adjusting his shorts. Under California law, prosecutors can tell jurors considering a death sentence of prior criminal activity even if no charges were filed. The niece's mother backed up the girl's claim, as did one of the detectives who said Westerfield told him about it, saying that it had been a misunderstanding. Others who testified were Brenda and Damon van Dam and their daughter's teachers—all of whom spoke about how lovely the child was, emotionally touching the jurors who had heard weeks of testimony about her corpse and death. Brenda spoke of the effect Danielle's murder had on her two brothers; that the older one was angry and felt he was to blame, and the younger one, now six, had reverted to baby talk and bed-wetting. Danielle's room was as she left it, and family members would go in there to "talk" to her, or just to feel or smell her, Brenda said. A video of snapshots and footage of Danielle was played, causing some of the jurors to weep openly.

For Feldman's side, he was determined not to let people think Westerfield was "the worst of the worst." He called Westerfield's sister and aunt—the latter was not recognized by the defendant—and his former girlfriend from 2000, as well as a high school crush he hadn't seen since the early 1970s. People familiar with Westerfield's inventions also testified, but the most heartbreaking witnesses were his son and daughter, Neal and Lisa, who both cried on the stand, causing Westerfield to also shed tears, his only display of sensitivity throughout the trial.[32] Neither child addressed their father's guilt but rather tried to humanize him by expressing his importance in their lives and their affection for him.

On January 3, 2003, Judge Mudd formally sentenced Westerfield to death in San Quentin State Prison, near San Francisco—the same complex that houses Scott Peterson, who was convicted of killing his pregnant wife, Laci. The sentencing hearing was delayed six weeks while Feldman prepared to argue the case. One of the points he made in seeking a life sentence for his client was that there was a chance Danielle was killed in her bed, which would eliminate the kidnapping charge and the special circumstances of the murder conviction. The legal loophole prompted van Dam family advocate and civil rights attorney Gloria Allred to push legislators for the passage of "Danielle's Law," which would make a death penalty "special circumstance" when a child is killed in his or her home. Mudd also rejected Feldman's claim that Westerfield's rights were trampled upon when he answered police questions without a lawyer; the judge responded that the jury never heard the disputed evidence.

Before Mudd pronounced his sentence, he let the van Dams speak their piece. As Westerfield sat stone-faced, Brenda snarled at him: "It disgusts me that your sick fantasies and pitiful needs made you think that you needed Danielle more than her family. You do not deserve any leniency, any mercy, because you refused to give it to Danielle." And Damon told the judge he would never get to see his daughter grow up, be a sister to her two brothers, or get married and have her own children. "As the years pass and these things don't happen, all I'll have are the memories of her . . . and having to know how brutal her last hours were," he said.[33]

San Diego taxpayers were billed more than a million dollars for the trial of Danielle's murderer—police costs topped $756,000, while the district attorney spent $270,000.[34] But I suspect few people would complain that the results were not worth the money. A civil suit settlement with Westerfield's insurance company paid the van Dams almost a half million dollars. "No amount of money can ever replace my daughter and no one can bring her back," said Brenda van Dam. The money was earmarked for the college educations of her sons and to pay back the state victims' fund for past counseling. The van Dams also formed the Danielle Legacy Foundation to advance child safety issues. Westerfield's motor home was repossessed, and his home was deeded over to his defense attorneys and sold for $435,000. A stock portfolio was emptied before its assets could be frozen and seized, and royalties from his inventions were transferred or sold.[35]

Jeff Dusek and Woody Clarke were, I think, appropriately named Prosecutors of the Year in 2003 by the California District Attorneys Association. Shortly thereafter, Dusek was chosen by District Attorney Bonnie Dumanis to preside over a new cold case unit to tackle the almost two thousand unsolved homicides and missing persons cases. Clarke was appointed to a judgeship on the San Diego County Superior Court.[36]

Steven Feldman and Robert Boyce are still practicing defense attorneys, likely busier than ever. In an interview in the December 2002 issue of the *San Diego Jewish Journal*, Feldman, finally free of the court-imposed gag order on the case, said his life would be different from now on, for defending Westerfield. "We've been inundated with e-mails, with letters, with faxes, with telephone calls, with threats, with anti-Semitic remarks . . . with letters that say my children should get AIDS, with letters that hope my wife gets gang-raped," he said. Even FOX News anchor Bill O'Reilly got into the act when he urged his TV viewers to file ethics complaints with the San Diego County Bar Association. He called Feldman and Boyce "sleazy" and said, "No American should ever talk to these two people again." Feldman told the magazine that his responsibility as a defense counsel is to keep the prosecution honest and to protect his client, while not necessarily believing him or her. "Whether or not an individual is guilty or not guilty is not my issue," he said. "I don't care. My job is to evaluate the case and assist the person as best as I possibly can. That is the ethical requirement of the criminal defense lawyer."[37] One person who didn't object to Feldman's often flamboyant courtroom dynamic was Jeff Dusek. "He promised a vigorous defense," he said of Feldman. "He did not say his guy was innocent."

In a coincidental sidebar, my co-author, Dawna Kaufmann, who covered the van Dam case from the disappearance of Danielle through the sentencing of Westerfield as a freelance investigative journalist for *Globe* magazine, never communicated with the attorneys during the trial, knowing there was a gag order. But one of her articles led to an important development that helped prosecutors. In March 2002, around the time of the preliminary hearing, Dawna learned that Danielle's passport photo was taken on Friday, February 1, hours before the girl went missing. She was also aware of a photo taken earlier of Danielle, with her hair a few inches longer.

Because hairs of similar color and appearance to Danielle's had been found in the sink trap of Westerfield's RV, Dawna wanted to know when the girl had had her last haircut. This was at a point when the forensic evidence against Westerfield was scant—there were only

Danielle's presumed hairs in the sink, her prints in the RV, and her blood on his jacket and on the RV floor. Since none of those items could be time-dated with scientific certainty, Westerfield could say they were from Danielle playing inside his motor home and, somehow, bleeding. His supporters on the Internet were already suggesting that he parked the vehicle in front of his home and left it unlocked, where it might seem like a fun playhouse to a little kid. But Kaufmann learned that the RV had not been parked in Sabre Springs for months and was kept eight miles away, including on the night in question. Therefore, if Danielle's recently cut hairs were found in the vehicle, she could not have deposited them innocently, on her own—she would have had to get a ride to the location from Westerfield. And even if the hairs had no roots for DNA comparison, their bluntly cut ends might still be helpful in identifying them as Danielle's.

So Dawna began phoning every hair salon in the immediate area to Sabre Springs, asking if anyone had cut Danielle's hair. Several calls later she reached Be Luong, of Camelot Hair Designs, who posed for a photo for the magazine outside her salon and spoke of the young girl whose hair she often trimmed. She said Danielle's last haircut was on the previous Saturday, and she had clipped about five inches.

When Kaufmann's *Globe* piece ran, it evoked a lot of discussion on the Internet crime chat forums where this, and other cases, are discussed and debated. The article, which showed Danielle's photos with short and long hair, included quotes from an FBI lab expert about how to estimate when a hair was cut by looking at it under a microscope. This chat-room topic was brought to the attention of Dusek and Clarke, who later admitted they had never thought about finding out when Danielle's hair was cut. The hair became its own little time line and a slam-dunk for prosecutors, who brought up the information in court testimony.[38]

The next year, at the annual meeting of the American Academy of Forensic Sciences, Dawna ran into Woody Clarke, whom she remembered from when she helped cover the O. J. Simpson trial for the *National Enquirer*. She told Woody about the haircut article and learned that they had heard about it from the Internet. He said he was pleased to talk to the woman behind the byline, and then called Jeff Dusek on his cell phone and handed the phone to Dawna. She repeated her story for Dusek and was thanked by him as well. Both told her to keep up the good work, which I think she is doing.

I'm often asked about this case and why I would consider assisting the defense of someone who committed such an act of depraved indifference. After all, his attorneys persuaded him to admit to killing the girl and telling them where he hid her body, in exchange for a sentence of life without parole. The pen was virtually in Westerfield's hand to sign the agreement when Danielle's body was recovered and the plea deal was abandoned. But, like the rest of the world, except for the handful of key personnel directly involved in the negotiation, I did not learn about that until after the trial ended. Steven Feldman had no obligation to inform me of his private communications with his client, since it had no relevance to my expertise as a forensic pathologist. My involvement in this case was limited, unlike my consulting on the Stephanie Crowe case, which was more far reaching as a medical detective.

If I had an opinion substantially different from that of the county medical examiner, I would have testified and let the jurors sort out what they believed, as they did with the entomological experts. And if I were testifying, it would be based on the medical and autopsy evidence, and I would hold my head up and testify the same way I would if I were a prosecution expert. I cannot let my personal disdain for a defendant interfere with my scientific analysis and presentation. There's also the reality that when a loathsome defendant gets a robust defense, his or her conviction will be unlikely to be overturned by a higher court.

MEMORIAL MEDICAL CENTER

I t's a popular misconception that the Latin maxim *primum non nocere*—first, do no harm—is mentioned in the Hippocratic Oath that many students pledge when they graduate from medical school. In fact, there is even doubt whether the father of modern medicine, the Greek Hippocrates, who lived in fourth century BCE, was responsible for the dictum, which was paraphrased by the Romans down through history.[1] Nevertheless, the widely accepted precept is one that should be recognized by every physician who has the privilege of attending to the sick. Let us do so with integrity, humility, and the sincere desire to, if at all possible, leave the patient in better condition than we found him or her—and to remember that the patients who entrust us to help are human beings and not just case numbers, maladies, or broken bodies.

This is why the suspicious deaths of nine patients receiving medical care in a New Orleans hospital in the aftermath of Hurricane Katrina provoked such a fiery debate in the medicolegal community, touching on such issues as end-of-life treatment, professional ethics, politics, compassion, and runaway healthcare costs. The questions that these deaths have posed are far from being resolved.

Hurricane Katrina was one of the deadliest natural disasters to ever hit the United States, claiming at least 1,836 lives in five states. It formed over the Bahamas on August 23, 2005, and then crossed over to southern Florida, where it caused flooding and took some lives but retained its moderate Category 1 classification. As it traveled over the Gulf of Mexico, it steadily built to Category 5, becoming history's strongest-ever hurricane at sea. The rains were torrential and the winds whipped up to one hundred seventy-five miles per hour, with a coastal storm surge of more than twenty feet above sea level. By Monday, August 29, when Katrina hit southeast Louisiana and the Mississippi border, it was downgraded to a Category 3 but still set forth destruction that effectively wiped out entire parts of New Orleans and many towns along Mississippi's Gulf Coast. On the books, it's the fifth-most powerful hurricane to ever hit the states, but the damage it wreaked— estimated at $81.2 billion—makes it the United States' costliest storm. It also left five hundred thousand residents homeless.

The devastation of New Orleans, in the wake of the hurricane, can mostly be blamed on the failure of the city's levee system, which breached in fifty places, causing severe flooding in 80 percent of the city and its neighboring parishes.[2] After the storm moved on, area residents thought the worst was over. The sun came out, and people began moving about the city again. But as the wind stopped pushing the water out of Lake Pontchartrain, north of the city, and Lake Borgne, east of the city, the returning tidal surges caused those levees to fail, one by one. It was almost to be expected that disaster would strike this picturesque city that sits in a bowl and is eight to twelve feet below sea level in some places. For years, engineers had warned about the levees, only to be ignored in the same way as the mythological prophet Cassandra had been ignored when she unsuccessfully tried to warn the city of Troy of its own imminent destruction.

It took only a few weeks for the water to subside, but the economic and human toll can still be felt years later. At least 1,079 deaths were logged in by the state coroner, and a couple of hundred people were reported missing and never found. Some might have drowned in the salt waters of giant Lake Pontchartrain, or were eaten in alligator-infested swamps or buried alive under collapsing structures. Floodwaters opened coffins from cemeteries with above-ground tombs, releasing ancient remains into the gruesome gumbo, with some eventually recovered thirty miles from where they were once buried.[3] While portions of bridges crumbled, many of the roads leading in or out of town were underwater but still navigable. Some thoroughfares were contraflowed for outbound traffic only, and the parade of cars was endless, rivaled only by the lines at the few operating gas stations. Temperatures spiked as high as 110 degrees and stayed that way for nearly a week.[4] Looting and violence were endemic throughout the city, but at one local medical center, where encroaching fetid waters had marooned hundreds of people, another kind of crime spree was going on.

I had been in New Orleans that February for the fifty-seventh annual meeting of the American Academy of Forensic Sciences, a weeklong event that brings together the best and brightest of all the disciplines of modern crime solving. My colleagues, Dr. Henry C. Lee—chief emeritus of the Connecticut Forensic Laboratory and State Police—and Dr. Michael M. Baden—director of the Forensic Sciences Unit of the New York State Police—and I delivered the key evening session before a full house. Our topic was "Complex Forensic Science Issues in Highly Controversial Cases," and we each made a Power-Point presentation about the high-profile cases we've worked, including the Scott Peterson and Jayson Williams murder trials, the rape accusation against Kobe Bryant, and many others. There was enthusiastic attendance for the whole conference, I suspect, because people especially enjoyed going to New Orleans. More spouses than usual showed up, as was evident in the French Quarter restaurants each evening.

The location for the conference was the Hyatt Regency Hotel, near the Superdome. Every ballroom, meeting room, conference area, and café was filled with registered AAFS members, most of whom also stayed at the hotel for the week. So it was a shock to watch the hurricane coverage on TV months later and see the Hyatt, devoid of electricity and running water, with every window facing east blown out by the winds and curtains flapping through the holes. The hotel was then closed to business but became the temporary headquarters for Mayor Clarence "Ray" Nagin and his staff, the hub for emergency workers and the media, and a haven for the families of employees who had nowhere else to go. At its peak, nine hundred displaced people called the Hyatt Regency home. The fancy ballrooms, which had held our forensic poster sessions and exhibits, now slept people on the floors, shoulder to shoulder. The ones who were more fortunate got service-able guest rooms that were dark and dank. The giant brass luggage carts that dotted the lovely atrium lobby were now transporting elderly or infirm people who didn't have their wheelchairs or walkers. The hotel sustained so much physical damage it is not scheduled to reopen until spring 2009. Someday, I hope to go back and enjoy it again.

The news coverage of the storm's devastation was overwhelming to me, in my comfortable home in Pittsburgh. I could only imagine what it must have been like on the streets of New Orleans, watching dead and bloated bodies floating past people's yards, where the hopeless-ness and stench of death would be all too real. Mayor Nagin predicted that as many as ten thousand lives might have been lost, and from the continuous, depressing news footage, that seemed feasible. Why was no one rescuing the people perched on top of their roofs, shouting to the canoes sailing by? What about the homes whose roofs were sheared off? Why wasn't anyone able to give these poor souls food or a sip of clean water? There were substantial resettlements in the Superdome and the Ernest N. Morial Convention Center, neither of which had electricity or running water. Some corporations had donated bottled water and food, which was better than nothing.

As the week went on and more homes were emptying out, it became apparent that the last evacuees were often the elderly who stubbornly refused to leave their homes and belongings to vandals. They worked too hard and for too long to let thugs rob them blind when they couldn't protect their property. And many of them just wouldn't abandon their pets after being told that only humans would be allowed onboard the rescue boats. Sadly, many of those senior cit-izens would drown, their bodies discovered in their attics, after the last pockets of air filled with water. There were gut-wrenching reports about the emergency shelters, the kinds of scary stories kids might tell around campfires, about people getting slaughtered for a candy bar or a cigarette, or rowdy crackheads assaulting the defenseless. One particularly brutal story was about a seven-year-old girl pulled away from her mother, gang-raped, and murdered. The appalling tale picked up more details with each telling until witnesses swore they saw the child's naked body in a restroom, with her throat slashed. After seeing footage around the clock of the worst kind of suffering, it wasn't such a leap to envision a crime of this nature against a little girl. It would take months before that story was exposed as a hoax. One wonders what kind of satisfaction it brought whoever wove that concoction out of whole cloth.

I considered contacting my old friend Frank Minyard, the coroner of Orleans Parish, and offering my assistance, but the area had no cell phone service, landlines, faxes, or Internet. It would be a while before Frank was able to tell me just what horrors he faced during that week and for months afterward. The deceased individuals on whom he performed post-mortems could not have asked for a more caring physician to try to identify them, find their cause of death, and return their bodies to their loved ones, whenever possible. In his youth Dr. Minyard was a tall, blue-eyed, handsome lifeguard, who placed second in the Mr. New Orleans bodybuilding contest. He went to medical school at Louisiana State University, and when he began his career, it was as an obstetrician, not a forensic pathologist. In the 1960s, he married, had a family, and lived the lush life in a ritzy home with a pool and a tennis court. Then one day he heard Peggy Lee sing, "Is That All There Is?" and he was prompted to ask himself that same question. He felt shallow just going after the Cadillac and country club membership; he desired to devote himself to serving the public. A nun who ran a breakfast program for poor children signed him up as a volunteer. She warned him that the kids' parents were likely prostitutes and shoplifters. Frank replied, "Well, Sister, nobody's perfect."

Together Frank and Sister Mary David started the city's first methadone clinic to help heroin addicts. Frank then went into prisons and treated addicts there, a revolutionary idea at the time. In 1974, he ran for the office of coroner and has never lost an election for the post since. He's in the ninth term of a job he loves and does well. Around town he's known as "Dr. Jazz," due to the trumpet he's prone to pull out and play at the drop of a hat. He has hired musicians as morgue assistants and has raised $800,000 for city charities through Jazz Roots, an annual concert he produces where the elite locals come to jam with Minyard's own band.[5] Minyard's favorite tune is one made famous by New Orleans–born Louis Armstrong, with its lyrics so meaningful to Frank: *"I went down to St. James Infirmary / Saw my baby there / Stretched out on a long white table / So sweet, so cold, so fair."*[6]

During this whirlwind of depressing activity that surrounded Hurricane Katrina, President George Bush appeared ridiculously slow to react, and FEMA (the Federal Emergency Management Agency) seemed to lose its map to New Orleans. Moreover, the Army Corps of Engineers deflected criticism for the levees by saying that Congress had underfunded them. And the National Guard and Blackwater USA security personnel toted weapons instead of food as they passed by the starving citizenry. Still, some heroes did emerge. Frank Minyard is one, and so is Dr. Louis Cataldie, the Louisiana state medical examiner. At the time I didn't know Lou but had heard of him. He's a general practitioner and emergency room physician in Baton Rouge and had served as a local coroner before he took the state job. He would write about his Katrina experience in a book titled *Coroner's Journal: Stalking Death in Louisiana.*[7]

Minyard and Cataldie set up a make-shift morgue in the tiny town of St. Gabriel, near Baton Rouge, about seventy miles west of New Orleans. For weeks they worked onsite, sleeping only three hours a night when they could calm their minds at all. The smell of death permeated the air and their clothes. They requested and got help from DMORT—the Disaster Mortuary Operational Recovery Team—a mobile squad funded by the Department of Homeland Security, which had provided manpower after the World Trade Center attacks and other catastrophes. But even the trained DMORT professionals were unprepared for the sheer enormity at "Camp Katrina." I would soon have the opportunity to see their work firsthand.

Memorial Medical Center, at 2700 Napoleon Avenue in the Uptown/Broadmoor part of New Orleans, was called Southern Baptist Hospital when it was founded in 1926. In 1969, the religious organization separated itself from the hospital, and the facility became an independent nonprofit entity. In the early 1980s, $100 million was spent to renovate the original building, and in 1990, it merged with Mercy Hospital to become a six-city-block campus. The combined hospitals were acquired in 1996 by Tenet Healthcare Corporation—a for-profit operation—and renamed Tenet HealthSystem Memorial Medical Center, Inc., or more simply, Memorial Medical Center. Dallas-based Tenet also owned four other facilities in the city. Since 1967, the New Orleans Saints football team deemed the hospital its official healthcare provider because the team's original orthopedic surgeon, Dr. Ken Saer, had his home base there.[8]

With its solid reputation and eight-story, red brick façade, Memorial seemed impenetrable—just the place to go for safety when Katrina hit. It had stood its ground against hurricanes in the past, without there ever being an evacuation. Now, with the streets eight feet deep in water, the hospital seemed like an island in the middle of an ocean.

Two nights before the hurricane, Father John Marse, the fifty-one-year-old hospital chaplain and Catholic priest, was awoken from a dead sleep by a voice he had never heard before. It was God, he later recounted, telling him to get to the hospital and help people there. Marse packed a bag with three days' worth of clothes and hurricane gear, grabbed six more hours of sleep, and then made his way to Memorial. He arrived in time to conduct Sunday mass at 8 a.m. for a smaller than usual crowd. Staffers knew the hurricane was coming and they were busy making preparations. Julie Campbell, who worked in the surgical intensive care unit, was one of seventy-five nurses who showed up for their twelve-hour shifts. She had returned to work from extended leave due to Hodgkin's disease, a lymphatic cancer, and now she was nine months pregnant. But she knew she would be automatically terminated if she failed to report to duty. She brought along her eighty-seven-year-old grandmother and an eighty-year-old great-aunt, feeling they'd be more secure with her than on their own. She wasn't the only employee who brought relatives—Memorial became the shelter of choice for many loved ones of the staffers and patients. A rough head count totaled two hundred sixty patients, five hundred hospital workers, and an assortment of kin and friends, to bring the hospital's population to about two thousand. And it wasn't just two-legged refugees: The medical records office had been turned into a kennel, with hundreds of cats and dogs, and one ferret, in pet carriers. The meowing and barking from that room was deafening for anyone who tried to get a little shut-eye in the nearby doctors' lounge.

As the countdown to Katrina continued, staffers pitched in to bring several tons of food from the basement kitchen to the fourth floor, which they hoped would stay dry. There were also plentiful supplies of five-gallon bottles of water. Caravans were made of stretchers, hospital beds, and wheelchairs for carrying the goods up the stairs. Other employees nailed plywood on dozens of upper-floor windows, where they feared cyclonic-force winds and rain might cause those walls and floors to buckle and become moldy. Like much of the city, Memorial lost electrical power, but generators on the second floor kicked in, allowing people to monitor TV coverage of the storm watch. The satellite images tracking Katrina through the Gulf Coast were all the inspiration they needed to keep battening down the hatches. As more folks kept arriving, the anxiety level heightened. Soon every hallway was filled with sobbing and frightened strangers, with Father Marse going from one to the next, offering prayers and gentle thoughts.

While nurses had to report for hurricane duty beginning Sunday, doctors had a less formal rotation. The only physicians whose presence was required that morning were the six department heads, including chief of medicine Richard E. Deichmann, who would also soon be one of the primary heliport evacuation organizers, and the emergency room doctors. The rest were free to make their own arrangements, as long as their patients were covered by a designee. Dr. Anna M. Pou, forty-nine, was on duty that morning, but before she came to work she stopped by the home of her eighty-three-year-old mother, Jeanette, who suffered from heart problems and arthritis. In 2004, when Hurricane Ivan had threatened New Orleans, another doctor had storm duty, so Anna was able to drive her mother out of harm's way. They spent ten and a half hours in the car, which was no fun for either lady. The elder Pou didn't want to leave her home, but her daughter insisted, or as Ms. Pou tells it: "She dragged me out of the house." But on this day, pre-Katrina, Pou's mom stuck to her guns and wouldn't budge, so Anna went off to Memorial alone. She was in good spirits when she left her mother. It would be days, however, before they would talk again.

Pou had recently moved back to her Big Easy birthplace after living in Galveston, Texas; being able to take care of her mother was worth the cut in pay she took when she joined the Memorial staff. Anna's father, Frederick, had been a physician for fifty years. But even when Anna went to medical school, Jeanette doubted her seventh child of eleven would make it as a doctor. "She was too tenderhearted," she told a reporter. When a laboratory test required Anna to kill a guinea pig, she refused. Even today her colleagues say that she's the kind of doctor who gives patients her cell phone number.[9]

Anna Maria Pou graduated with a bachelor of science degree in 1978 from Louisiana State University in Baton Rouge and earned her medical degree in 1990 from its School of Medicine in New Orleans. She served a two-year residency as a general surgeon at the University of Tennessee in Memphis and a four-year residency at the University of Pennsylvania in Pittsburgh. It was at their Department of Otolaryngology that she began to specialize in reconstructive surgery for patients who have been disfigured by cancer. She followed up with a one-year fellowship in Head and Neck Surgery at Methodist Hospital of Indiana in Indianapolis. In 1997 she moved to Galveston where she became an assistant professor, then an associate, at the University of Texas Medical Branch. She served that school's Department of Otolaryngology first as a co-director, with a fellowship in Advanced Head and Neck Oncologic Surgery, and then as the director of the department's Head and Neck Surgery division. In September 2004, she moved back to New Orleans and became an associate professor of Louisiana State University Health Sciences Center's Otolaryngology–Head and Neck Surgery, and in 2006, she also became the school's director for resident education—both are titles she still holds. She's given lectures around the world and published papers, monographs, and book chapters in numerous scientific publications and is a member of all the appropriate medical and scientific societies.[10] According to public documents, at the time of Hurricane Katrina, she earned a combined $230,000 per year, with $105,000 of that paid by LSU and the balance from Louisiana Medical Center and grants.[11]

When Dr. Pou arrived at Memorial that Sunday morning to supervise residents, she checked into the command center where administrators took down her cell phone number and room assignment. Then she received the wristband all employees had to wear so that security guards would grant them full access to the facility.

By Sunday evening, between twenty-five and forty doctors were present. Dr. Roy Culotta, an internist, was given a bed on the seventh floor for his eighty-nine-year-old grandmother, Nathalie Andree. Much of that floor had been leased from Memorial's owner, Tenet, by LifeCare Holdings, Inc., a Plano, Texas–based long-term acute care corporation. LifeCare's patients were chronically ill or suffering from calamitous accidents or ailments, requiring full-time care until they were healed enough to be discharged to their homes, a nursing home, or wherever they came from. As the storm approached, LifeCare transferred nineteen patients, some on ventilators, from their facility in Chalmette, Louisiana, to Memorial's seventh floor, filling fifty-five of the eighty-two beds. Dr. Culotta had moved Ms. Andree from a nursing home in neighboring Metairie, so that he and LifeCare's nurses could keep an eye on her. "It was great, because all the nurses knew she was my grandmother so they took wonderful care of her," said Culotta. "But they also knew I'd be coming up to see her, and if they needed anything, I'd be there to help. . . . I think I spent more time up there than the other physicians."

A furniture maker named Mark LeBlanc felt relieved that his eighty-two-year-old mother was on the seventh floor, where floodwaters surely wouldn't reach her. Elvira LeBlanc had Parkinson's disease and cancer, and had had her colon removed days before. Before Mark and his wife, Sandy, left town on Sunday afternoon, they stopped to check on Elvira and the private-duty nurse assistant they had hired to stay with her. The LeBlancs brought them a cooler with food, a flashlight, batteries, and a cell phone. Mark became concerned when he learned that his mother's doctor, John Wise, the director of the Life-Care unit, had already evacuated and, according to Mark, wasn't returning several calls LeBlanc had made to him. Sandy bluntly asked if her mother-in-law should be evacuated now, but, Sandy told a reporter, a nurse said it wasn't necessary; besides Elvira was too frail for something risky like that. There were doctors throughout the building and, on that floor alone, forty nurses and four administrators, so Elvira was in good hands. Assured, they kissed Elvira and told her they'd be back for her soon.[12]

Kathryn Nelson was also a registered nurse, but she didn't work at LifeCare—she was just there to be with her ninety-year-old mother, Elaine. The Metairie resident had checked into the facility in July after having heart problems and ulcers on her back and face. Kathy didn't want her mother to wake up and not see her there, so as long as Elaine had a pulse, her daughter was going to be there.[13]

Monday, August 29, the hurricane slammed New Orleans, turning the city into one humongous steam bath and giving its Day of the Dead décor and voodoo gift shops a new and ominous meaning. The "Cat 3" winds and rain were really hammering Memorial's eighth floor. Even though plywood boards were nailed to the inside of the windows, staffers wondered if they would hold up against the horizontal gales.

The glass could be heard breaking and the boards were bending inward. Post-surgical patients from the intensive care unit had been moved up there where it was considered safer, and while most of them slept through the chaos, their bedside relatives were panicking and wanting to know if their loved ones could be moved again. It wasn't an easy task since many of the patients were on life-support machines or hooked up to oxygen. By morning, Memorial's roof began to leak, and soon puddles formed on the linoleum, which made the carpeted areas soggy. When the electricity blew, the backup generators took over, but the pneumatic system for sending prescriptions back and forth was lost, as were most of the elevators and some phones. The metal skeleton of the building was creaking, making it sound like the ship in the movie *Titanic* right before it sank. Possibly the most popular folks in the building were head chef Scott Perry and his kitchen staff, improvising meals on the fourth floor. Eggs, grits, sausage, rice, beans, and muffins kept coming, all of it served in Styrofoam cups to the lines of grateful employees and visitors.

Dr. Richard Deichmann, Memorial's chief of medicine, assigned one physician to each of the entire hospital's twelve nursing stations. The exception was the seventh floor, where LifeCare ran its own hospital-within-a-hospital. Deichmann later explained that he lacked the authority to send his doctors there since the floor had its own personnel. I never quite understood that remark, because all of the Memorial doctors had privileges to work on the LifeCare floor, and during an emergency one would expect them to fill in wherever they were needed. LifeCare's medical director did not report for hurricane duty, the company acknowledged after the fact, later contending that Memorial's doctors would cover its fifty-five patients. That afternoon, when LifeCare's nurses called a "Code Blue"—signaling that a patient was in a life-threatening crisis—one of the doctors who responded was Anna Maria Pou, even though she had no patients on the floor. The seventy-three-year-old patient could not be saved, however. Over the next three days, twenty-three more of the critically ill LifeCare patients would also die.

Around 3 p.m., the first reports of levees breaching surfaced on

Internet sites, such as www.nola.com, a discussion board supported by New Orleans' hometown newspaper, the *Times-Picayune*. Though news photos showed some neighborhoods taking on water, many people thought Memorial's district was probably safe—and besides, help from the federal government would surely be on the way. FEMA, Homeland Security, the National Guard, the Red Cross—all of America's finest crisis response organizations—would soon be on the scene to get the citizens to higher ground and deal with the hurricane. By dusk, hospital staffers walked their dogs and some even drove home. The worst seemed over. It wasn't.[14]

The levee system continued to fail, bringing down entire neighborhoods like tumbling dominos. Restaurants and businesses boarded up and closed, and people in homes with multiple stories brought heirlooms, food, and pets upstairs as the muddy floodwaters rushed uninvited through their doors and windows. Dr. Deichmann knew that much of that water would end up at Memorial, with its especially low elevation. However, Deichmann, an avid triathlete with a wife and three daughters, chose to command operations at the hospital instead of scrambling to get out of town with his family. "I felt a moral obligation to stay," Deichmann told reporter Jeffrey Meitrodt of the *Times-Picayune*. "I also felt a strong moral obligation to go with my family. I don't know if I made the right decision, but I know I did a lot of good there." While other staffers abandoned the facility, Dr. Pou stayed put, even after her husband, Vince, showed up Monday night and urged her to leave.

Tuesday started pretty well, with doctors making their rounds, nurses changing bedding, and meals being served to workers. Chef Perry served what he called his "breakfast parfait," with scrambled eggs, bacon, and grits layered in a cup, and later Father Marse conducted a mass for about fifty people. Tenet executives in Dallas were keeping tabs on their hospital, but due to unreliable phone lines, communication was difficult. Memorial's chief executive officer Rene Goux did get an e-mail from the Texas brass, telling him to close the facility immediately and prepare to get everyone out. Tenet also contacted Cynthia Matherne, the regional coordinator for emergency services at City Hall, whose territory included New Orleans and three other parishes. Though sympathetic—two of her grandchildren were stuck at Memorial with their mother, who was a nurse there—there wasn't much she could do. Boats and helicopters were in short supply and the priority was to get residents off roofs, not to take care of hospitals, which were considered safe environments. Roy Culotta, the visiting doctor who decided to stay with his mother on the LifeCare floor, saw nurses hovering over critically ill patients, waving cardboard fans to create a little airflow. "To see these debilitated patients struggling for their lives in this heat was just really nauseating," he said.

Dehydration was a real concern, with one patient later saying she was only given one teaspoon of water every hour.[15] But I never could balance that statement against what I learned investigators found when they were finally able to go back in the building—there were unopened five-gallon plastic bottles of water on each floor. Although it's accurate that there was no running water, there didn't need to be any water rationing. I was also told that investigators discovered that the vending machines that dotted the building had not been broken into, which is what might have been expected after the electricity went down, if people were starving. I'm not saying that Memorial was any kind of a vacation paradise, but it was made clear to me when I worked on the case that any suggestion that there was an acute food and water shortage misstates the facts.

At the afternoon's crisis team meeting, it was decided that patients and family members would be evacuated separately, even mothers and their newborns. There was only so much room on the helicopters and it had to be designated for those who could not sail away on a boat. Trucks and cars couldn't be used, since their engines would just become flooded. Deichmann announced that the first to go would be the most at-risk patients, including those on dialysis who had already missed treatments. Soon eighteen ailing or premature babies, and some critical care patients, were choppered to safety. But on two occasions, when the pilots didn't see the patients and had orders not to wait, helicopters took off without loading anybody.

Last on the evacuation list were the "Do Not Resuscitate" patients, many of whom were on the LifeCare floor. The goal was to evacuate everyone, but priority had to go to those who were most viable. The going was slow, with each patient having to be carried on a stretcher down flights of pitch-black stairs, then passed through a three-foot hole in the wall to the parking garage where a vehicle would ferry the person up the nine levels to the top of the structure, and then there would be another two flights of stairs before reaching the helipad. By 11 p.m. on Tuesday, only twenty-five patients had been flown out. Another handful had died.

Father Marse had spent the day performing emergency baptisms on the newborns who would go in the copters and last rites on the dying elderly who wouldn't make it. There were two morgues in the hospital—one on the third floor and one on the eighth—and as the body count grew, corpses were placed two on each slab. The helicopters that were bringing food and medical supplies were also now asked to bring body bags, although there never seemed to be enough of them. Before the ordeal was over, Marse would sacrifice his chapel, a room he considered sacred, and turn it into a makeshift morgue to house even more bodies.

Tuesday night had been dreadful inside the facility. Toilets overflowed, spilling feces and filth down the hallways, and there was no running water and scant communication between floors. Memorial was used to flooding each year, which is why, long before, its generators had been moved to the second floor. But no one ever ordered that the electrical grids be moved out of the basement, and, around 1 a.m. on Wednesday, those grids began failing. Cell phones could not be recharged and computers fell silent. People who didn't have flashlights would have to slowly stumble down the hallways or stairs, hoping not to trip over a sleeping or dead body. By 5 a.m., there was a total blackout, including the life-support systems of some patients. Hospital workers reminded patients, and themselves, that the outside world knew they were in the facility, so surely help would be coming.[16]

On Wednesday morning, August 31, a brigade of private citizens in seven boats showed up and whisked away hundreds of patients and guests. Many patients had to be moved in their wheelchairs, and two who could not walk each weighed as much as four hundred pounds. But internist Dr. John J. Kokemor, who was helping to organize the evacuations, was worried. More than one thousand people were still trapped inside the facility and supplies were running short. Electrical power kept going off, and the air conditioning was shut down so as not to strain the system.[17] I was told that there was power from a separate generator in the cancer center, which was connected to the main hospital via an overhead walkway, and the hushed talk among staffers was that that area still had air conditioning and was a good place to go to catch a few hours of rest.

By Wednesday morning, word of the critical conditions arrived at Tenet's corporate headquarters in Dallas. Bob Smith, a senior vice president with the firm, was shocked and dismayed to learn that the federal government wasn't on the spot with an evacuation plan. It's my understanding that Tenet bosses convened in a crisis room and were making minute-by-minute decisions and probably regretting that the corporation didn't have its own plan in place already. Smith called Cynthia Matherne, who told him there were no helicopters or boats that she could dispatch that day. If Tenet wanted a faster response, she said, it should use private assets. Smith had no clue where to start looking for help.

Mark and Sandy LeBlanc, who had left town on Sunday, had had second thoughts about leaving his mother, Elvira, on the LifeCare floor, even though she had a private nurse assistant. They decided to return to New Orleans, but the closest they could get was a triage center, several miles away. They slept in their truck in a line of other vehicles pulled to the side of one of the unflooded roads. Someone told them about a massive boat rescue leaving the next morning, and the LeBlancs decided to take part in it.

At 8 a.m., the hospital crisis squad ordered the staff to bring the remaining two hundred or so patients down to the first two floors to implement the mass evacuation. The only exceptions would be those patients who were dying or too ill to move—they would be brought down last. This time the evacuees would be lined up on the emergency room ramp and near the heliport—so there would be no way to miss them. Three miles away, also at 8 a.m., one hundred boats and pilots prepared to take off on rescue missions, but not one of them was assigned to go to Memorial. Elvira's sitter had called Mark several times to report the dire conditions at LifeCare, including deaths on the seventh floor overnight, so he found someone in charge at the launch and pleaded his case. Three airboats were redirected for the medical center; Mark and Sandy LeBlanc, who was an emergency medical technician, were onboard one of them. When their flotilla arrived about 10 a.m. and rounded a corner to the hospital, a cheer went up from the dozens of patients and personnel who had been waiting on the ramp. Memorial administrators, who had hit-or-miss contact with their bosses in Tenet headquarters in Dallas, had been under the impression an armada of government rescue boats would be there. Their zeal would turn to crushing anguish when they realized this wasn't the full-blown rescue they had hoped for. But were it not for LeBlanc's insistence and the help of the private sector, the eventual death toll at Memorial would have been far greater.

When Mark LeBlanc walked into Elvira's room, she whispered, "You came back." "Yeah, Mom, I told you I'd be back," he replied. He asked how she was, and she responded that she was "hanging in there." The old woman was badly dehydrated and it was impossible to know when she had last eaten or had anything to drink. On her chart, someone had scrawled, "Disaster Mode." LeBlanc cornered a Life-Care administrator and handed over his cell phone, making the staffer call the corporate office in Plano. The executive in Texas said the company had made arrangements with private transportation companies. Helicopters were expected to start arriving soon. Relieved that his fragile mother wouldn't have to be evacuated in an airboat, LeBlanc went downstairs and began helping load other patients into the boats.

"We knew we had a monumental task on our hands," he said, "so we started rolling people out immediately."

One of the first people onto the boats was Julie Campbell, the pregnant intensive care nurse who had gone into labor the day before. She was perturbed at leaving behind her grandmother and great-aunt, but her supervisors and some of the ICU nurses urged her not to risk having her baby at Memorial. Two of the nurses who persuaded her were Lori L. Budo, forty-two, and Cheri A. Landry, forty-eight, whose names would later become well known. "They said they'd look after Grandma and Aunt Mildred. Lori and Cheri made sure they took their medicine," Campbell told a reporter. Julie and a nurse who was five months pregnant made it safely to land where a fleet of ambulances met the boats; the ladies were sped to a Baton Rouge hospital. Doctors there stopped Julie's contractions and she gave birth to a son, John Luke, on her natural due date of September 20. Her grandmother, however, had a minor stroke the day after Campbell left her; she was safely evacuated but would die a few months later.

Five new mothers and their babies were also among the day's initial evacuees, accompanied by a nurse. The boat ride through the flooded streets terrified them. "There were people on the neutral grounds begging for food and water," said Stella Eisenman, who carried her five-day-old daughter. "We had heard about the lootings and the shootings and I was scared that someone was going to take the boat away from us. We had no protection. I had a diaper bag full of formula. That is what the nurse kept saying: 'All we have is formula.' Fortunately, nobody tried to approach us."

Dr. Glenn Casey, head of anesthesia, and the other doctors involved with the boat rescue were not pleased at the pace of the evacuation. Each boat needed more than an hour to make the six-mile round-trip voyage. At this rate he feared it would take a week to clear out Memorial. After consulting with the pilots, it was decided a better place to deposit evacuees was at the corner of Napoleon and St. Charles avenues, about twelve blocks from the hospital. No ambulances were there though—all of the ambulances in the city seemed to be in use elsewhere. The intersection became the drop-off point for other evacuees from homes throughout the various flooded neighborhoods; by 3 p.m., some two thousand displaced people were waiting for transportation. The federal government had put out a call for vehicle operators to help out, and James Pafford, from Hope, Arkansas, and his son Greg, brought four boats, eight ambulances, fuel, and water. They were held back from helping by gun fights in the area between looters and police, but when they were finally able to get to the waiting throng, they realized there were just too many people for their modest vehicles. They talked a couple of young men into hot-wiring two school buses, a van, and several other cars, and the Audubon Zoo contributed a shuttle.

LeBlanc's and Pafford's groups were responsible for moving about five hundred people from Memorial, most of whom wound up at a triage center a few miles away, then were bused out of town. An unlucky fifteen ended up at the Convention Center, which was a hotbed of criminal activity, with no amenities. Rather than go inside with her elderly parents, Olga de la Vega slept with them outside. It was humiliating, she said, when they had to go to the bathroom in the open, but better than facing the violence inside. Mark LeBlanc finally gave up on the promised LifeCare rescue vehicles, which he said never did show up. His last chore was to put his frail mother, Elvira, and her minder on a boat. Elvira made it to a Baton Rouge nursing home but died days later of complications that her son will always believe were Katrina-related.

All over town, police officers were fighting outbreaks of looting. Near Memorial, thieves had swarmed a Wal-Mart and a Winn-Dixie supermarket, and nurses saw looters try to crash a boat into a credit union and commandeer a drug store. Many people in the streets carried firearms, and the sounds of gunshots permeated the air, day and night. Trees and power lines were down everywhere, cars flooded out and were ditched, and the heat was so oppressive people wished some of the rain and wind would come back. And over at nearby Tulane University Hospital, helicopters were kept from landing on the rooftop because punks in the street were firing automatic weapons at their rotors.

Afraid that Memorial might also be hit by troublemakers, hospital administrators told security guards not to allow anyone else on the premises, unless they were in dire need of medical care. This policy didn't sit well with one young doctor named Bryant King, who had worked at Memorial for about a month. He confronted CEO Rene Goux in the lobby. According to Dr. Kokemor, who overheard the exchange, King asked Goux about Memorial's new priorities. "What are you doing, man?" King asked incredulously. "You've got four hundred animals in this hospital and you're turning human beings away?" But Goux explained the issue wasn't pets versus humans, but security. "We don't have food, we don't have water, we aren't functioning as a hospital—we aren't going to take care of people we aren't responsible for," Goux replied. Kokemor's account was later confirmed by officials with Tenet.[18]

King wasn't satisfied with the answer or much of what he saw. The following message appeared on a real-time discussion board at nola.com. It's undated but was likely written on Wednesday, August 31, or Thursday, September 1, after the power went out:

> Begging for Baptist Hospital!!!
> From: Rachelle King
>   Doctors, patients and staff are stranded at Baptist Hospital (extended campus of Memorial Hospital). My brother, Dr. Bryant King, is stranded there and has been sending occasional text messages to let us know the situation. . . . He explained that management at the hospital decided to selectively withhold food and water from patients. Doctors are being forced to decide who gets to live and who will starve to death. The hospital is surrounded by 8 feet of floodwater; there is no more electricity, food or water. Windows are

broken out and people are starving. There has been very little press about this hospital, but conditions are deplorable and they need to be evacuated. My brother asked that we please get them out of there.[19]

An oncology nurse named Joanne Lalla somehow got word to her sister who spoke to a CNN reporter for an August 31 broadcast. Lalla's sister said Memorial staffers could hear looters break into cars in the parking structure, and when one nurse walked outside to get some air, she was robbed at gunpoint. Hospital administrators had locked everyone in the building and were saying it might take five days before they could be rescued. National Guard troops were outside the building but were reassigned to quell an uprising at a prison.[20]

More than one hundred patients were now on the second floor, on wall-to-wall cots. Dr. Pou ministered to the LifeCare/Tenet group, who were at particularly high risk; she dispensed medicine and listened to their cries. Dr. Culotta watched in admiration as Pou treated his grandmother. He recalled thinking: "Here is Anna Pou, who does these complicated, twelve-hour neck surgeries, and she's down here taking care of these debilitated medical patients." Pou even monitored patients' glucose levels, a task generally performed by nurses. "It was kind of out of her area, but she wasn't complaining," Culotta said. A lady visitor had failed to get doctors to give pain medication to her husband who was recovering from heart surgery, but Pou ordered him Percocet straightaway and earned thanks from the wife.

To make more room for human evacuees, no animals were allowed in the rescue vehicles, so the owners of the hundreds of pets still in cages at Memorial were among the last to vacate. They were aghast at the notion of leaving their cats and dogs alone in an empty hospital with nothing to eat but dead bodies and only putrid water to drink. "That is when I first heard of euthanasia," Culotta told a reporter. "It was pretty clear that the animals weren't getting evacuated, and people were very upset. There were several people I know of who euthanized their dogs." Dr. Kokemor witnessed a cat being tossed out the window into the raging waters. When the animal struggled to swim, someone ran downstairs and brought it back inside; the next time the cat was thrown out the window it had a broken neck. While Kokemor didn't personally euthanize any animals, he was aware that other doctors were doing so. "One man wanted to put his fifteen-year-old dog down, and I told him I don't know where that was taking place, but if he talked to some of the other doctors, they might have something to help him," Kokemor said, adding: "The next time I saw him, he didn't have his dog with him. He said they gave him something."

It is unknown how many animals were given lethal injections and how many were left to starve to death in their cages. Kokemor stated that he never heard discussion about putting humans out of their misery. "None of us thought of euthanizing anybody," he said. "We were disappointed and beginning to get scared for the people who were under our responsibility. But we were concerned about how many we were going to lose, not about how inconvenient it was to be there, or what was the most expedient way of getting out of there."

Among those who had left the Memorial premises were its security guards, so janitors and volunteers were deputized and given guns, and even the hospital's CEO strapped on a firearm. There was a real fear that armed thugs would try to enter the building to rob people and steal drugs, so the last holdouts wanted to be prepared.[21]

At their 7 a.m. briefing on the emergency room ramp on Thursday, September 1, Kokemor and a small group of other medical personnel vented their frustrations. They were sleep deprived, haggard, sweaty, and operating on automatic pilot. They had been told that Tenet Healthcare was planning to mount a private rescue, but the head nurse and incident coordinator, who had been in touch with Tenet executives, dropped a bombshell when she purportedly told them there was no longer assurance of any boats or helicopters. The group was on its own, and there was a lot of work to do—by 5 p.m., all living patients had to be out of the building.

Father Marse could only offer a shoulder for people to cry on and more prayers. "It really was doomsday, almost," Marse said. "At that point, we were beginning to ration the food because we didn't have much left. Some staff members started losing it. The big question was: "When are we going to get some help?"[22] Marse also described a heartbreaking encounter he had had the day before with an elderly patient: "There was one old lady in her wheelchair. She was crying. She wanted to go home. I said, 'You can't go home. Look at all the water.' She said, 'You can put me on your back and swim.' I told her, 'Honey, I can't swim.' She more or less cried herself to sleep."

The group went back into the hospital to share the bad news with the other staffers. Eyes were red and voices were strained as they explained to their colleagues that they might not survive this nightmare.[23]

They had to keep trying, come hell or high water. And that's what they had in spades—hell and high water.

Nine seriously ill LifeCare patients—four men and five women, ranging in age from sixty-one to ninety—remained on the seventh floor, five of whom had Do Not Resuscitate orders on their charts. In my view, having studied their autopsy reports and medical records, none of these individuals were immediately terminal. However, all of them died that day—with high levels of painkillers in their systems.

In a January 2008 issue of the *New England Journal of Medicine*, Dr. Anna Maria Pou provided written answers to questions by author Susan Okie, MD "The standard of rescue [had] changed from Tuesday to Thursday; initially the sickest patients were evacuated first. When we realized that help was not imminent . . . the standard of rescue changed to that of reverse triage," Pou wrote. "It was recognized that some patients might not survive, and priority was given to those who had the best chance of survival. On Thursday morning, only category 3 patients [the most gravely ill] remained on the LifeCare unit." Someone must have told that to Pou because except for the Code Blue earlier in the week, she had not been on the seventh floor.

Okie describes a conversation on Wednesday between the chief of medicine, Dr. Richard Deichmann, and the head nurse and incident commander, Susan Mulderick, who had been the point person for Tenet executives in Dallas. Deichmann wrote about the conversation in *Code Blue*, his book about the Memorial disaster. Mulderick is said to have asked him if euthanasia should be considered for any of the patients with DNR orders, which Deichmann says he decisively rejected. When Okie requested a statement from Mulderick, no response was offered. Deichmann, however, told Okie that the topic of euthanasia never arose at any of the twice-a-day meetings he held— evacuation was the only sanctioned goal. Like a good ship's captain, he watched as the last surviving patients were loaded onto choppers before he boarded one himself. Weeks later, when the allegations of euthanasia hit the media, he was surprised. "I just can't reconcile that," he told Okie.[24] But I was told that Deichmann spent most of his time on the helipad and may not have been fully aware of all that was happening down below.

In a September 2007 interview with *Newsweek* magazine, Pou described the deplorable conditions at the facility, with death around every corner and a smell so bad "it would burn the back of your throat." She said a hospital administrator announced that no help would be arriving, but she didn't name the individual. Pou further said that staffers then convened to determine the best way to help the patients who were least able to be evacuated. The group decision, she said, was to provide "sedation" for them. Pou claimed to the magazine that she didn't volunteer to administer drugs to the patients, but "it was a group decision."[25]

Who was part of that group?

Perhaps the most telling interview was given just days after the patients died and all survivors had been safely evacuated. In the British newspaper the *Mail on Sunday*, the authors withheld the name of the doctor they interviewed because, as they wrote, "euthanasia is illegal in Louisiana." The article was about a religious, female physician at Memorial who administered lethal injections to nine extremely ill patients. The exclusive story explained that the doctor willfully broke every rule of medical ethics to end the lives of the patients the hospital's staffers had been trying for days to save. Her remarkable, purported confession included the following quote: "I didn't know if I was doing the right thing. But I did not have time. I had to make snap decisions, under the most appalling circumstances, and I did what I thought was right. I injected morphine into those patients who were dying and in agony. If the first dose was not enough, I gave a double dose. And at night I prayed to God to have mercy on my soul."

The doctor continued: "This was not murder, this was compassion. They would have been dead within hours, if not days. We did not put people down. What we did was give comfort to the end. I had cancer patients who were in agony. In some cases the drugs may have speeded up the death process. We divided patients into three categories: those who were traumatised but medically fit enough to survive, those who needed urgent care, and the dying. People would find it impossible to understand the situation. I had to make life-or-death decisions in a split second. It came down to giving people the basic human right to die with dignity. There were patients with Do Not Resuscitate signs. Under normal circumstances, some could have lasted several days. But when the power went out, we had nothing. Some of the very sick became distressed. We tried to make them as comfortable as possible. The pharmacy was under lockdown because gangs of armed looters were roaming around looking for their fix. You have to understand these people were going to die anyway."[26]

A total of forty-five dead bodies—including eleven from before the hurricane hit—were discovered at Memorial once the sealed building was reentered on September 11.[27] Yet, there was not an immediate outcry for an investigation. In this shell-shocked city with its population scattered around the country or missing, and its courthouses, jails, and businesses destroyed or in need of repair, and where looting and violence were still major concerns, probing these deaths took a backseat. After his "Brownie, you're doing a heck of a job" remark (referring to the head of FEMA, Michael D. Brown), President Bush finally addressed the abysmal lack of organization: "Katrina exposed serious problems in our response capability at all levels, and to the extent that the federal government didn't fully do its job right, I take responsibility," he said. "I want to know what went right and what went wrong. I want to know how to better cooperate with state and local government to be able to answer that very question that you asked: 'Are we capable of dealing with a severe attack or another severe storm?' And that's a very important question and it's in our national interest that we find out exactly what went on so we can better respond."[28]

In reality, Katrina revealed just how the whole Gulf Coast and Hurricane Alley had been hanging on by the skin of their teeth for way too long. What mattered now was getting the levees fixed, and engineers and workmen had begun the job. But just as Mayor Nagin was planning to declare the city safe again on September 19, Hurricane Rita looked like it might hit New Orleans. While it did compromise more levees, the brunt of that storm was in Texas, Florida, and western Louisiana; Rita's death toll was seven, including one in Louisiana.[29]

There were rumbles of discontent over the happenings at Memorial, including an article published on September 13, in Scotland's national newspaper, the *Scotsman*. An unnamed male nurse accused Memorial's management of deserting patients and staff. Standing in the muddy street outside the shuttered brick building, he railed to the reporters: "It was hard. It was hell. It was hot, life-threateningly hot," he said. "It was bad in there, I find it hard to think about. We were left here to die, all of us—the patients and staff. We had no communication, we had no help from those you'd have expected to help. It was just volunteers coming in, trying to help us get people off on boats." To add insult to injury, the nurse complained that Tenet announced it was cutting off benefits and paychecks, "abandoning us again now, just like they did after the storm."[30]

CNN sent a team to New Orleans to check into rumors of euthanasia at Memorial Medical Center. A riveting report aired on the *Anderson Cooper 360* show on October 13, but I only found out about it much later. An internist named Bryant King—the same one whose sister asked for help on the nola.com bulletin board—and a nurse manager named Fran Butler described to correspondent Jonathan Freed how the hospital was functioning as a shelter, under battlefield conditions. In the CNN piece, there was open and repeated discussion of euthanizing the patients who some—unnamed by the network—felt might not survive to be evacuated. Butler said her nurses asked if there was a plan to end the patients' lives. Because of her own personal beliefs, Butler refused to participate, and she didn't see anyone take part in such an act. But Dr. King bluntly told Freed: "Most people know that something happened that shouldn't have happened."

In the CNN exclusive, King said that on Thursday morning, September 1, a doctor told him of a conversation between a hospital administrator and a third doctor who suggested that patients be put out of their misery. King's response was "You've got to be ****ing kidding me that you think that that's a good idea," and the doctor he was speaking with said the third doctor would be willing to do it. King said the doctor who told him this was also against the plan, but about three hours later, King became aware of an uneasy quiet in the triage section, on the second floor. All relatives had been told to leave, and only the patients, a second hospital administrator, and two doctors—including the one who had first raised the question of mercy killing—were present. The administrator asked if the group wanted to join in prayer, something that had not been done in any of the previously hellish days—neither when the storm hit nor when they lost electrical power.

"I looked around, and one of the other physicians—not the one who had the conversation with me, but another—had a handful of syringes. I don't know what's in the syringes," Dr. King told correspondent Freed. "The only thing I heard her say is, 'I'm going to give you something to make you feel better.' I don't know what she was going to give them. But we hadn't been giving medications like that to make people feel better or any sort of palliative care—or anything like that. We hadn't been doing that up to this point." King said he saw the female doctor go from one patient to the next, presumably to inject them, although he never saw the actual injections. He stated that it was odd that a physician would be injecting any patient—that was a nurse's duty. And he wondered why all of the patients seemed to be getting the same medication.

Dr. King told CNN that he realized something untoward was happening and he wanted no part of it. He grabbed his bag and one of the doctors hugged him, then King got on a boat and left Memorial. Nurse Butler said the doctor who was resistant in the conversation with King also spoke to her about euthanasia. "She was the first person to approach me about putting patients to sleep," Butler told the CNN reporter. "She made the comment to me on how she was totally against it and wouldn't do it." King said the numbers alone proved there was euthanasia: "There's only one person that died overnight. The previous day, there were only two. So for there to be—from Thursday to Friday, for there to be ten times that many just doesn't make sense to me."

CNN's Freed announced that King had spoken to the state attorney general's office—and now attorney general Charles C. Foti Jr. was asking coroner Frank Minyard to perform autopsies and toxicology screenings on all forty-five deceased patients from Memorial. They ran a clip of Minyard saying, "Well, they thought someone was going around injecting people with some sort of lethal medication."

The news story continued with Freed saying he spoke to the three people King alleges he was with in the triage section. The hospital administrator said, "I don't remember being in a room with patients or saying a prayer," and added that King must be lying—and the doctor who King said was against euthanasia said she wouldn't talk to the media. But the doctor who King allegedly saw with the syringes had several phone conversations with the CNN reporter, emphasizing how everyone inside the hospital felt abandoned. "We did everything humanly possible to save these patients," the doctor told Freed, who withheld her name in his report. "The government totally abandoned us to die, in the houses, in the streets, in the hospitals. Maybe a lot of us made mistakes, but we made the best decisions we could at the time." When told about King's allegation, this doctor responded that she would not comment either way. Nurse Manager Fran Butler says that while some nurses did discuss euthanasia, they never stopped caring for the patients: "The people who were still there, they really and truly took and put their heart and souls into every patient—whether that patient lived or died." The story ended with general statements from Tenet and LifeCare, citing the heroism of their personnel and their cooperation with the investigation.[31]

While I missed that CNN program, other media coverage about post-Katrina Louisiana reinvigorated my desire to speak with Frank Minyard, my longtime friend who was the coroner of Orleans Parish. I reached him on his cell phone at the temporary morgue he was operating in St. Gabriel, since his own New Orleans facility and lab were flood damaged. We had spoken earlier after he had arrived at the field location, and I had offered to come down and help, but he said there wasn't a place for me or any outsiders to stay. The red tape was worse than the job, he sighed. It took him a month to even get a working phone, and for a long time he didn't have a medical transcriptionist who could type out the autopsy reports. But FEMA finally seemed to be stepping up to the plate, including bringing in trailers for housing.

Frank told me that he and the state medical examiner, Lou Cataldie, had dead bodies from all over the state—at that point the number was over a thousand—and that his meager crew was only one-third of the way through autopsying and identifying the remains. There were also more than six hundred disinterred caskets from flooded cemeteries that had to be handled. This time when I volunteered to help, Minyard accepted my offer; I would be their first outsider. I canceled some work engagements and on October 27 headed south for the next three days. From Pittsburgh I flew to Atlanta, and then took a short flight to Baton Rouge—all at my own expense, which I was only too happy to bear.

Biblical scholars view Gabriel as the "archangel of death," who sounded his trumpet outside the gates of heaven. In the Jewish faith, he was the voice who told Noah to gather animals before the great flood. So perhaps St. Gabriel was an inspired choice as the site for the interim morgue for Katrina victims.

My years as a captain in the US Air Force Medical Corps, in the early 1960s, were good preparation for what I saw at St. Gabriel. There was a military precision that I appreciated and the esprit de corps was as tight as in any war zone unit. Volunteers from every state in the union, including Alaska and Hawaii, were deployed to the area. The DMORT squad was storing the bodies in refrigerator trucks that were parked four miles away in Carville, a city that also happens to be the home of the only Hansen's Disease museum—or leprosarium—on the continental United States. Carville is also the hometown of political consultant James Carville, whose grandfather was the town's postmaster. Blackwater USA security guards, working pro bono, accompanied each truckload of bodies, an honor befitting the precious cargo.

The temporary morgue was a tent-like, white warehouse about two football fields in size. It wasn't fancy on the outside, but inside scientific magic was being performed. Only workers wearing special "Morgue Ops" badges were allowed on the premises. Each Katrina corpse was given a number to track its progress, with the goal being an identification and release to its next of kin. Bulletin boards with constantly changing information tried to match bodies with family members looking for missing people, while other boards just listed partial data. Some cases would be promptly solved, others would remain a mystery. There was a lot of respect for the victims; one of the medical examiners hung up a sign that read: *Mortui vivis praecipant.* It means "Let the dead teach the living."

As soon as I arrived, I dropped off my bag on the cot in my trailer, changed into scrubs, and asked Minyard where he wanted me. Over the next three days I would perform thirty autopsies, with as much detail as possible under such challenging circumstances. While some of the younger forensic pathologists could only do four or five cases a day, my experience enabled me to complete about ten autopsies per day—a fact that I took great pride in. Forty percent of the victims appeared to be over the age of seventy, and scores were evacuees who died out of state and were brought back. In most cases it was impossible to determine an exact cause or manner of death. Many dates of death were listed as August 29, 2005, the day Katrina struck US soil, while others were left blank. Sexual assaults, had they taken place, could not be proven, because of the deterioration of the bodies. Mental stress probably played a role in many deaths, and heart attacks were prevalent. I had one female victim who had a head wound from a gunshot, but whether she was murdered or committed suicide would be impossible to determine. Of all the dead bodies that were autopsied at St. Gabriel, only seven deaths were by gunshot.

When a new body would arrive, the first stop would be to look for a wallet or information card with a name and address—although anything found would have to be verified. In many cases, those primary clues didn't exist. Clothing and personal effects would be removed from the corpse, with notes chronicling each item of jewelry, footwear, or apparel—including any T-shirt logos. Personal items were stored for safe-keeping or given to whomever claimed the body.

Next, a number of steps would be followed—in no particular order, as long as everything on the master checklist was eventually marked off. Photographs would be shot at each point along the way. The body would be washed and decontaminated, and an external visual inspection would be made. Attention would be paid to existent surgical scars, historic bone fractures, missing body parts, and tattoos and/or piercings. The body would then be wheeled to the radiology station, where head-to-toe X-rays would be taken. Heart pacemakers and hip and breast implants all have serial numbers on file with their manufacturers, which could be useful in identifying their owners. In the autopsy arena, medical examiners and assistants would receive the corpses—none of them embalmed, but all of them in varying stages of decomposition, including partial mummification. The individuals would be cut open and examined, with samples extracted for toxicology testing. Since Minyard's in-house lab was gone, he was shipping samples to National Medical Services' laboratory in Willow Grove, Pennsylvania. Pieces of tissue—liver, kidney, or brain—would be tested since there was no blood, bile, urine, or vitreous humor. Later the bodies would be sewn up and placed in caskets.

Efforts would be made to establish gender, race, and an approximate age, which was not always possible in some extreme cases. Forensic anthropologists would study the bones to help answer those questions. In some cases there was just a solo body part to work with.

Determining eye color was often unfeasible due to the postmortem decomposition that makes eyes turn cloudy very rapidly, but head and facial hair were described with as much detail as possible. Because many of the faces were swollen and discolored, and some even gnawed away by rodents or insects, forensic odontologists would look to a victim's teeth for clues by making X-rays of the mouth. Families looking for loved ones would furnish a photo—even an old yearbook image would suffice since, in most cases, a gap between the teeth, or some other dental oddity, would likely follow the individual through his or her life. Technicians would try to lift fingerprints to put into the federal database, but sometimes the skin would slip off like a glove, foiling that plan.

DNA testing was overseen by the Louisiana Department of Health and Hospitals and the Louisiana State Police Crime Laboratory. All tests were run in duplicate to ensure quality control. Numerous labs across the country were employed to hasten the testing, including Reliagene Technologies in New Orleans; Orchid Cellmark, Inc., in Nashville, Tennessee; and the University of North Texas Health Science Center Laboratory in Fort Worth. The inside of each victim's mouth was swabbed for buccal cells and, when possible, matched against a missing person's hairbrush, toothbrush, nail clippers, or clothing from his or her residence, providing the items weren't contaminated from the floodwaters. Family members were also swabbed and asked to contribute greeting cards or mail sent by the deceased in the hope that DNA could be extracted from the glue on the envelope or on the stamp. A software program titled DNAVIEW was accessed to locate "cold hits," or lucky matches.

The more puzzling cases required additional handling—for those, DNA would be extracted from tibias, or shinbones. These samples would then be cataloged, packaged, and sent to two different laboratories. One lab was Bode Technological Group in Virginia, and the other was the International Commission of Missing Persons laboratory in Bosnia, where scientists had voluminous experience in identifying corpses retrieved from mass graves. Geneticists from the National Institute of Health and other major universities also contributed expertise in contacting families and establishing connections.

When new data would come back, it would be screened all over again. Once a body was identified, the coroner, Frank Minyard, would sign the death certificate, and the state medical examiner, Louis Cataldie, would authorize release of the remains. About two hundred of the dead were claimed, in no condition for open-casket funerals. In many instances, Lou would later tell me, finding addresses for some of the people would be pointless because not only would their homes be lost, but many of their streets and neighborhoods would be gone, too.

At dusk we would knock off work and join in the mess hall for conversation and pretty good grub. "In the history of this country, there had never been such a forensic challenge," Minyard remarked one night. It was a subject that still made him emotional. "These are my people, every one of them. This devastation—not only of our people, but our lives—will be with us forever. We will never be the same." He was angry at the way some people reported salacious rumors without checking their facts. The story about the little girl who was raped and murdered especially rankled him. "If something like that would have happened, we would have known about it. It never happened," he said. "You know how people are, they exaggerate. At times like this, people hallucinate. People are not themselves now. They think they saw things; they're not lying but they think they saw things that never happened." Then he grabbed his trumpet and some other musicians and played another song made famous by Louis Armstrong: "Do You Know What It Means to Miss New Orleans?"

FEMA had anticipated that as many as five thousand bodies would be in need of processing and had funded and built a $17 million morgue to replace the St. Gabriel temporary operation. In December of 2005— weeks after I had left Louisiana—the new "Carville Victims Identification Center" opened for business. The seventy thousand square-foot, state-of-the-art facility—complete with a full laboratory, a cafeteria, and a fitness center—was so imposing Dr. Minyard referred to it as the "forensic Taj Mahal." The space was designed to decontaminate and examine one hundred fifty bodies per day, and there was living space for six hundred workers. But when the number of state-wide Katrina deaths remained at about thirteen hundred, FEMA decided to close the new headquarters and mothball all of the equipment—it was only in operation for less than three months. I understand it's now just being used for training, although it would be a cinch to get it up and running should there be another massive disaster with high casualties.

Minyard and his coroner's staff returned to New Orleans and a new office rental in an unused funeral home. A special mausoleum was also built nearby to house the unclaimed remains. So successful was the six-month-long endeavor, fewer than thirty bodies went unidentified. And throughout the entire time, mental health professionals were also present to help grieving families and friends either come to terms with their loved one's demise or provide a sympathetic ear to those for whom there was never any closure.

In November, after my return to Pittsburgh, staffers of Louisiana Attorney General Charles Foti's office contacted me. Assistant Attorney General Arthur "Butch" Schafer of the Criminal Division, Medicaid Fraud Control Unit, was heading the inquiry. Butch explained that he and special agent Virginia Rider were presently interviewing witnesses and investigating a number of possibly suspicious deaths at Memorial Medical Center. Later Victoria Sweeney and Elizabeth C. Engels, both of whom were also registered nurses, joined the team. A total of fourteen dedicated individuals would serve on this task force.

The top-secret investigation had begun when Schafer asked Coroner Minyard to send him the toxicological results of all the deceased Memorial patients. As Butch looked at the data from the National Medical Services lab, he needed an expert to verify his suspicion that some patients had been given a purposeful, lethal dosage of medication. I agreed to review the medical and toxicology charts and I was floored by the results. At least nine victims had seemingly received a deadly cocktail of, primarily, morphine and midazolam hydrochloride, a hypnotic benzodiazepam marketed under the named Versed. According to the documentation, the two drugs were mixed together into one injection for most of the patients.

I learned that the attorney general's office was pushing for homicide or manslaughter charges to be filed against a physician, Dr. Anna Maria Pou, and possibly some nurses. The attorney general's investigators had witnesses who claimed they knew the patients had been injected. The concept of a medical worker giving unsuspecting patients injections that would surely end their lives was antithetical to everything a licensed doctor should hold dear. There was no way such an action could rightly be defined as "euthanasia," since that would require a patient approving of, and specifically asking for, help to die. And while these LifeCare patients all had major medical problems, none was terminally ill—another requirement for legal euthanasia in the few jurisdictions where it is permissible around the world.

I asked Schafer what could possibly be the defense. He replied that, as he understood it, the intention was to sedate these nine very sick patients. But I pointed out that morphine and midazolam hydrochloride are strong painkillers, not sedatives to calm an individual. Together these drugs would produce an increase in delta activity in the brain, which would depress the central nervous system and lead to death, usually within minutes. I asked Butch why the patients were not evacuated, and he told me that no good reason had been discerned. It seemed that a person, or persons, had made the decision to terminate, not evacuate, these people. There was no way to sugarcoat it—a terrible crime had been committed. These deaths were clearly homicide, which is what I wrote in my report.

Louisiana law states that on original jurisdiction, the attorney general has the power to investigate and arrest, but the district attorney of any parish takes over the case, unless there is a recusal or an assist is requested. The district attorney then convenes a special grand jury, and if probable cause to indict is found, a "true bill" is handed down and the case goes to trial. Conversely, if a grand jury finds "no true bill," the case is dismissed. The Orleans Parish was covered by New Orleans District Attorney Eddie Jordan—previously a US attorney in the area—who was apprised of the Schafer investigation. Because his community was still so distraught, with residents not yet moved back and neither businesses nor the courts operating at peak levels, he seemed grateful to accept the state's grasp of the facts. Jordan also liked that I was involved. He knew I had no personal stake in the matter and would react solely to the evidence.

As I waited to hear what was next, I kept in phone contact with Frank Minyard and began to notice that he seemed to be rethinking the deaths. He wondered if the extreme decomposition of the bodies might be cause for the spike in the morphine and Versed readings. The bodies had been left in the hospital for ten days, the temperature topped 100 degrees, and there was ungodly moisture in the air—if all of that created an extraordinary set of circumstances that produced false readings, would it be appropriate to charge anyone with a crime? It was a fair question, and one that deserved a scientific experiment.

I took blood and liver tissue samples from three Pennsylvania residents whose autopsies I performed—after they had died of drug overdoses—and I sent the samples to National Medical Services for toxicological analyses. Then I took a second set of samples and exposed them to conditions that replicated those during Katrina at Memorial Medical Center. The temperature in Pittsburgh at the time was unusually warm, over 90 degrees. I put the samples into three environments for three weeks—room temperature, refrigerated, and outdoors—then I also sent those samples to National Medical Services. The results I got back were most convincing: There was no significant variation in the opiate levels over time in any of the samples. I sent an organized summary of the test results to Minyard, with copies to Butch Schafer and Victoria Sweeney of the attorney general's office, and hoped it would guide them in their research.

On July 17, 2006, arrests were made of Dr. Anna M. Pou and two nurses, Lori L. Budo and Cheri A. Landry, for allegedly injecting Memorial patients with pharmaceutical drugs that took their lives. Attorney General Charles Foti, the former longtime sheriff of Orleans Parish, stated at a press conference, "This is not euthanasia. This is homicide. We're talking about people who pretended that maybe they were God." Second-degree murder charges were filed on behalf of only four patients—Emmett Everett, Rose Savoie, Hollis Alford, and Ireatha Watson—not nine. I was told prosecutors narrowed the cases to those most likely to net convictions. Often in cases with multiple victims, prosecutors will hold back on some of them, so that in case there is an acquittal, they can come back for a new trial with different victims and the same defendants. This avoids the constitutionally protected double jeopardy rule that disallows a person from being tried twice for the same offense. But I'm told that wasn't a factor here.

The four patients had fatal doses of morphine and Versed in their bloodstreams, and then water was carefully flushed into the patients' IVs to ensure that the drugs circulated. None of the patients were receiving the two drugs on a regular basis, Foti said, adding: "When you use both of these drugs it becomes a lethal cocktail and it guarantees you're going to die." The patients would have survived had they not been injected, Foti told the crowd. Asked for a reason for the deaths, he answered: "It is not my job or duty to say what the motive was." And he hinted that there might be more arrests.[32]

The affidavit, which was released to the press, was filed outlining the charges that the state of Louisiana was making against the three women, which listed their addresses, license numbers, and dates of birth. For the most part, other employees were designated only by their initials, and while the names have since been publicly disclosed, I'll use initials here. The affidavit began by stating that LifeCare, through its attorneys, self-reported the "possible euthanasia of patients following Hurricane Katrina by personnel working at Memorial Medical Center," then explained that LifeCare leased space from Memorial, which was owned and operated by Tenet. Next, K. J., the director of physical medicine for LifeCare, described the Thursday morning meeting where Memorial's incident commander, S. M., stated that the LifeCare patients were very sick and "we don't expect them to make it." Two hours later, according to the document, K. J.; S. H., LifeCare's director of pharmacy; and LifeCare's assistant administrator, D. R.; asked S. M. what Memorial planned to do about the seventh-floor patients, to which S. M. apprised them that they "were not going to leave any living patients behind." S. M. instructed them to find Dr. Pou, and S. H. and D. R. went to look for her. K. J. returned to the seventh floor to try to persuade LifeCare patients' family members to evacuate from the facility.

Later, the affidavit states, T. M., a nurse executive and director of education for LifeCare, found K. J. downstairs and told K. J. the Life-Care patients were going to receive a "lethal dose." The two women walked upstairs to the seventh floor, and K. J. observed Pou and two nurses in the charting room drawing liquids from vials into syringes. Dr. Pou seemed nervous and stated that she was going to tell patient Emmett Everett that she was going to give him something for his dizziness. One of the nurses asked Pou if she wanted accompaniment, but Pou said no and went into Mr. Everett's room herself and closed the door. K. J. was then asked to show Pou and the two nurses where the remaining LifeCare patients on the floor were, which she did. K. J., Pou, and Budo entered the room occupied by patients Rose Savoie and Alice Hutzler. Out of the corner of her eye, K. J. saw Budo inject Savoie with something and heard the first woman say, "That burns."

K. J. then accompanied the nurses and Pou to all the patients' rooms and identified each. Pou instructed K. J. to make a list of all patients, because they didn't want to miss anyone; she also told K. J. to cover each expired patient's head with a sheet. At the same time, K. J. was instructed to tell the remaining LifeCare staff to evacuate, that Life-Care patients were "in our hands now," and "you've done everything you can." K. J. then went down to the second-floor evacuation area but was not allowed to check on the LifeCare patients who were in that floor's triage section.

T. M. says, as set forth in the affidavit, that Pou had told her that morning the seventh-floor LifeCare patients were "probably not going to survive" and that "a decision had been made to administer lethal doses" to them. When T. M. asked "doses of what?" she said that she believes Pou answered morphine and Ativan. T. M. asked Pou if the LifeCare patients were the only ones who would receive the doses, and T. M. said Pou responded that that was not the case. Pou added that the LifeCare staffers were not involved in this at all and that "there was no telling how far it would go." According to T. M., Pou further advised her that nurses from another part of the hospital would be assisting her; then she advised T. M. to leave the hospital with the other LifeCare staffers. As T. M. was rounding up workers to leave with, she noticed two nurses she didn't know and assumed them to be Pou's assistants. T. M., D. R., and S. H. joined K. J. on the second floor and were also stopped by Memorial staffers from going into the triage section.

D. R.'s statement, as written in the affidavit, matched K. J.'s and T. M.'s but added that Pou did not seem to be familiar with the medical conditions of the LifeCare patients. Pou told her that she was under the impression the patients were unaware of what was happening, but D. R. pointed to Mr. Everett as someone who was quite alert, even though he was paralyzed and weighed three hundred eighty pounds. Pou allegedly then made the decision that he would not be evacuated, despite the fact that two other four-hundred-pound patients who could not walk had been safely evacuated in the previous days.

Pou asked that D. R. find a nurse who could sedate Everett. They spoke to a nurse about it, but D. R. then decided she didn't want one of her nurses involved. D. R. soon saw two nurses she didn't recognize and figured Pou had brought them in.

Pou instructed D. R. to bring her a tray and assemble the remaining LifeCare staff. Pou then told D. R., "I want ya'll to know I take full responsibility and ya'll did a great job taking care of the patients." On the second floor, when D. R. tried to look in on the Life-Care patients in triage, a Memorial staffer gave her an e-mail address and said she could inquire about her patients that way; because no one had paper, the person jotted the e-mail address on T. M.'s scrub shirt.

S. H.'s account in the affidavit conformed to the others with the addition that, as the pharmacy director, he furnished Pou with more than one hundred vials of morphine. She also requested and was given syringes and saline flushes—saline flushes follow an intravenous administration of medication to ensure the medicine does not stay in the IV port and enters a patient's system. As S. H. was leaving the seventh floor, he noted Pou and her two nurses going in and out of the LifeCare patients' rooms. S. H. then went downstairs and was also barred from seeing the LifeCare patients in the triage section.

In a subsequent interview, the affidavit states, S. H. was shown photos of various Memorial staffers. He positively identified Dr. Anna Pou. On December 5, 2005, he accompanied a representative of the attorney general's office to the seventh floor of Memorial to complete an inventory of the LifeCare pharmacy. Also there were Lori Budo and Cheri Landry, who were doing a walk-through with their attorneys. S. H. then positively identified them to the attorney general staffer as the two nurses who accompanied Pou on September 1.

The affidavit listed patients Hollis Alford, Rose Savoie, Ireatha Watson, and Emmett Everett, and stated that they were brought from Memorial to the DMORT facility on September 11. DMORT doctors performed their autopsies, and various tissue samples were collected and delivered to National Medical Services for testing. The tests came back positive for morphine and midazolam. It also stated that the results and patient medical records were reviewed by a forensic pathologist—me, unnamed in the affidavit—who advised that "in all four cases it appeared that a lethal amount of morphine was administered" and that none of the patients' normal medication protocols included those drugs.

Finally, the affidavit listed the charge of four counts of second-degree murder against all three women, citing Louisiana Revised Statute 14.30.1 as "the killing of a human being when the offender has a specific intent to kill or inflict great bodily harm."[33]

Pou was arrested at 9 p.m., after a thirteen-hour day of surgery. She was still in her scrubs, alone in her Baton Rouge home, eating a lettuce and tomato salad, when four armed agents from the attorney general's office arrived, handcuffed her, and brought her to the East Baton Rouge Parish Prison. Several hours later she was again handcuffed, then driven to Orleans Parish Prison. "The whole way, I was asking God to help my family get through this," she told *Newsweek*.[34] She was especially concerned that several of her hospitalized patients were now without a primary care physician. Landry was arrested at the hospital where she worked, and Budo's arrest was at her home, in front of her children. Though arrested, they were all quickly released on their own recognizance, subject to a small bond to be filed later.

Pou's supporters felt the arrest was overly dramatic since her attorney and the attorney general's office had a "firm agreement" that she would be allowed to present herself to authorities without a formal and public arrest.[35] I would have to agree that an honorable surrender to custody might have been more appropriate. After all, I doubt that she was much of a flight risk. And as much as I felt the arrests were apt, I was also mindful that Attorney General Charles Foti was in a tight reelection bid.

On August 13, 2006, I flew to Louisiana, where Frank Minyard's New Orleans coroner's office was again up and running in the temporary quarters of an old funeral home. Over the next two and a half days, I attended several roundtable meetings with Minyard; Assistant Attorney General Butch Schafer and members of his team; Dr. Robert A. Middleberg, lab director and chief forensic toxicologist from National Medical Services; and my friend New York forensic pathologist Dr. Michael M. Baden. Michael had also performed some volunteer work at the St. Gabriel DMORT facility, and Minyard asked him to consult on the Memorial deaths. Although District Attorney Eddie Jordan never came to our meetings, two of his assistants popped in briefly. The sessions were very productive in bringing us up to date on the ongoing investigation. Now it seemed that in addition to the four initial patients whose deaths I had reviewed, there were five others whose demises seemed suspicious. I agreed to take home the five newest cases and prepare reports, as did Dr. Baden.

On a side note, as I waited to fly back to Pennsylvania on August 16, I saw on an airport television the arrest in Thailand of John Mark Karr, who claimed to have killed tiny beauty queen JonBenét Ramsey in her Boulder, Colorado, home in 1996. I had written a book on the case several years ago and instantly recognized what few in the media or the Boulder district attorney's office seemed to be thinking—that Karr was a false confessor. Within days his story would fall apart after there was no DNA, handwriting, or trace evidence linking him to the case.

Schafer's staff spoke with family members of the LifeCare victims, all of whom had been under the impression that their loved ones had died of natural causes. The relatives were helpful in giving background on the patients' medical histories and each was thunderstruck when shown evidence of the medications found in the bodies at autopsy. In almost every case, these drugs were not part of the patients' therapeutic regimen.

Schafer's investigators had also been interviewing Memorial employees who each had a small piece of the puzzle that they weren't sure added up to anything but wanted to contribute because they felt something sinister had occurred. Even more significant data came from Dr. Bryant King, the internist who had spoken to CNN. While he held back from naming names and giving titles on the broadcast, he made a more complete disclosure to the authorities about what he observed on that last eventful day. He stated categorically that Anna Maria Pou was the doctor with the handful of syringes preparing to inject people on the second-floor triage section and mentioned the two nurses with her—he didn't know their names but recognized them from around the hospital. King told Schafer's people that he left when he heard talk of euthanasia, stating that he would rather be a physician who abandoned his patients than one who took their lives. He left in a boat, then had a three-and-a-half-hour walk home where he tormented himself by wondering if he should have been more forceful in protesting what he assumed was about to happen. He was an athletic man who had rescued many people that day—could he have used his strength to physically intimidate the first doctor who mentioned that patients were to be put out of their misery? King again maintained that he never actually saw Pou inject anyone. However, had he stayed behind, he wondered, could he have fought against something he believed was a termination plan?

The patients Dr. King left in that triage section were distinct from the seventh-floor LifeCare patients who were never brought downstairs because there was no one to carry them—recall that there was no electricity for lights or the elevators. Those nine patients all died in their beds.

Dr. Minyard briefed District Attorney Jordan about our three-day meeting and said that Michael Baden and I would both be doing reports on what were nine deaths. Jordan asked that we increase the number of experts on our team, which I viewed as a good thing. The more scientific proof we could offer, the more assured we would be. I brought in my friend Arthur L. Caplan, PhD, chair of the Department of Medical Ethics at the University of Pennsylvania, in Philadelphia, and Dr. James Young, former chief coroner of the province of Ontario, Canada, who was the current president of the American Academy of Forensic Sciences, a post I had held some years before. Minyard also brought in a colleague, Dr. Frank Brescia, a Charleston, South Carolina, expert in end-of-life issues.

With a minimum of discussion beforehand, each of the other team members was given the exact set of physical material I had—nine patients' medical records, autopsy reports, and toxicology results—and asked to review and write an analysis. I'm not so egomaniacal that I expected everyone's findings to echo mine. In fact, I probably would have enjoyed the intellectual exercise of differing opinions, but that's not what we got. Over the next several weeks, as the results of these independent thinkers—each with decades of experience—became known, their opinions aligned with mine, in that we felt that homicides had been committed. There was no other interpretation for the unnecessary and fatal injections of drugs given to these victims. Whatever explanation this supposed "Angel of Mercy" might have would need to be brought before a jury.

As word got out that we five were working on the Memorial Hospital case, someone good-naturedly referred to us as "The Forensic All-Stars," which made us sound like the world's worst softball team. That was amusing, but we were serious in our vow to stand by our findings, first to a grand jury and later at trial. For the Orleans Parish, which had suffered so greatly and would need years to recover, our gift would be unanimous encouragement for District Attorney Jordan to present what we saw was an easily winnable case. What better way to prove that New Orleans was back on track than to seek justice on behalf of the most vulnerable victims imaginable? Eddie Jordan would go on to convene a grand jury all right—but a big surprise lay ahead.

On October 3, 2006, I sent three reports to Butch Schafer, with copies to Frank Minyard. The first was an analysis of the deaths of five Life-Care patients: Harold Dupas, George Huard, Alice Hutzler, Wilda McManus, and Elaine Nelson. In all cases I determined the patients died of "acute combined drug toxicity." At this juncture I was only looking for the presence of morphine and midazolam (Versed) in the patients' systems; later I would get back reports that disclosed the presence of other medications in these patients. I further explained that in a review of the patients' hospital charts, neither morphine nor midazolam had been properly and officially ordered by an attending physician for Mr. Dupas, Mr. Huard, or Ms. Hutzler. Morphine had been previously ordered for Ms. Nelson, I wrote, but it had been discontinued days earlier. Morphine had been ordered in a therapeutic dosage for Ms. McManus, but there was nothing in the record to indicate that it was ever administered.

I could find no "appropriate and reasonably necessary clinical basis" for either morphine or midazolam to have been prescribed and administered to any of these patients. And I noted that it would have been physically and procedurally impossible for any of these patients to have obtained and administered morphine and Versed to themselves, which led me to assert that the drugs were administered to these patients by one or more third parties. "In light of all of the above described physical and clinical circumstances relating to these patients at and around the reported times of their respective deaths, the manner of death would be classified as homicide," I wrote.

My second report was with regards to patients Hollis Alford, Emmett Everett Sr., Rose Savoie, and Ireatha Watson, all four of whom had been on a number of medications for a variety of ailments—but none of whom were being administered either morphine or midazolam for their routine pharmaceutical care requirements. Only Mr. Alford had a physician's order, dated August 31—the last day any charting was done—stating that the patient "*may* have morphine sulfate one to four mg [emphasis mine]" every hour as needed to counter agitation. "Postmortem analysis of tissues and fluids from these individuals showed the presence of morphine in liver, brain, and purge fluid," I wrote. Three cases also had muscle tissue analyzed, showing presence of morphine, and three had midazolam present. Then I made a chart of which patient had what drugs and the amounts. I noted that the toxicological analysis of the tissues also showed the presence of some of the routine drugs the patients had been administered during their Life-

Care stay, and those levels were in the routine and therapeutic category. I then drafted another chart showing the significant morphine quantities in each person's liver, brain, and muscles—levels that I felt were consistent with a lethal overdose. I found that Mr. Alford and Ms. Watson had midazolam quantities in their tissues that appeared to be in greater concentrations than would be expected from therapeutic doses.

There was not a lot of literature written about tissue concentration for midazolam lethality, but I cited one textbook, titled *Disposition of Toxic Drugs and Chemicals in Man*, by analytical toxicologist Dr. Randall C. Baselt. It explained that purge fluid is not identical to blood; rather, it is fluid that develops in the body during decomposition. Purge fluid, however, will contain quantities of the same drugs that are in the blood. The purge fluid in each of the four cases I outlined also contained significant quantities of morphine and midazolam, I offered. In summary, I stated that a lethal amount of morphine was present in all four cases. Mr. Alford's liver had a lower concentration of the morphine than the other three, but he still had significant levels in his muscle, brain, and purge fluid—the dosage was "much greater" than what had been ordered in his medical record. And in three of the cases, the midazolam was greater than therapeutic. I wrote that there was intent to produce a lethal outcome in these patients.

The third report listed eleven different LifeCare patients who also died, I found, from acute drug toxicity. Six patients died with midazolam, alone, in their systems: George Baumgartner, Sonia Beard, Warren Clifton, Wilmer Cooley, Carrie Hall, and Martha Hart. Donna Cotham had only methadone in her system. Marcus Grant had only morphine and Dilaudid—and Lawrence Batiste, Essie Cavalier, and Merle Lagasse had combined levels of morphine and midazolam. I wrote that none of these drugs had been properly and officially ordered by an attending physician for any of these patients and that there was no appropriate and reasonably necessary clinical basis for any of these drugs to have been prescribed and administered to the eleven. As with my first report, I stated that these patients could not have dosed themselves and had to have received their medications from one or more third parties. "In light of all the above described physical and clinical circumstances relating to these patients at and around the reported times of their respective deaths, the manner of death would be classified as homicide," I wrote. Unfortunately, I was later informed that these eleven cases were not going to be considered for prosecution, although I never learned the reasoning for that decision.

After receiving more detailed toxicological analysis on the first group of LifeCare patients—Harold Dupas, George Huard, Alice Hutzler, Wilda McManus, and Elaine Nelson—on October 20, I sent Schafer a new report. I informed him of the precise medications in each patient and in what parts of the body I detected the presence of drugs and in what quantities. Again, I prepared a chart. Harold Dupas had received morphine, midazolam, and sertraline, or, as it is marketed, Zoloft. George Huard had morphine, midazolam, and metoclopramide, which is sold under the name Reglan. Alice Hutzler had morphine, midazolam, paroxetine—which is sold under the name Paxil—and citalopram escitalopram, also known as Celexa or Lexapro. Wilda McManus had morphine, midazolam, hydromorphone—which is known as Dilaudid—and lorazepam, which is sold under the name Ativan; she also had desmethylsertraline, a metabolite of Zoloft, in her blood. And Elaine Nelson had morphine, fentanyl, and meperidine, which is also known as Demerol.

A summary of our five expert reports on the nine LifeCare patients follows and was posted by a CNN employee at its Internet site. Due to the advanced decomposition of these patients, the various medical examiners who performed their post-mortems offered only minimal details in the autopsy reports, but each patient's physical maladies were listed. Here, I've deleted the patients' medical backgrounds for their privacy. Attached to each autopsy report was the full toxicological screening from the National Medical Services laboratory.

HOLLIS ALFORD, sixty-six, male; race was not stated. No order for midazolam (Versed). Toxicology results showed he had morphine and midazolam in his system at autopsy.

HAROLD DUPAS, seventy-eight, black male. No documented use of morphine, midazolam, or lorazepam (Ativan). Toxicology results showed he had morphine, midazolam, and sertraline (Zoloft) in his system at autopsy.

EMMETT EVERETT, sixty-one, male; race was not stated. Toxicology results showed he had morphine and midazolam in his system at autopsy.

GEORGE HUARD, ninety-one, male; race was not stated. No orders for morphine or Versed. Toxicology results showed he had morphine, midazolam and metoclopramide (Reglan).

ALICE HUTZLER, ninety, white female. No orders for morphine or Versed. Was given both Lexapro and Paxil (with a note asking why she was prescribed both). Toxicology showed she had morphine, midazolam, paroxetine (Paxil), and citalopram escitalopram (Celexa or Lexapro). Toxicology results showed she had morphine and midazolam in her system at autopsy.

WILDA S. McMANUS, seventy, black female. Morphine and Ativan prescribed on August 31, but not documented; Vicodin given. No Versed order. Toxicology results showed she had morphine, midazolam, hydromorphone (Dilaudid), lorazepam (Ativan), and desmethylsertraline (a metabolite of Zoloft) in her system at autopsy.

ELAINE NELSON, ninety, white female. Last morphine dose on August 22. Demerol prescribed. Toxicology results showed she had morphine, fentanyl, and meperidine (Demerol) in her system at autopsy.

ROSE SAVOIE, ninety, white female. No documentation of morphine or Versed. Toxicology results showed she had morphine in her system at autopsy.

IREATHA B. WATSON, eighty-nine, female; race was not stated. No order for morphine or Versed. Toxicology results showed she had morphine and midazolam in her system at autopsy.[36]

A couple of weeks after the evacuation, on September 20, 2005, CNN correspondent Jonathan Freed had reported on some of the difficulties posed in evacuating the Memorial patients in a timely way. But he also stated that the fleet of helicopters that rescued people on Thursday, September 1, was provided by Tenet Healthcare and that the corporation also hired private security to guard the empty building until it was safe to bring out the dead bodies.[37]

On December 21, CNN's *Anderson Cooper 360* featured correspondent Drew Griffin interviewing the daughter of one of the "Memorial Nine." Angela McManus had been with her critically ill mother, Wilda, since the hurricane hit, but on that final Thursday she said that she noticed a change in the demeanor of the seventh-floor nurses. She heard them discussing which patients would be left behind, and it was decided that patients with DNRs—who did not want to be resuscitated by unnatural means—would not be rescued. Wilda, recovering from an infection due to rectal cancer, was one such patient, but she was alert, her daughter said. Angela wanted to believe her mother died peacefully from her illness, but after hearing Dr. Bryant King's comments about possible mercy killings, she was puzzled. "I think she died from the infection. I don't know. I really don't know," she told Griffin. "And, you know, hearing—this doctor was saying about euthanasia—euthanasia at the hospital, I just don't know where to go." The death certificate didn't help—Minyard had all of these first causes of death as "hurricane-related."

I believe this news piece was also the first time Dr. Anna Pou's name was made public on national television. Griffin did his own interview with Dr. King, who said it was Pou he saw in the triage section:

KING: This is on the second floor in the lobby. This—and
across that walkway, there's a group of patients. And
Anna is standing over there with a handful of syringes.

GRIFFIN: Dr. Ann Pou.

KING: Talking to a patient. And the words that I heard her
      say were, "I'm going to give you something to make you feel
      better." And she had a handful of syringes. I don't—and that
      was strange on a lot of different levels. For one, we don't
      give medications; the nurses give medications. We almost
      never give medications ourselves, unless it's something crit-
      ical. It's in the middle of a code or—even in the middle of a
      code, the nurses give medications. Nobody walks around
      with a handful of syringes and goes and gives the same
      thing to each patient. That's just not how we do it.

Griffin also played a clip of an undated TV interview Dr. Pou had
given to a Baton Rouge news broadcast:

POU: There were some patients there that—who were critically
     ill, and, regardless of the storm, were—had the orders of,
     do not resuscitate. In other words, that if they died, to allow
     them to die naturally and not to use any heroic methods to
     resuscitate them. We all did everything within our power to
     give the best treatment that we could to the patients in the
     hospital, to make them comfortable.

Griffin made the point that in several conversations with CNN, Pou
would not comment on the euthanasia allegations and had hired an
attorney, Rick Simmons, who provided this written statement: "The
physicians and staff responsible for the care of patients, many of whom
were gravely ill, faced loss of generator power, the absence of routine
medical equipment to sustain life, lack of water and sanitation facilities,
extreme heat, in excess of 100 degrees, all occurring in an environment of
deteriorating security, apparent social unrest, and the absence of governmental authority. Dr. Pou and other medical personnel at Memorial Hospital worked tirelessly for five days to save and evacuate patients, none of
whom were abandoned. We feel confident that the facts will reveal heroic
efforts by the physicians and the staff in a desperate situation."

Griffin finished his report by stating that Tenet Healthcare, which owns the hospital, and LifeCare, which leases space on the seventh floor, whose patients died from possible excessive amounts of morphine, declined to comment except to state they are cooperating with the attorney general's investigation.[38]

Later on, National Public Radio obtained sealed court documents regarding the ongoing investigation that indicated four key witnesses allegedly told authorities of the decision to end the lives of Memorial patients, but none could be sure who gave the order. On February 16, 2006, the correspondent for the NPR program *All Things Considered*, Carrie Kahn, interviewed Angela McManus about her mother's death. Angela said that she had been staying with Wilda on the LifeCare floor for two weeks before Katrina and that her mother was making good progress. On the day after the hurricane, hospital staffers told her that Wilda would soon be evacuated by helicopter and that Angela should leave right then and there on a boat. She got as far as the first floor and then was locked in because of looting outside.

The next day when she returned to the seventh floor she saw that her mother hadn't been evacuated as promised—and she said that she noticed her mother was far more lethargic than she had been. Nurses admitted sedating Wilda, which Angela didn't feel was necessary. She sang gospel songs to her mother as the older lady slept. Angela refused nurses' requests to leave the area, which is when she said that she first heard the discussion about leaving behind the DNR people. "DNR means 'do not resuscitate.' It does not mean do not rescue, do not take care of," McManus said on the radio report. She tried to rescind her mother's DNR order, to no avail. That evening, McManus said three New Orleans police officers approached her with guns drawn and told her she would have to leave. Her mother screamed and cried, but Angela was forced out. She would later find out her mother died with a high level of drugs in her system. Kahn's report stated that McManus had hired an attorney to look into the matter because she "wants answers."

NPR's look at the sealed documents also revealed that on Thursday morning, at an incident-command meeting on the emergency room ramp, a nurse reportedly told LifeCare's pharmacy director that the remaining patients were not expected to be evacuated. That pharmacist, plus the director of physical medicine, and an assistant administrator, all purportedly told the attorney general's investigators that the plan for the seventh floor was to "not leave any living patients behind" and that "a lethal dose would be administered." According to NPR, the pharmacy director allegedly said he saw Dr. Pou in the medical charting area and that she, and two unnamed nurses, informed him of the decision to administer the lethal doses. The court documents do not make clear where the instruction came from. When the pharmacist asked which medication was to be given, the paperwork reportedly stated that Pou showed him a big pack of morphine vials. Before he left the floor and was evacuated, the pharmacist alleged that he saw Pou and the two nurses enter the rooms of the remaining LifeCare patients. NPR's Kahn stated that no arrests have been made to date and no other person is known to have witnessed the injections being given. The attorney general's spokesperson, Kris Wartelle, would only say that her office had subpoenaed seventy witnesses and was proceeding with its investigation. Dr. Pou's attorney offered the same written statement he gave to CNN, and Tenet officials declined to comment, although their corporate Web site posted praise for the doctors and staff and regret for the loss of life. LifeCare's spokesperson offered a similar comment.

Frank Minyard would not disclose to NPR whether any of the tissue samples he sent for testing had morphine in them. He would only say that the bodies were not retrieved from the hospital until two weeks after the storm and were in advanced stages of decomposition. That, he said, undermines the accuracy of toxicology tests. "If these people had been treated for their pain prior to the storm, they are going to have it in their system. And they are sick people, and their system is not working like it should work," Minyard said.[39] When he made this statement, he had had the report of my scientific experiment for two weeks already.

My co-author, Dawna Kaufmann, had heard a similar account to what happened with Angela McManus. Early on in the writing of this book, Dawna spoke to Kathryn "Kathy" Nelson, the daughter of another Life-Care patient, Elaine Nelson. Kathy had been with her mother before, during, and after Katrina hit. A registered nurse who used to work in the intensive care unit of Houston's Methodist Hospital while legendary cardiac surgeon Dr. Michael DeBakey saved lives, she had moved back several years before to her family's Metairie, Louisiana, home to give full-time care to her mother. Kathy said her mother had been doing fairly well while at Memorial, but when she developed a bladder infection, then pneumonia, she was transferred to LifeCare. From July 11 forward, Kathy moved into Elaine's various rooms and stayed around the clock, although nurses still performed the feeding tube and clean-up duties.

In the days after Katrina hit, Kathy was repeatedly pressured to evacuate Memorial, until she was the last remaining nonessential personnel on the LifeCare floor. Soon Elaine began breathing heavily, and a nurse gave her some medication, telling Kathy, "Sometimes this dosage is just enough to push the patient over the edge." Kathy explained to Dawna that she wasn't sure what the medication was, but her mother was never the same after that. By Thursday morning, a nurse told Kathy to leave because Elaine was dying, but that only made the younger woman want to stay longer. Finally, a security guard ordered her out. "I kissed my mother and told her what a wonderful mom she was. She was the center of my life," she told Dawna.

Kathy walked down the seven floors of stairs to where the boats were launching and had to wait a couple more hours before she could board one. Eventually a staffer lined up behind her, asked if she was Kathy Nelson, and said, "Your mama died twenty minutes ago." It would be weeks before Ms. Nelson's body was collected from Memorial and sent to the St. Gabriel DMORT facility.[40]

Tenet got a fresh zapping on March 8, 2006, when Drew Griffin appeared on Paula Zahn's CNN program to recap the Memorial case. But he also mentioned the corporation's troubled history. According to

Griffin, in 1995, Tenet's predecessor, National Medical Enterprises, was involved in a medical insurance fraud, and since then Tenet has settled dozens of lawsuits when the company was charged with over-billing and practicing medicine that harmed patients. In 2005, Tenet paid out $31 million to cardiac patients at a Florida hospital where twenty patients died. Those who sued claimed dirty conditions led to patients getting infections. An FBI probe in 2002 charged that a Red-ding, California, hospital owned by the group was performing unnec-essary open-heart surgeries. Though Tenet admitted no wrongdoing, it paid $60 million to settle federal and state claims, and another $395 million to seven hundred fifty patients who claimed they were victims. The CNN report said that civil attorneys have accused the corporation of cost cutting and breaking rules to make increased profits. Griffin said since the Katrina deaths, more people have contacted CNN with complaints about Tenet.

My friend bioethicist Arthur Caplan was interviewed for the seg-ment and stated: "I think at the end of the day, if you look at it over the past fifteen, twenty years of this company, you'd have to say that management has been pushing the bottom line, telling the doctors to cut corners. Basically saying we're going to evaluate you and promote you on how well you make money. Not on how well you take care of the patients." Caplan also said that Tenet management had been making a policy of not acknowledging allegations of wrongdoing in the Memorial matter—and then a clip was played from September 2005, when Memorial's CEO, Rene Goux, denied having heard about the euthanasia charges and said he was only involved with the evacu-ation part of the disaster, not the healthcare part.

Griffin had posted a preview of his report on CNN's Web site, and Tenet executives sent him a letter, which he showed on the air. The com-pany stated it was informed by the attorney general's office it was not a target of the investigation, which was true, initially. The attorney gen-eral's office told Tenet it was looking into allegations of various things, not just at Memorial, but at all local hospitals. Tenet also stated in its letter that its hospitals were prepared for the hurricane and functioned appropriately. And the corporation also maintained that new management took over in 2003, and a decision was made to resolve its past legal problems and regain the public's trust with honesty and integrity.[41]

Kathleen Johnston, Griffin's senior producer, was sent a pointed letter from Tenet executives, stating the same.[42] And one week later, a similar letter was sent to Johnston's executive vice president for news standards and practices, with copies to the top two executives at Time Warner, Inc., CNN's parent company.[43] In June 2006, it was announced that Tenet Healthcare was selling Memorial Medical Center, three other hospitals in the New Orleans metro area, and seven elsewhere. Ochsner Health System would soon become the new owner of Memorial.[44]

In all of the media accounts I saw at the time, and all of those since that I came upon while researching this chapter, only one Tenet executive with the Dallas home office was named in connection with the Memorial deaths: Robert L. Smith, who in 2005, was the corporation's senior vice president of operations for the Tenet Texas–Gulf Coast region.[45] In 2006, Smith was named to the American Heart Association's Texas Affiliate Board and was described then as the regional senior vice president for Tenet's twelve Texas hospitals, having joined the corporation in 2003 when it was doing business as National Medical Enterprises.[46] In 2007, Smith, as senior vice president of operations for Tenet's hospitals in Texas, welcomed a new partnership with Blue Cross and Blue Shield of Texas.[47] But the only place I could find his name invoked with regard to Memorial was in a *Times-Picayune* article in August 2006, where he was referred to as the Tenet boss who got the bad news on Wednesday, August 31, 2005, the second-to-last day of the evacuation. Smith was "shocked and dismayed" when he took a phone call from Cynthia Matherne, New Orleans' regional coordinator for emergency services, and learned that the federal government was not on the scene with an evacuation plan. She told him there were no available boats or helicopters and that if Tenet wanted a quicker response it should "use private assets."[48] Shortly thereafter, according to the *New England Journal of Medicine*, Susan Mulderick, Memorial's head nurse and incident commander, spoke to someone at Tenet headquarters, then had a conversation with the hospital's chief of medicine, Dr. Richard Deichmann. She allegedly asked him whether euthanasia should be brought up with any patients who had Do Not Resuscitate orders, and he claimed to have immediately rejected the idea.[49]

One positive aspect of the arrests was that it evoked public discussion of end-of-life issues. Is it ever acceptable for a physician to take the life of a patient? Should "assisted suicide" be legalized, and if so, what restrictions should be in place? What if the patient is suffering and otherwise terminal? Is a severely depressed person even capable of making such a decision? On talk shows and in OpEd pieces, two doctors' names were often mentioned: Jack Kevorkian and Harold Shipman.

Kevorkian, born in 1928, is often called "Doctor Death." In the late 1980s, he became an advocate for the critically ill and devised a mechanism that an individual could use to release drugs to end his or her life, which Kevorkian would witness. The doctor claims to have helped one hundred thirty patients die. Even though the state of Michigan eventually rescinded his medical license, and Kevorkian would serve eight years in prison, he never regretted helping people euthanize themselves, which he felt was his "duty." He also made sure that the individuals seeking to die were truly terminal and suffering, and they had to sign documents attesting to that. It's Kevorkian's hope that states will accept the premise of doctor-controlled assisted suicide, but so far only Oregon has decriminalized the act.[50] Some forms of euthanasia are legal in Belgium, Luxembourg, The Netherlands, Switzerland, parts of Spain, and Thailand.[51]

The other controversial doctor was British general practitioner Harold Shipman, who hanged himself in his prison cell in 2004 at the age of fifty-four. Unlike Kevorkian, Shipman had no altruistic impulse—he was a drug-addled fiend who may have killed as many as two hundred fifty patients, at least one of whom he injected with heroin and forged a will, making himself the sole beneficiary. While convicted for fifteen deaths, his motivations were never made clear, but I feel comfortable in describing him as a "serial killer."[52]

If the compassionate Kevorkian is at one extreme of the spectrum and the sociopathic Shipman is at the other, where would Dr. Anna Maria Pou belong, if she were indeed pronounced guilty of the crime? Ultimately, that is up to society—and you, the reader—to determine.

Due to Katrina, the burden upon Louisiana's court system has been staggering. In August 2006, one New Orleans judge began releasing prisoners who had waited behind bars for a year without being able to meet with counsel or get their shot at justice. The number of public defenders was insufficient before the hurricane—it's much worse now, just as violent crime is at a record high in the area.[53]

While the criminal matter percolated, civil suits began hitting the courts, with families of patients who died at Memorial suing both Tenet and LifeCare. In time, all nine families would file independent civil suits, most of which are still pending. A common theme was that the medical center failed to provide backup electrical power, which was responsible for the deplorable conditions. LifeCare attorneys fired back with a claim that once the Federal Emergency Management Agency and the US Coast Guard became aware of the evacuations, the patients became wards of the government and not LifeCare's liability.[54]

On September 24, 2006, Dr. Pou took advantage of one of America's best opportunities to defend herself in the public eye—by being interviewed on CBS's *60 Minutes*. Correspondent Morley Safer listened attentively while Pou stated about herself and her nurses, "I want everyone to know that I am not a murderer, that we are not murderers." Attorney General Foti limited his participation to the briefest of comments, apparently feeling it would seem unethical to try the people's case on the airwaves, which allowed Pou to explain her side with little interference. About her arrest, she said: "It completely ripped my heart out, because my entire life, I have tried to do good. And my entire adult life, I have given everything that I have within me to take care of my patients." She was able to set the scene of Memorial over those horrid days—the stench, the heat, the squalor. Landry and Budo were also on the broadcast, with Landry making the point that neither she nor the other two women even considered leaving on the evacuation boats themselves. "Not until everybody else was out as far as patients or visitors or families. I mean, we were there for the duration," she said.

While Safer read from the attorney general's affidavit, it lacked the emotion of the women talking of their experience. Safer brought up to Foti that many of the patients were very ill and had DNR orders, but Foti countered that he thought there were as many as nine patients who were murdered. "Would you not think that in [a] case of murder, the perpetrators would try to conceal their actions?" Safer asked. To which Foti replied: "Maybe they just didn't think that anybody would ever find out."[55] That was an astute comment—the floodwaters were expected to be there for six months, which would have left the corpses skeletonized, with little way of proving how or why the victims died. But the waters had receded early, and the bodies—and all the evidence they held—were found.

Citing the criminal case for which a conviction could bring a life-long prison term, plus the civil cases, attorneys for the women told Morley Safer they would not permit their clients to talk about the injections or specific actions. That meant a slam-dunk for the defense, ratcheting up sympathy for the trio without their having to answer tough questions. Pou ended the segment by assuring Safer that she did not kill anyone. "I do not believe in euthanasia. I don't think that it's anyone's decision to make when a patient dies," Dr. Pou declared. "However, what I do believe in is comfort care. And that means that we ensure that they do not suffer pain."[56]

I wondered why Orleans Parish district attorney Eddie Jordan, who was to prosecute the case, did not appear on the program. I recall turning to my wife, Sigrid, and musing that this criminal case just might never see the inside of a courtroom. I was wrong about that, actually. The hour-long, lighthearted ABC TV series *Boston Legal* fashioned an episode on the case, which aired in January 2007, with one of the cast regulars defending an Anna Pou–type doctor. I should have specified to my wife that I felt the criminal case might never see the inside of a *New Orleans* courtroom—obviously it was nicely represented in Hollywood's soundstage courtroom.

In October 2006, CNN reported that coroner Frank Minyard had indicated that a special grand jury would be looking into the Memorial deaths—news that Jordan's office would neither confirm nor deny.[57] Five months later, word leaked out that Jordan had indeed convened a panel. Fourteen jurors and two alternates were seated, with nine needing to agree in order to indict Pou and the nurses or clear them of wrongdoing. Assistant district attorney Michael Morales was heading the case, with help from Craig Famularo of his office and Julie Cullen, who sat in from the attorney general's staff. Hearings did not get under way until May 2007.[58] The work of any grand jury is secret, so we don't know what was discussed, or what wasn't. But local news reporters spotted individuals who seemed to be affiliated with the case as they entered the courthouse. I kept waiting for a phone call, asking me to fly to New Orleans and give testimony, but it never came. My four colleagues who wrote reports were also not contacted. District Attorney Jordan didn't seem interested in having us explain our findings to the grand jurors.

I would guess that Dr. Minyard testified, but he had never formally declared his opinion on the question of homicide. In fact, on the autopsy reports of the Memorial patients, where the coroner was expected to list classification of death, there was only a blank line for each of the patients. Later Minyard would get sued by the *Times-Picayune* for not filling in these blanks, but, as far as I know, that case has not gone to court, and I don't see much chance of it prevailing for the newspaper. "We did everything we were asked to do," Minyard told a Reuters reporter. "We took toxicology and sent it up to one of the best labs in the country for them to analyze . . . but as we stand now, with all of the consultants we have used in our investigation, the classification is undetermined."[59] Minyard might have been more focused on the Katrina-related deaths he was still seeing in his community. "People with pre-existing conditions that are made worse by the stress of living here after the storm. Old people who are just giving up. People who are killing themselves because they feel they can't go on," Minyard told an Associated Press reporter.[60] I could understand how that would overwhelm anyone.

There was no set deadline for the vote on whether to indict, but in June the two nurses were offered an immunity deal to testify against Pou and avoid prosecution themselves. Pou's attorney, Rick Simmons, issued a statement that his client "had had no role in the grand jury proceedings," which I took to mean she never testified. "We remain confident that once all the facts are known, all medical personnel will be exonerated of any criminal charges," Simmons wrote. "The fact that certain witnesses may or may not be talking to the grand jury does not change that fact."[61] I believe it was appropriate that charges against the nurses were dropped—nurses follow orders of doctors, not the other way around.

On July 16, 2007, Simmons, on behalf of Pou, filed a lawsuit in Baton Rouge against Louisiana Attorney General Charles C. Foti Jr., accusing him of playing politics with her life and demanding that the state provide her with a legal defense in the mounting lawsuit by patients' families.[62] Although her case against Foti has not yet gone to court, Simmons successfully argued to be paid to defend Pou, since he knows the case better than any other attorney. The attorney hired to defend his client against prosecution by the attorney general's office was now being paid by that office to defend her. I anticipate that the civil judge assigned to this case will dismiss it since I don't see that there was malice on Foti's part, a necessary ingredient for that claim to go forward.

The bigger news would come on July 24 with the announcement that the grand jury declined to indict Dr. Pou on any of the counts of second-degree murder. When she heard the news, Pou fell to her knees and thanked God, she told reporters. Reading from a prepared statement, she added: "This is not a triumph, but a moment of remembrance for those who lost their lives during the storm and those who stayed at their posts to serve those in need," she said. Her attorney, perhaps in hinting at the defense he'll use in the civil suits, said that he would like the death certificates to be amended to list the cause of death as "government abandonment. Anyone with a television set knows the cause of death." Pou refused to criticize the attorney general, stating, "I'm putting Mr. Foti in God's hands—he has to live with the decisions that he made." And when asked if she would resume her medical practice, Pou answered, "In a heartbeat . . . as soon as possible, as far as I'm concerned."

There were swift responses from the Louisiana State Medical Society and the American Medical Association, both rejoicing in Pou's verdict. An AMA statement called Pou and the other doctors who stayed behind "bright lights during New Orleans' darkest hours."[63] And a WDSU-TV news report, showing the doctor celebrating her victory, ran a poll that asked: "Do you agree with the grand jury's decision to decline charges against Dr. Anna Pou?" Of the 3,435 votes that were counted, 3,122, or 91 percent, said yes, and 313, or 9 percent, said no.[64]

District Attorney Jordan told reporters: "I think justice has been served with due process. I think the grand jury did the right thing. The grand jury considered all the evidence—carefully considered. They concluded no crime had been committed."[65]

I have no doubt the jury carefully considered what was presented to them. But Jordan's team did not present important witnesses. Not only were we experts not called to testify, no family members of the victims were permitted to speak at the hearings. And unbelievably, Dr. Bryant King, the internist—who said that he was so angry about the euthanasia plan that he left the hospital and later spoke to CNN—was not asked to tell his account to the jurors. In fact, according to what he told my co-author, Dr. King was never interviewed by anyone on Eddie Jordan's staff.[66] We'll never know how much time was spent on the case by the grand jury members—hours, days, or weeks. I have heard that while the panel began with twelve members, it concluded with ten, as one member died and another went missing.

Three days after Pou was not indicted, *USA Today* published an anonymous OpEd piece titled: "Our View on Medical Ethics: Katrina Survivors Say Doctor Wasn't a Killer. Enough Said," which reflected on Dr. Pou's two years of anxiety and the miserable conditions she faced in the post-Katrina hellhole that was Memorial Medical Center. It asked the good question: "When is it appropriate to give a terminal patient medication at levels that can hasten death?" then answered with a mention of the murderous Dr. Harold Shipman and nurses in our own country who were found to have killed patients. "If the attorney general had proof Pou acted in this manner, he was right to pursue the case," the article stated. It further went on to compare Pou's situation with a war zone, citing the Feres doctrine, a battlefield provision that shields doctors from prosecution. The piece concluded with the pronouncement that "the jury heard the evidence" and its judgment deserves respect: "Foti should move on, and so should everyone else. The jury has spoken."[67]

That was their opinion. Mine is that had any of these medical personnel injected the patients deliberately to kill them, it should not have been considered "euthanasia" or "assisted suicide," since the patients involved did not ask to be injected with fatal drugs and all nine could have lived had they been evacuated. There's also the role of managed healthcare in a time of crisis. With the increased life span of Americans today, and more people lingering from diseases that would have ended their lives sooner in years past, our hospitals and nursing homes have more elderly patients. There is indisputably a financial element at play when prolonged hospice care exceeds reimbursement limits. Add in a natural disaster, such as we saw with Katrina, and hospital owners have an incentive to end suffering—their own. A jury trial would have uncovered which, if any, entity—Pou, Tenet, and/or Life-Care—was to blame and to what degree.

CNN, which did such stellar work on this case, was not giving up. On August 26, Drew Griffin showed the reports we five experts issued, which the network received through a public records request. He told viewers that our unanimous conclusions of homicide were never brought to the jury's attention. Further, Griffin promised that while Tenet and some medical personnel are seeking to keep further records sealed, CNN, along with the *Times-Picayune* newspaper, intends to keep fighting for the information. He also said that Eddie Jordan had refused repeated requests from CNN to discuss why the five experts were never called. But the district attorney supplied an e-mail response that read: "It is inappropriate to disclose what the grand jury did or did not consider. The Orleans Parish grand jury concluded that there was insufficient evidence to indict Dr. Poe [*sic*] on any violations of criminal law."[68] Eddie Jordan spent all of that time on preparing his substantive case, yet misspelled the name of the defendant.

In an unrelated incident to the Memorial case, the district attorney's office was hit with a lawsuit charging workplace bias. A federal judge awarded the dozens of plaintiffs a total $3.7 million judgment, and Eddie Jordan resigned his position on November 1, 2007, with slightly more than one year left on his six-year term.[69] Jordan's handpicked successor, Keva Landrum-Johnson, was disinclined to reopen the Memorial investigation and resigned in August 2008 to take a judgeship at the criminal district court. Her replacement, Robert L. Freeman Jr., agreed to hold the post on an interim basis. Two candidates are facing off in an election that will be held in November 2008—after this book has gone to press. I have no idea what their respective views are on the Memorial matter, but who knows what could happen if a district attorney who wants to dig deeper is ever elected? Attorney General Foti lost his bid for reelection and was replaced by Buddy Caldwell in January 2008.[70] Butch Schafer and his agents in the Medicaid Fraud Control Unit remain in place, in case charges are ever filed again.

On December 6, 2007, CNN posted another scathing report about the case on its Web site. Correspondent Drew Griffin and senior producer Kathleen Johnston obtained a document that spelled out even more details about the attorney general's investigation than I had known. I had seen a six-page summary of the report, called "Memorial Medical Center, Case #59-2652," but the CNN team had the full sixty-eight-page account. The investigative report chronicles incidents beyond the LifeCare seventh floor, including "for the first time, the deaths of other patients, elsewhere in the building, who may have been given lethal injections." Witness statements were taped and transcribed, says the report, and the names and titles of all people interviewed or discussed at the hospital were provided. One doctor—whose name was not revealed by CNN, likely for legal reasons—told a LifeCare employee that "only the strong would survive" and that "Mother Nature would take its course and that they might have to hasten Mother Nature along." A source told CNN that "Pou was believed to have controlled more than one hundred twenty-seven vials of morphine on the day the patients died, based on pharmacy inventories, toxicology reports, and eyewitness accounts."

Griffin and Johnston also cited a doctor in the report who claimed he observed Pou "administer a syringe of medicine into one of the patient's femoral area." The report mentions another doctor—besides Bryant King—who objected to the alleged plan to euthanize patients. Additionally, the document describes a male nurse who alleges that he did not feel comfortable sedating one of the patients, and how Pou reportedly said to him: 'If you don't feel comfortable, or if you are not ready to do it, don't, because it will come back to haunt you. I know the first time I did it, it haunted me for two years.'"[71] I think that comment will haunt *me* for the rest of my life! I certainly would have liked to know what she meant by that.

The report mentioned that LifeCare's director of physical medicine told investigators about Angela McManus, who said she was rushed off the seventh floor at gunpoint. CNN's report charged that the director heard Dr. Pou talking to Angela's mother, a patient named Wilda McManus. Pou was purportedly overheard telling the senior citizen, "I'm going to give you something that's going to make you feel better." The director told CNN that she later heard Pou say: "You know, I had to give her three doses, she's fighting." Pou's attorney,

Rick Simmons, told CNN that the report was just an assemblage of "witnesses and alleged statements that have not been cross-examined or verified"—which is accurate. But one wonders how Eddie Jordan could have ignored it when he decided to pull the plug on his own case. It's entirely possible that a jury, grand or petit, might have heard all of the evidence against Dr. Pou and concluded that no crime had been committed. I would have accepted that and not looked back. But withholding key evidence was an intolerable affront to the victims and their loved ones.

Most maddening, at least to me, was a statement in the report that said, in August 2006, when Foti's office was in full swing on the probe, then District Attorney Jordan wrote a letter, asking that the investigation be halted. "Upon review of the documents presented to my office, I am now of the opinion that such an investigation would not be advantageous to the case," Jordan wrote in the letter, which was obtained by CNN and mentioned in an article on its Web site. "Therefore, I am requesting that the investigation by your office of such deaths cease until the Grand Jury investigations begin in earnest." Butch Schafer confirmed to CNN, "Yes, we got that letter and yes, it told us to stop investigating. And through other phone calls we already knew we were being told to stop, they didn't want any more information."[72]

That was the same month that I attended the three-day conference in New Orleans. Little did I know then that there was no intent to go forward. Butch later told me that he had worked day and night for eighteen months on the case and was frustrated by its ending. He was particularly disappointed in the former district attorney's behavior since when the case was being so thoroughly investigated by Schafer's office, Jordan informed them that he was taking over and said, "This is the kind of case the people of New Orleans would expect their district attorney to prosecute." It's Schafer's hope that the public gets to hear what really happened in the case, and he is closely watching two separate scheduled proceedings, one in the Louisiana Supreme Court and the second in the Louisiana First Circuit Court of

Appeals, where attempts to seal documents or limit access to them are being weighed.

Some excellent news for CNN is that its entire Katrina team—senior investigative producer Kathleen Johnston, producer Coleen Kaman, correspondents Jonathan Freed and Drew Griffin, and managing editor Steve Robinson—was nominated for an Emmy award by the National Television Academy, for their documentary "Death at Memorial Hospital."[73] And quite deservedly, Griffin received a National Press Foundation award for his hard-hitting reportage on Memorial and other stories.[74]

Dr. Bryant King, who spoke out about the shameful situation he witnessed, moved to Indiana University, where he is two years into a fellowship in nephrology.[75] He has both talent and compassion, the hallmarks for a successful career in medicine.

I wasn't stunned to learn that a jury had acquitted the owners of a St. Bernard's Parish nursing home where thirty-five people perished. Sal and Mabel Mangano, who operated St. Rita's home, just outside New Orleans, evacuated themselves but left behind their patients, some of whom drowned in their beds. Yolanda Hubert's seventy-two-year-old mother, Zerelda Delatte, was one of the deceased. Hubert attended the trial and complained to a reporter about the Manganos: "They still have never said they were sorry. They never said, 'I'm sorry I let your mother drown like a rat.' They're guilty as hell." The prosecution put on forty witnesses, including then governor Kathleen Blanco, who testified that she left the decision to evacuate to local officials. St. Bernard's never called for mandatory evacuation. Thirty-six of the fifty-seven nursing homes in Katrina's path never evacuated, but the jury never heard that—they did hear that three homes close to St. Rita's successfully evacuated. The attorney general's office investigated at least one hundred forty deaths in hospitals and nursing homes, but when local district attorneys took over, there were no convictions. One case is still pending, where twenty-two people died at Lafon nursing home, in eastern New Orleans, which is in the Orleans Parish.[76]

Craig R. Nelson—the attorney son of Elaine Nelson, one of the Life-Care Nine patients—wanted more information about why his mother never made it out of Memorial. While he accepted that his mother was very ill, he couldn't understand why she wasn't evacuated—and why she died so suddenly. Nelson had a local forensic pathologist/toxicologist, Emil M. Laga, review his mother's medical records and autopsy results. I have never met Dr. Laga, although I have heard of him and I certainly found his report very thorough and professional. I also did a concurring report for Nelson, based on my analysis of his mother's autopsy and toxicological reports. Nelson filed a wrongful death action against both Tenet and LifeCare, but I have heard that he has since settled the claims. I suspect most, if not all, of the civil court actions will end with confidential settlements and no admission of wrongdoing on the part of Tenet and LifeCare.

Angela McManus has retained the Geoffrey Feiger law firm out of Michigan to sue on behalf of her mother who died at Memorial, and if any lawyer actually enjoys taking a case to court, it's Fieger. But I can't fault any family members for wanting to put this nightmare behind them and moving ahead with their lives.

Almost exactly three years after Katrina, Hurricane Gustav blew through the Gulf region, causing forty-three deaths in Louisiana. There was an organized five-day evacuation in New Orleans that prevented more damage and loss of life. But because the levees held, there was essentially no flooding and much less devastation than occurred in 2005. Gustav put a damper on the 2008 Republican National Convention in St. Paul, Minnesota, when President George Bush, Vice President Dick Cheney, and Louisiana Governor Bobby Jindal chose to stay home and take care of business instead of celebrating with their Grand Old Party.[77]

It is important to understand that Dr. Anna Maria Pou was not acquitted or cleared of any crimes against the Memorial/LifeCare patients. She was simply not charged. A capital case can be brought against her at any time since there is no statute of limitations for murder.

This case profoundly affected me, from how these defenseless victims died to the manner in which the grand jury was handled. Someone has to speak for the victims, and I will do all that I can to continue to educate the public. On March 1, 2008, at the forty-eighth annual meeting of the American College of Legal Medicine in Houston, Texas, I gave a ninety-minute presentation titled "Memorial Hospital Deaths (Hurricane Katrina): Forensic, Medical, Legal, Ethical, and Societal Perspectives," which was very well received. Of course, I shall be available, report in hand, should the criminal case ever be reopened.

AFTERWORD

The nature of high-profile cases like these is that they generate discussion and debate for years to come. Members of Anna Nicole Smith's inner circle will perpetually be blamed for the blonde bombshell's death and that of her young son, Daniel. Despite all the reasons for declaring these cases accidental deaths—officially and by my investigation—people with too little information and too vivid imaginations will believe that murders were committed. Some weird need is satisfied by keeping the mystery alive, even though real people who cared for Anna and Daniel are still mourning their loss. That is a pity.

Richard Raymond Tuite and David Westerfield still have their defenders.

As of January 2008, ten years after Stephanie Crowe's murder, Tuite's mother and sister continue to insist he was wrongly convicted. I'm sure the women, who attended every day of his trial and much of the preliminary hearing, are legitimately heartbroken, even as I'm certain they are wrong about his innocence. And the Crowe family, who suffered so greatly, are still struggling for a remedy in the legal system—I hope they find it soon.

For some time after he moved onto San Quentin's death row, Westerfield would write letter to friends, complaining about the prison conditions while maintaining that he was framed. As he moves closer to his guaranteed appeal, his supporters will undoubtedly try to spin things in the media to his favor. Frankly, though, I would be surprised if there are any grounds for appeal. I can't think of one mistake made in the prosecution case that might open that door. In the meantime, he'll have plenty of opportunity to reflect on his callous disregard for a young child's life that caused him to end up behind bars.

How sad that the Crowe and van Dam families won't get to experience the joy of their daughters growing up and blossoming into their own personalities. They and we have all been robbed of seeing what these girls would have become.

As for the Memorial Medical Center case, there's a piece of me that thinks of it every day. I lament the loss of the victims and rail against the lack of justice, which I believe diminishes us all. Perhaps there will be some accountability in the matter, via civil suits. It's not the same, but it's a way to say that these people mattered and they were unfairly taken from us.

My co-author, Dawna Kaufmann, and I thank you for spending this time with us. If this book has taught you something about forensic pathology and how it connects to the legal system and the media, our goal has been met.

Cyril H. Wecht, MD, JD

NOTES

CHAPTER ONE: DANIEL WAYNE SMITH

1. David K. Li, "Grief After Joy: Anna Nicole Son, 20, Dies After Sis Born," *New York Post*, September 12, 2006.
2. "Anna Nicole Smith's Mother Speaks Out," transcript of *The Nancy Grace Show*, Cable Headline News, September 12, 2006.
3. Gina Serpe, "Anna Nicole's Son's Death Unnatural," *E! Online*, September 12, 2006.
4. Transcript of *Larry King Live*, CNN, September 12, 2006.
5. Jessica Robertson, "Official: Smith's Son's Death Suspicious," Associated Press, September 13, 2006.
6. Paul Turnquest, "Suspicious Death of Celebrity's Son Gets More Suspicious," *Bahamas Tribune,* September 14, 2006.
7. Robertson, "Official: Smith's Son's Death."
8. Transcript of *Inside Edition*, syndicated, CBS, September 13, 2006.
9. David K. Li, "Death of Sexpot's Son 'Suspicious,'" *New York Post*, September 14, 2006.
10. Robertson, "Official: Smith's Son's Death."
11. Paul Turnquest, "Inquest into Smith's Death Set," *Bahamas Tribune*, September 14, 2006.
12. Dawna Kaufmann, "Anna Nicole's Son: Why She Ordered Second Autopsy," *Globe*, October 2, 2006.
13. David Giancola (Edgewood Studios, director/co-producer of *Illegal Aliens*), in interview with author.
14. Transcript of *Entertainment Tonight*, syndicated, CBS, December 14, 2007.
15. Tosheena Robinson-Blair, "Doctors Tell of Frantic Efforts to Revive Son of Anna Nicole Smith," *Bahama Journal*, November 20, 2007.
16. Lloyd Grove, "A Photo Op Pays Off for Anna Nicole," *New York Daily News*, September 19, 2006.

17. Ibid.

18. Notes of Cyril H. Wecht, MD, JD, re: Daniel Wayne Smith.

19. Ibid.

20. Robinson-Blair, "Doctors Tell of Frantic Efforts."

21. Wecht, re: Daniel Wayne Smith.

22. Robinson-Blair, "Doctors Tell of Frantic Efforts."

23. Quincy Parker, "Foreign Pathologist's Report into Smith's Death Won't Affect Local Process," *Bahama Journal*, September 29, 2006.

24. "Anna Nicole Smith's Will and Assets Made Public," transcript of *The Nancy Grace Show,* Cable Headline News, May 15, 2007.

25. Don Gentile, "Anna Nicole Turns Tragedy Into Cash," *National Enquirer*, November 20, 2006.

26. Transcript of *On the Record with Greta Van Susteren*, FOX News, September 13, 2006.

27. Ibid.

28. Tosheena Robinson-Blair, "Inquest Resumes into Death of Anna Nicole Smith's Son," *Bahama Journal*, January 30, 2008.

29. Tosheena Robinson-Blair, "Testimony Continues in Coroner's Inquest," *Bahama Journal*, November 21, 2007.

30. Wecht, re: Daniel Wayne Smith.

31. Transcript of *Larry King Live*, CNN, September 26, 2006.

32. Jack E. Harding (private investigator), in interview with author.

33. Transcript of *Entertainment Tonight*, CBS, November 3, 2006.

34. Harding, in interview with author.

35. "Anna Nicole Smith's Mother Speaks Out," transcript of *The Nancy Grace Show,* Cable Headline News, October 12, 2006.

36. Robinson-Blair, "Inquest Resumes."

37. "Anna Nicole's Touching Tattoo Tributes," *Globe*, January 22, 2007.

38. "Anna Nicole Smith's Mother Speaks Out."

39. Ibid.

40. Ibid.

41. Bob Burns, "R.I.P. Daniel: 20-Year-Old Laid to Rest in His Favorite Clothes," *Globe*, November 6, 2006.

42. Rush & Molloy gossip item, *New York Daily News*, October 20, 2006.

43. Transcript of *Controversy TV*, Bahamian television program hosted by Lincoln Bain and Utah Taylor.

44. Bob Burns, "'I'm Sorry! I'm Sorry': Anna Nicole Wails at Tragic Son's Funeral," *Globe*, November 6, 2006.

45. Candia Dames, "Bar Association President Wants Public Hangings," *Bahama Journal*, March 20, 2006.

46. "Decision Expected Soon in Death of Anna Nicole's Son," Associated Press, January 11, 2007.

47. Natalie Finn, "Inquest Set in Daniel Smith's Death," *E! Online*, January 16, 2007.

48. Transcript of *On the Record with Greta Van Susteren*, FOX News, March 27, 2007.

49. Ibid.

50. Ibid.

51. "Daniel Smith Inquest Already Has Stalled," Associated Press, March 28, 2007.

52. Quincy Parker, "Daniel Smith Inquest Scheduled," *Bahama Journal*, September 25, 2007.

53. "Daniel Smith Inquest Delayed by Tropical Storm," TMZ.com, October 30, 2007.

54. Tosheena Robinson-Blair, "Jurors Selected in Smith's Inquest," *Bahama Journal*, October 31, 2007.

55. Robinson-Blair, "Doctors Tell of Frantic Efforts."

56. Inderia Saunders, "Raju: Only One of Eight Drugs Was Prescribed to Daniel," *Nassau Guardian*, December 11, 2007.

57. Tosheena Robinson-Blair, "Officer Testifies Gibson, Wife Were in Hospital After Smith Died," *Bahama Journal*, December 12, 2007.

58. Tosheena Robinson-Blair, "Expert: Smith's Son Died from Methadone," Associated Press Online, December 12, 2007.

59. Artesia Davis, "Daniel Smith Might Have Killed Himself," *Nassau Guardian*, February 1, 2008.

60. "Bahamas Jury Rules Anna Nicole's Smith's Son Died of Accidental Overdose," Associated Press, March 31, 2008.

61. Donna Leinwand, "Report Flags Rise in Deaths by Methadone ODs," *USA Today*, December 6, 2007.

62. *National Household Survey on Drug Abuse & Health*, 2007, Department of Health and Human Services.

CHAPTER TWO: ANNA NICOLE SMITH

1. Official autopsy and toxicology reports of Marilyn Monroe, Los Angeles County Coroner's Office, August 27, 1962.

2. Mark Bellinghaus, PR-Inside.com, February 9, 2007.

3. http://marilynmonroepages.com/index.html.

4. Gaby Wood, "Chronicle of a Death Foretold," *London Observer*, May 13, 2007.

5. http://www.playboy.com/magazine/features/remembering-anna-nicole-smith/cover-anna-nicole-smith-5.html.

6. Official autopsy and toxicology reports of Marilyn Monroe.

7. "Anna Nicole Smith Diary Auction," *Us*, March 19, 2007.

8. "Exposed! New Diary Bombshell," *Globe*, June 4, 2007.

9. Official autopsy and toxicology reports of Marilyn Monroe.

10. http://www.cityofmexia.com.previewyoursite.com/index.php/content/view/49/70/.

11. http://www.freewebs.com/sassy-silly/ansnamelist.html.

12. Wood, "Chronicle of a Death Foretold."

13. R. Daniel Foster, "Bombshell: Anna Nicole Smith Comes Clean on Dad, Sex Symbols, Hell, and Drinking Beer Texas Style," *Los Angeles Magazine*, January 1994.

14. http://www.freewebs.com/sassy-silly/ansnamelist.htm.

15. Randall Paterson and Aisha Mori, "Hungry Girl: The Potted Plant Lady's Strange Tale of Sex, Money, and Feeding Anna Nicole Smith," *Dallas Observer*, December 2, 1999.

16. Foster, "Bombshell: Anna Nicole Smith Comes Clean."

17. http://www.absolutenow.com/mugshots/anna_nicole_smith.html.

18. Foster, "Bombshell: Anna Nicole Smith Comes Clean."

19. Anne Maier and Laurel Brubaker Calkins, "Anna Nicole Smith Buries Husband," *People*, August 21, 1995.

20. Wood, "Chronicle of a Death Foretold."

21. Transcript of *Larry King Live*, CNN, May 29, 2002.

22. Transcript of *Primetime*, "Fame and Infamy Surround Anna Nicole Smith," ABC News, November 17, 2005.

23. http://www.bankruptcylitigationblog.com/archives/us-supreme-court-cases-239-the-courtship-of-anna-nicole-smith-part-ii-pierce-marshalls-appellate-arguments-reviewed.html.

24. http://www.imdb.com/name/nm0000645/bio.

25. Paterson, "Hungry Girl."

26. http://www.bankruptcylitigationblog.com/archives/us-supreme-court-cases-239-the-courtship-of-anna-nicole-smith-part-ii-pierce-marshalls-appellate-arguments-reviewed.html.

27. http://www.imdb.com/name/nm0000645/bio.

28. http://www.celebitchy.com/3547/look_inside_anna_nicoles_diaries_her_handwriting_looks_like_paris_hiltons/.

29. Paterson, "Hungry Girl."

30. http://www.imdb.com/title/tt011622/.

31. http://www.imdb.com/title/tt0110074/.

32. http://www.imdb.com/name/nm0000645/.

33. http://youtube.com/watch?v=ydcbKRVp8oI&feature=related.

34. http://www.imdb.com/name/nm0000645/bio.

35. http://youtube.com/watch?v=noxgsfJcwis&feature=related.

36. http://www.freewebs.com/sassy-silly/ansnamelist.htm.

37. Wood, "Chronicle of a Death Foretold."

38. Official autopsy and investigative report for Anna Nicole Smith, AKA Vickie Lynn Marshall, Broward County Medical Examiner's Office, March 2007.

39. Transcript of *Extra*, 1997; rebroadcast on February 9, 2007.

40. Anne Maier and Laurel Brubaker Calkins, "Anna Nicole Smith Buries Husband."

41. http://www.bankruptcylitigationblog.com/archives/us-supreme-court-cases-239-the-courtship-of-anna-nicole-smith-part-ii-pierce-marshalls-appellate-arguments-reviewed.html.

42. "Anna Nicole Smith Weds J. Howard Marshall II," *People*, August 1, 1994; reprinted online February 9, 2007.

43. Rush & Molloy, "The Anna Nicole Tapes," *New York Daily News*, April 30, 2007.

44. Nadine Brozan, "Chronicle," *New York Times*, October 21, 1994.

45. http://www.bankruptcylitigationblog.com/archives/us-supreme-court-cases-239-the-courtship-of-anna-nicole-smith-part-ii-pierce-marshalls-appellate-arguments-reviewed.html.

46. Transcript of *Primetime*, "Fame and Infamy Surround Anna Nicole Smith."

47. http://www.bankruptcylitigationblog.com/archives/us-supreme-

court-cases-239-the-courtship-of-anna-nicole-smith-part-ii-pierce-marshalls
-appellate-arguments-reviewed.html.

48. Maier and Calkins, "Anna Nicole Smith Buries Husband."

49. Page Six gossip column, "Anna Nicole's Dumb-Ash Stunt," *New York Post*, August 12, 2002.

50. Maier and Calkins, "Anna Nicole Smith Buries Husband."

51. Paterson, "Hungry Girl."

52. Wood, "Chronicle of a Death Foretold."

53. http://www.freewebs.com/sassy-silly/ansnamelist.htm

54. http://members.calbar.ca.gov/search/member_detail.aspx?x=159567.

55. Mark Bellinghaus, PR-Inside.com, February 9, 2007.

56. Transcript of *Extra*, syndicated, February 9, 2007.

57. Transcript of *Extra*, September 11, 2006.

58 http://fl1.findlaw.com/news.findlaw.com/hdocs/docs/annanicole/ansmith030702mem.pdf.

59. http://www.youtube.com/watch?v=0CbQAx8mI60.

60. "Anna Nicole: Bar Mitzvah Babe," TMZ.com, March 1, 2007.

61. http://www.imdb.com/name/nm0000645/.

62. http://www.youtube.com/watch?v=f-MrZWmdUGc.

63. Libby Copeland, "The Anna Enigma: Who Is Howard K. Stern?" *Washington Post*, March 7, 2007.

64. Paterson, "Hungry Girl."

65. http://video.msn.com/video.aspx?mkt=enUS&brand=msnbc&vid=e1262320-62d5-478a-b9d4-6b89ca855588.

66. Transcript of *Primetime*, "Fame and Infamy Surround Anna Nicole Smith."

67. Bill Murphy and S. K. Bardwell, "Smith, Stepson Have No Share of Estate," *Houston Chronicle*, March 8, 2001.

68. Charles Lane, "Anna Nicole Smith's Supreme Fight," *Washington Post*, March 1, 2006.

69. Jane Roh, "Anna Nicole Smith Wins Supreme Court Appeal," FOX News, May 1, 2006.

70. "IRS About to 'PWN' Stern," *Splash News*, March 21, 2007.

71. Lynette Rice, "The Boob Tube: Move Over, Ozzy!" *Entertainment Weekly*, July 26, 2002.

72. Marianne Goldstein, "Anna Nicole Smith Loved the Limelight," ABC News, February 8, 2007.

73. http://imdb.com/title/tt0328732/.

74. Tim Goodman, "Anybody Home?" *San Francisco Chronicle*, July 11, 2002.

75. "Anna Nicole Walks Out on Howard Stern Radio Show," *Extra,* May 4, 2004.

76. Alex Goen (TrimSpa founder and CEO), in interview with author.

77. Jeannette Walls, "Anna Nicole Smith, Kid Rock Face Off at Kentucky Derby," MSNBC News, May 4, 2004.

78. "Anna Nicole Walks Out on Howard Stern Radio Show," *Extra.*

79. Kanye West, "The New Workout Plan," *College Dropout*, BMI, 2004.

80. http://youtube.com/watch?v=Sk0j_Ih4dko&feature=related.

81. http://www.furisdead.com/feat/annanicole/.

82. "Anna Nicole Flashes Crowd at MTV Event," FOX News, April 3, 2005.

83. A. J. Hammer and Karyn Bryant, "Anna Nicole Wordsmith," *Showbiz Tonight*, CNN, April 7, 2005.

84. http://www.edgewoodstudios.

85. David Giancola (director/co-executive producer of *Illegal Aliens*), in interview with author.

86. http://www.edgewoodstudios.com.

87. Jeannette Walls, "Anna Nicole Smith Still Parties Hearty," MSNBC News, July 18, 2005.

88. Transcript of *On the Record with Greta Van Susteren*, FOX News, February 12, 2007.

89. "Anna Nicole Is Pregnant," Associated Press, June 1, 2006.

90. Larry Birkhead, in interview with author.

91. Transcript of *On the Record with Greta Van Susteren*, FOX News, February 12, 2007.

92. http://youtube.com/watch?v=cqioG2lV6ug&feature=related.

93. http://cdn.digitalcity.com/tmz_documents/110206_birkhead_smith _email.pdf.

94. Transcript of *Geraldo at Large*, FOX News, October 21, 2007.

95. Todd Venezia and Tom Liddy, "Anna Paperwork Is New Drug Clue," *New York Post*, March 16, 2007.

96. "Methadone Okay for Pregnant Anna," TMZ.com, February 16, 2007.

97. Transcript of *Larry King Live*, CNN, September 12, 2006.

98. http://youtube.com/watch?v=Bq1dPi1eNjc.

99. David Wright, "Anna Nicole Died Broke," *National Enquirer*, June 4, 2007.

100. Transcript of *Larry King Live*, CNN, September 26, 2006.

101. Transcript of *The Nancy Grace Show*, "Anna Nicole's Mother Speaks Out," Cable Headline News, October 12, 2006.

102. Roger Friedman, "Anna Nicole Smith: RX Shrink Was Next-Door Neighbor," FOX 411, March 27, 2007.

103. Dawna Kaufmann, "Anna Nicole Eviction Drama," *Globe*, November 20, 2006.

104. "Scandals Are Still Under Police Investigation," *Nassau Guardian*, October 3, 2007.

105. http://www.freewebs.com/sassy-silly/ansnamelist.htm.

106. http://www.youtube.com/watch?v=xMgJCJRrTmA&feature=related.

107. Inderia Saunders, "Rampant Corruption Surrounds 'Horizons' Case," *Nassau Guardian*, August 23, 2007.

108. http://www.freewebs.com/sassy-silly/ansnamelist.htm.

109. Larry Birkhead, in interview with author.

110. Jeannette Walls, "Is Anna Nicole Using Baby as Cash Cow?" MSNBC News, January 22, 2007.

111. http://www.broward.org/medical/final_press_release.pdf.

112. "Smith's Last Hours Spent in the Other Hollywood," Associated Press, February 13, 2007.

113. http://www.broward.org/medical/investigative_report.pdf.

114. Transcript of *Larry King Live*, "[Anna's] Bodyguard Speaks Out," CNN, February 23, 2007.

115. http://www.broward.org/medical/070223_2_scene.hardrock.pdf.

116. Wood, "Chronicle of a Death Foretold."

117. http://www.broward.org/medical/070223_2_scene032107_er.pdf.

118. http://www.youtube.com/watch?v=qYzszhP6kMA&NR=1.

119. http://video.msn.com/video.aspx?mkt=en-US&brand=msnbc&vid=e1262320-62d5-478a-b9d4-6b89ca855588.

120. Prince Frédéric von Anhalt, in interview with author.

121. Wood, "Chronicle of a Death Foretold."

122. Transcript of *Access Hollywood*, "Did Anna Choke on Her Own Vomit?" February 8, 2007.

123. Richard Luscombe, "After a Life of Controversy, Court Battles and Sadness, Anna Nicole Smith Is Found Dead," *Guardian Unlimited*, February 9, 2007.

124. Alex Goen, in interview with author.

125. Transcript of *Dateline*, "The Death of a Centerfold," NBC, February 10, 2007.

126. Transcript of *Good Morning America*, "Virgie Arthur Talks Exclusively," ABC News, February 9, 2007.

127. Transcript of *20/20*, "Interview with Virgie Arthur," ABC News, February 10, 2007.

128. Press conference with Seminole Police Chief Charlie Tiger and Broward County Medical Examiner Joshua Perper, February 9, 2007.

129. http://youtube.com/watch?v=6dlx3qRbr-s.

130. Transcript of *On the Record with Greta Van Susteren*, FOX News, February 2, 2007.

131. Alex Goen, in interview with author.

132. Transcript of Ford Shelley's testimony before Judge Larry Seidlin, Florida's 17th Judicial District Circuit Court of Broward County.

133. http://www.artharris.com/2007/12/29/bald-truth-exclusive-seminole-tribe-v-stern-hard-rock-cops-want-hks-subpeona-quashed/#more-664.

134. Transcript of *Larry King Live*, CNN, February 23, 2007.

135. Tosheena Robinson-Blair, "Inquest Resumes Into Death of Anna Nicole Smith's Son," *Bahama Journal*, January 30, 2008.

136. G. Ben Thompson, in interview with author.

137. http://i.a.cnn.net/cnn/2007/images/02/16/pleadings021607v2.pdf.

138. Dawna Kaufmann, Bob Burns, and Jim Nelson, "Anna Nicole's Will Forged, Experts Say," *Globe*, April 23, 2007.

139. http://en.wikipedia.org/wiki/Larry_Seidlin.

140. Jim Avila and Chris Francescani, "Exclusive: Judge's Wife: People Say He Should Have His Own TV Show," ABC News, February 22, 2007.

141. Hoda Kotb, "The Battle for Her Body," *Dateline*, February 24, 2007.

142. Transcript of Howard K. Stern's testimony before Judge Larry Seidlin, Florida's 17th Judicial District Circuit Court of Broward County.

143. http://youtube.com/watch?v=AuOD3S9sFQg&feature=related.

144. Transcript of Virgie Arthur's testimony before Judge Larry Seidlin, Florida's 17th Judicial District Circuit Court of Broward County.

145. Transcript of Larry Birkhead's testimony before Judge Larry Seidlin.

146. Kotb, "The Battle for Her Body."

147. Transcript of Larry Birkhead's testimony before Judge Larry Seidlin.

148. Transcript of Ford Shelley's testimony before Judge Larry Seidlin, Florida's 17th Judicial District Circuit Court of Broward County.

149. Transcript of Judge Seidlin's commentary during the Anna Nicole Smith burial hearing.

150. Transcript of the *Today Show*, NBC, March 4, 2007.

151. "Marijuana Charge Dropped Against Judge in Anna Nicole Simpson [*sic*] Case," Associated Press, November 18, 2007.

152. Bob Norman, "In the Bag: Judge Seidlin Heads Off to La-La Land with Collateral Damage to His Image," *Broward-Palm Beach New Times*, June 28, 2007.

153. "Anna Nicole Smith May Have Suffered from Lupus," Associated Press, March 1, 2007.

154. "Birkhead Sues Opri for Fraud, Malpractice," TMZ.com, June 1, 2007.

155. http://www2.dca.ca.gov/pls/wllpub/WLLQRYNA$LCEV2.Query View?P_LICENSE_NUMBER=37980&P_LTE_ID=789.

156. http://www.newsmeat.com/fec/bystate_detail.php?zip=91604&last =Eroshevich&first=Khristine.

157. http://www.imdb.com/name/nm0410469/.

158. http://cdn.digitalcity.com/tmz_documents/0301_ans_burial_wm.pdf.

159 "Family, Friends Say Goodbye to Anna Nicole," Associated Press, March 2, 2007.

160. Transcript of *On the Record with Greta Van Susteren*, FOX News, March 7, 2007.

161. Transcript of *Larry King Live*, CNN, March 2, 2007.

162. Transcript of *Access Hollywood*, "Birkhead Reveals His Anna Nicole Tattoo," March 2, 2007.

163. "Why Coroner Is a Real Conehead!" *Globe*, April 16, 2007.

164. Affidavit of Laurie Payne, filed on November 1, 2006, with the Los Angeles Superior Court.

165. Roger Friedman, "How Anna Nicole Smith's Shrink Got Her Pink Slip," FOX 411, March 7, 2007.

166. "Kapoor Excuse," TMZ.com, March 9, 2007.

167. David Bianculli, "L&O Bombshell Saga Just Bombs; Kristy Swanson as An All-Too-Familiar Doomed Celebrity," *New York Daily News*, May 8, 2007.

168. http://imdb.com/name/nm0969651/.

169. Transcript of *The Nancy Grace Show*, "Private Eye Says Anna Nicole's Son Dreamed of Her Death," Cable Headline News, March 14, 2007.

170. http://www.aolcdn.com/tmz_documents/0316_kapoor_letter.pdf.

171. Roger Friedman, "Anna Nicole Smith's Doctor: She Ordered Drugs," FOX 411, March 16, 2007.

172. Roger Friedman, "Anna Nicole Smith's Shrink Ignored Drug Expert's Warning," FOX 411, March 20, 2007.

173. "Tune In Next Week for ID of Dannie's Daddy," *New York Daily News*, April 3, 2007.

174. http://www.broward.org/medical.

175. Emmanuella Grinberg, "Jury Seated in Coroner's Inquest Into Daniel Smith's Death, But There Is Another Delay," Court TV News, March 300, 2007.

176. Transcript of *On the Record with Greta Van Susteren*, FOX News, March 31, 2007.

177. "Drugs That Killed Anna Rx'ed to Howard K., Others," TMZ.com, March 31, 2007.

178. Roger Friedman, "Anna Nicole Smith's Doctor in The Hot Seat," FOX 411, April 5, 2007.

179. Transcript of *The Nancy Grace Show*, "Anna Nicole Psychiatrist Investigated by California Medical Board," CHN, April 5, 2007.

180. http://www.law.cornell.edu/ethics/ca/narr/CA_NARR_1_08 .HTM#1.8:210.

181. Roger Friedman, "Anna Nicole Wrecked Everything," FOX 411, December 28, 2007.

182. Stephen M. Silverman, "DNA Test: Birkhead Is Dannielynn's Father," *People*, April 10, 2007.

183. "Birkhead Named Baby's Dad: Stern Won't Fight for Custody," CNN, April 10, 2007.

184. Silverman, "DNA Test: Birkhead Is Dannielynn's Father," *People*.

185. Transcript of *On the Record with Greta Van Susteren*, FOX News, May 2, 2007.

186. Transcript of *On the Record with Greta Van Susteren*, FOX News, April 3, 2007.

187. Thomas Francis, "Curse of the Dead: Anna Nicole's Ghost Could Go Home at Last, If Some Trial Hotshots Get Their Way," *Broward-Palm Beach New Times*, October 4, 2007.

188. Geoffrey N. Fieger, Esq., in interview with author.

189. Transcript from the *Today Show*, NBC, April 4, 2007.

190. Jennifer Fermino, "Daddy Larry's Li'l Girl: Tells of Joy with Anna's Dannielynn," *New York Post*, April 18, 2007.

191. "Grandma Virgie Loses Out Again," Associated Press, April 28, 2007.

192. Page Six, "Birkhead, NBC in Secret Deal," *New York Post*, April 29, 2007.

193. "Anna's Louisville Filly: Larry Takes Baby to Old Ky. Home," *New York Post*, May 2, 2007.

194. http://www.tmz.com/2007/05/14/anna-nicole-smiths-will-officially-filed/.

195. Transcript of *On the Record with Greta Van Susteren*, "Stern Files Anna Nicole's Will in California," FOX News, May 14, 2007.

196. Transcript of *The Nancy Grace Show*, "Anna Nicole Smith's Will and Assets Made Public," CHN, May 15, 2007.

197. Wright, "Anna Nicole Died Broke."

198. Bob Burns and Dawna Kaufmann, "Anna Nicole's Missing Millions," *Globe*, June 4, 2007.

199. Don Clark (legal strategist), in interview with author.

200. Transcript of *20/20*, ABC News, February 10, 2007.

201. Transcript of *The Nancy Grace Show*, "Anna Nicole Smith's Will and Assets Made Public."

202. "Exclusive: Stern Files Claim Against Anna Nicole's Estate," celebtv.com, October 22, 2007.

203. http://www.orato.com/node/2487/&page=1.

204. Linda Deutsch, "Anna Nicole Left Everything to Dead Son," Associated Press, June 19, 2007.

205. "Criminal Probe into Anna's Prescriptions," TMZ.com, July 6, 2007.

206. "Six Locations Raided in Anna Nicole Probe," Associated Press, October 12, 2007.

207. Cathy Burke, "Larry A '1'-der Dad: Throws Anna's Girl a 'Royal' Birthday Bash," *New York Post*, September 9, 2007.

208. http://www.emmys.org/inmemoriam/inmemoriam59list.php?page Num_getInmemoriamML=2&totalRows_getInmemoriamML=50.

209. Transcript of *Access Hollywood*, "Anna's Bodyguard Dishes About Stern," October 19, 2007.

210. "Anna Nicole's Lover Howard K. Stern Tells Us: I'm Broke!" *Us*, November 14, 2007.

211. http://www.artharris.com, "Anna Nicole FBI Probe," November 21, 2007.

212. http://www.edgewoodstudios.com/.

213. "Larry Birkhead Sued by Ex-Lawyer Debra Opri," *Us*, September 24, 2007.

214. "Richard Milstein Says His Final Payment Will Be Determined by the Court," *ET Online*, October 16, 2007.

215. "Anna's Lawyers Want Estate to Pay Up," TMZ.com, November 9, 2007.

216. "Anna Nicole Sued Over Unpaid Legal Bills," celebtv.com, November 26, 2007.

217. http://www.artharris.com, "Seminole Tribe V. Stern? Hard Rock Cops Want HKS Subpoena Quashed," December 29, 2007.

218. Tracy Gilchrist, "He's Larry, the Cable TV Guy: Raising Dannielynn to Become a Reality Show," *National Enquirer*, September 24, 2007.

219. "Is Anna Nicole and Larry Birkhead's Baby Headed for Surgery?" *Insider Online*, January 12, 2008.

220. "Larry and Dannielynn Birkhead Visit the Final Resting Place of Anna Nicole Smith on the One Year Anniversary of Her Death," *ET Online*, February 5, 2008.

221. Tosheena Robinson-Blair, "Howard Stern Remembers Anna Nicole," *Bahama Journal*, February 9, 2008.

222. http://www.annanicolesmith.com.

223. "Anna Nicole Smith's Baby Daughter Named Sole Heir," Associated Press, March 5, 2008.

224. Lea Goldman and David M. Ewalt, "Top-Earning Dead Celebrities," *Forbes*, October 29, 2007.

CHAPTER THREE: STEPHANIE CROWE

1. Notes of Cyril H. Wecht, MD, JD, re: *Crowe, et al., v. City of Escondido, et al.*

2. Mark Sauer and John Wilkens, "Haunting Questions: The Stephanie Crowe Murder Case," *San Diego Union-Tribune*, May 11, 1999.

3. Wecht, re: *Crowe.*

4. Sauer and Wilkens, "Haunting Questions."

5. Wecht, re: *Crowe.*

6. Sauer and Wilkens, "Haunting Questions."

7. Wecht, re: Crowe.

8. Sauer and Wilkens, "Haunting Questions."

9. Wecht, re: *Crowe.*

10. Mark Sauer, "Tuite Defense Theory Assailed: Expert Derides Blood Transfer Explanation," *San Diego Union-Tribune*, April 30, 2004.

11. Wecht, re: *Crowe.*

12. "Book: Tuite Should Not Be Convicted for Killing Crowe," NBC San Diego, June 17, 2003.

13. "Crowe Civil Suit to Move Forward Now That Tuite Charged," NBC San Diego, May 23, 2002.

14. Mark Sauer and John Wilkens, "Items in Tuite's Pockets May Show He Was in Girl's Home," *San Diego Union-Tribune*, February 5, 2003.

15. Mark Sauer, "New Evidence Against Tuite Ruled Admissible," *San Diego Union-Tribune*, January 15, 2004.

16. "Judge Says Tuite Defense Can Use Statements from Stephanie's Brother," *San Diego Union-Tribune*, February 6, 2004.

17. Mark Sauer, "Defendant in Girl's Slaying Caught After Massive Three-Hour Manhunt," *San Diego Union-Tribune*, February 2, 2004.

18. Mark Sauer, "Ex-Cop Defends Grilling of Teen in Crowe Killing," *San Diego Union-Tribune*, March 25, 2004.

19. "Crowe Case Detective: May Have Been Wrong About Blood on Knife," *San Diego Union-Tribune*, March 25, 2004.

20. Mark Sauer and John Wilkens, with Greg Moran, Onell R. Soto, and J. Harry Jones, "Tuite Found Guilty of Manslaughter," *San Diego Union-Tribune*, May 27, 2004.

21. Teri Figueroa, "Judge Throws Out Most of Crowe Civil Suit," *North County Times*, March 1, 2005.

22. Teri Figueroa, "Crowe Family Can Sue Makers of Lie-Detector Tests," *North County Times*, April 11, 2005.

23. Onell R. Soto, "Interrogation Machine's Maker Settles Crowe Suit," *San Diego Union-Tribune*, May 24, 2005.

24. http://www.cvsa1.com/index.htm.

25. Greg Moran, "Tuite's Conviction Is Upheld; Appellate Court Rules in '98 Crowe Slaying," *San Diego Union-Tribune*, December 15, 2006.

26. Teri Figueroa, "State's High Court Declines Review of Tuite's Case," *North County Times*, March 28, 2007.

27. Teri Figueroa, "Fallout from Slaying of Escondido Girl Continues Ten Years Later," *North County Times*, January 20, 2008.

28. Greg Moran, "Suit Over Girl's '98 Slaying Is on Appeal; Interrogation Tactics Focus of US Hearing,"*San Diego Union-Tribune*, June 11, 2008.

29. Figueroa, "Fallout."

CHAPTER FOUR: DANIELLE VAN DAM

1. Brian Hazle, "Search on for Missing Girl," *San Diego Union-Tribune*, February 3, 2002.

2. http://www.signonsandiego.com/news/metro/danielle/20020607-9999_1n7brenda_911.html.

3. Anne Krueger, "Rarity of Abductions Outside Family Raises Interest in Such Cases," *San Diego Union-Tribune*, February 10, 2002.

4. Joe Hughes and Brian E. Clark, "Police Believe Girl Was Abducted," *San Diego Union-Tribune*, February 5, 2002.

5. Transcript of *Larry King Live*, CNN, February 6, 2002.

6. Alex Roth, "Westerfield Failed Polygraph Test Badly," *San Diego Union-Tribune*, January 9, 2003.

7. Joe Hughes, "Anxiety, Worries Grip Missing Girl's Parents," *San Diego Union-Tribune*, February 7, 2002.

8. Alex Roth, "Westerfield Hinted at Suicide," *San Diego Union-Tribune*, January 8, 2003.

9. Joe Hughes and Elizabeth Fitzsimons, "Imperial County Dunes Scoured for Missing Girl," *San Diego Union-Tribune*, February 8, 2002.

10. Bruce Lieberman, "Tow Driver's Account Wrong," *San Diego Union-Tribune*, February 10, 2002.

11. Transcript of *Larry King Live*, CNN, February 11, 2002.

12. Joe Hughes, with David E. Graham and Pauline Repard, "Police Return to the Homes of Missing Girl and Neighbor," *San Diego Union-Tribune*, February 14, 2002.

13. Kristen Green, "Parents Believe Daughter Taken While They Slept," *San Diego Union-Tribune*, February 8, 2002.

14. "Parents Drug Use, Sex Lives Steal Focus" Court TV News, March 14, 2002.

15. Green, "Parents Believe Daughter Taken While They Slept."

16. Michael Stetz and Kristen Green, "Van Dam Neighbor Had Been Focus for Investigators Almost from Start," *San Diego Union-Tribune*, February 23, 2002.

17. Jeff McDonald and Joe Hughes, "Kidnap Suspect Jailed," *San Diego Union-Tribune*, February 23, 2002.

18. J. Harry Jones, "D.A. to Seek Murder Charge in Danielle's Disappearance," *San Diego Union-Tribune*, February 25, 2002.

19. Jeffrey J. Rose, "Testimony: DNA, Fingerprints from Motor Home Link Westerfield to Danielle," *San Diego Union-Tribune*, March 12, 2002.

20. J. Harry Jones, "Plea Deal 'Minutes Away' When Body Found," *San Diego Union-Tribune*, September 17, 2002.

21. Notes of Cyril H. Wecht, MD, JD, re: *The People v. David Westerfield.*

22. http://www.courttv.com/trials/westerfield/keyplayers.html.

23. Preston Turegano, "Gavel to Gavel: Cable's Court TV Brings Trials into Our Homes and Finds There Are Plenty of 'Friends of the Court,'" *San Diego Union-Tribune*, September 10, 2002.

24. "Blood, Hair, Fingerprints, Point to Westerfield, Prosecutor Says," *San Diego Union-Tribune*, June 4, 2002.

25. Kristen Green, "Attorney an Advocate of Legalizing Marijuana," *San Diego Union-Tribune*, June 13, 2002.

26. "Parents Drug Use, Sex Lives Steal Focus," *Court TV News*, March 14, 2002.

27. http://www.signonsandiego.com/news/metro/danielle/witnesses.html.

28. Wecht, re: *The People v. David Westerfield.*

29. http://www.signonsandiego.com/news/metro/danielle/defensewitnesses.html.

30. Kristen Green, "Defense Could Pin Hopes on Insect Life," *San Diego Union-Tribune*, June 30, 2002.

31. Harriet Ryan, "Westerfield Convicted, Will Face Death," *Court TV News*, August 21. 2002.

32. http://www.signonsandiego.com/news/metro/danielle/witnesses _penalty.html.

33. Jeff Dillon, "Westerfield Sentenced to Death for Kidnap-Murder of Danielle Van Dam," *San Diego Union-Tribune*, January 3, 2003.

34. Mark Arner, "Total Cost of Westerfield Case Surpasses $1 Million," *San Diego Union-Tribune*, February 22, 2003.

35. "Judge OKs Van Dam-Westerfield Civil Suit Settlement," NBC San Diego, May 14, 2003.

36. J. Harry Jones, "Westerfield Prosecutor Picked to Lead New Unit on Unsolved Homicides," *San Diego Union-Tribune*, May 13, 2003.

37. Alex Roth, "Attorney Breaks His Silence on Defending Westerfield," *San Diego Union-Tribune*, December 1, 2002.

38. Alex Roth, "A Chat Room Helped Westerfield Prosecutors," *San Diego Union-Tribune*, December 12, 2002.

CHAPTER FIVE: MEMORIAL MEDICAL CENTER

1. http://en.wikipedia.org/wiki/Hippocratic_Oath.

2. http://en.wikipedia.org/wiki/Hurricane_Katrina.

3. "Death Toll from Katrina Likely Higher Than 1,300," Associated Press, February 10, 2006.

4. http://en.wikipedia.org/wiki/Hurricane_Katrina.

5. Shaila Dewan, "For Trumpet Playing Coroner, Hurricane Provides Swan Song," *New York Times*, October 17, 2005.

6. "St. James Infirmary Blues," traditional American song, in the public domain, circa 1928.

7. http://www.npr.org/templates/player/mediaPlayer.html?action=1 &t=1&islist=false&id=5281495&m=5281496.

8. http://en.wikipedia.org/wiki/Ochsner_Baptist_Medical_Center.

9. Jeffrey Meitrodt with Michelle Krupa, "For Dear Life: How Hope Turned to Despair at Memorial Medical Center," *Times-Picayune*, August 20, 2006.

10. http://www.medschool.lsuhsc.edu/Otorhinolaryngology/faculty _detail.asp?id=1138.

11. Public documents citing employment salary of Dr. Anna Maria Pou.

12. Meitrodt with Krupa, August 20, 2006.

13. Kathryn Nelson, interview with author.

14. Meitrodt, "For Dear Life," August 21, 2006.

15. Meitrodt, "For Dear Life," August 22, 2006.

16. Ibid.

17. Meitrodt with Krupa, August 20, 2006.

18. Meitrodt, "For Dear Life," August 23, 2006.

19. John M. Glionna and David Pierson, "Dispatches from the Desperate," *Los Angeles Times*, September 5, 2005.

20. Transcript from *CNN Live Today*, "Hurricane Relief Floods to Gulf Coast," CNN, August 31, 2005.

21. Meitrodt, August 23, 2006.

22. Meitrodt with Krupa, August 20, 2006.

23. Meitrodt, August 23, 2006.

24. Susan Okie, MD, "Dr. Pou and the Hurricane: Implications for Patient Care During Disasters," *New England Journal of Medicine*, January 3, 2008.

25. Julie Scelfo, "A Doctor Says She Didn't Murder Her Patients," *Newsweek*, September 15, 2007.

26. Caroline Graham and Jo Knowsley, "We Had to Kill Our Patients," *London Mail*, September 11, 2005.

27. "Nursing Home Owners Acquitted of Katrina Deaths," Associated Press, September 8, 2007.

28. Jacqui Goddard and Richard Luscombe, "They Left Us to Die: It Was Hell," *Scotsman*, September 13, 2005.

29. http://en.wikipedia.org/wiki/Hurricane_Rita#Louisiana.

30. Goddard and Luscombe, "They Left Us to Die."

31. Transcript of *Anderson Cooper 360*, "Possible Mercy Killings after Katrina," CNN, October 13, 2005.

32. Adam Nossiter and Christine Hauser, "Three Arrested in Hospital Deaths after Katrina," *New York Times*, July 18, 2006.

33. Affidavit filed by the State of Louisiana, Orleans Criminal District Court, Parish of Orleans, versus Anna M. Pou, Lori L. Budo, and Cheri A. Landry, July 17, 2006.

34. Scelfo, "A Doctor Says She Didn't Murder Her Patients."

35. http://www.supportdrpou.com/.

36. http://i.a.cnn.net/cnn/2007/images/08/27/memorial.medical.center.pdf.

37. Transcript from *Newsnight with Aaron Brown*, "New Orleans Evacuates," CNN, September 10, 2005.

38. Transcript from *Anderson Cooper 360*, "New Orleans Hospital Murders?" CNN, December 21, 2005.

39. http://www.npr.org/templates/story/story.php?storyId=5219917.

40. Kathryn Nelson, in interview with author.

41. Transcript from *Paula Zahn Now*, "President Bush Visits Gulf Coast," CNN, March 8, 2006.

42. http://www.tenethealth.com/TenetHealth/PressCenter/PressReleases/Tenet+Letter+to+CNN+March+8+2006.htm.

43. http://www.tenethealth.com/TenetHealth/PressCenter/PressReleases/Tenet+Responds+to+CNN+Broadcast+of+March+8.htm.

44. "Four Area Hospitals for Sale," WDSU-TV, June 19, 2006.

45. Janeen Browning, "Gary Stokes Named CEO of Tenet's East Texas Facilities," Nagadoches Medical Center Press Release, March 16, 2005.

46. "Tenet's Robert L. Smith Named to American Heart Association's Texas Affiliate Board," *Business Wire News*, July 12, 2006.

47. "Blue Cross and Blue Shield of Texas Sign New Agreements with Tenet," *Business Wire News*.

48. Meitrodt, August 23, 2006.

49. Okie, "Dr. Pou and the Hurricane."

50. http://en.wikipedia.org/wiki/Jack_Kevorkian.

51. http://en.wikipedia.org/wiki/Euthanasia.

52. http://en.wikipedia.org/wiki/Harold_Shipman.

53. Amy Goodman, "New Orleans Judge Slated to Release Prisoners Citing Breakdown in Criminal Justice System," *Democracy Now!* August 29, 2006.

54. James Varney, "Katrina Deaths at Memorial Lead to Lawsuits," *Times-Picayune*, July 30, 2006.

55. "Was It Murder?" *60 Minutes*, CBS News, September 24, 2006.

56. Ibid.

57. Kathleen Johnston and Drew Griffin, "Coroner: Katrina Hospital Deaths Going to Grand Jury," CNN, October 4, 2006.

58. Gwen Filosa and John Pope, "Grand Jury Refuses to Indict Anna Pou; Medical Community Cheers, Foti Jeers Decision," *Times-Picayune*, July 25, 2007.

59. "New Orleans' Coroner Ruling Won't End Murder Case," Reuters, February 1, 2007.

60. "Debate Rages Over Whether Katrina Is Still Killing," Associated Press, June 3, 2007.

61. Drew Griffin, Kathleen Johnston, Susan Roesgen, Belinda Hernandez, and Eric Marrapodi, "Katrina Nurses Offered Immunity to Testify," CNN, June 22, 2007.

62. Gwen Filosa, "Foti Sued by Doctor Accused in Memorial Hospital Deaths," *Times-Picayune*, July 16, 2007.

63. Gwen Filosa and John Pope, "Grand Jury Refuses to Indict Anna Pou; Medical Community Cheers, Foti Jeers Decision," *Times-Picayune*, July 25, 2007.

64. WDSU-TV poll of July 24, 2007.

65. Filosa and Pope, "Grand Jury Refuses."

66. Bryant King, MD, in interview with author.

67. "Our View on Medical Ethics: Katrina Survivors Say Doctor Wasn't a Killer. Enough Said," *USA Today*, July 27, 2007.

68. Drew Griffin and Kathleen Johnston, "Medical Experts Never Testified in Katrina Hospital Deaths," CNN, August 26, 2007.

69. "New Orleans District Attorney to Resign," Associated Press, October 31, 2007.

70. "Caldwell Elected Louisiana Attorney General," KTBS-TV, November 12, 2007.

71. Drew Griffin and Kathleen Johnston, "Report Probes New Orleans Hospital Deaths," CNN, December 6, 2007.

72. Ibid.

73. http://www.emmyonline.org/emmy/docu_27th_nominees.html.

74. http://www.nationalpress.org/info-url3520/info-url_show.htm?doc_id=114052.

75. Bryant King, MD, in interview with author.

76. "Nursing Home Owners Acquitted of Katrina Deaths," Associated Press, September 8, 2007.

77. http://en.wikipedia.org/wiki/Hurricane_Gustav_(2008).

INDEX